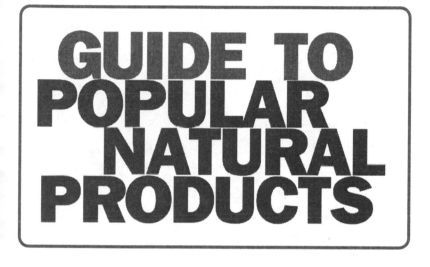

GUIDE TO POPULAR NATURAL PRODUCTS

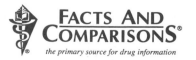

FACTS AND COMPARISONS®

the primary source for drug information

A Guide to Popular Natural Products, First Edition, 1999

Adapted from *The Review of Natural Products* loose-leaf drug information service.
© 1996-1999 by Facts and Comparisons®
© 1989-1996 *The Lawrence Review of Natural Products* by Facts and Comparisons®

Photography by Martin Wall Botanical Services
Pleasant Garden, North Carolina

ISBN 1-57439-063-5

Printed in the United States of America

Published by

Facts and Comparisons®
111 West Port Plaza, Suite 300
St. Louis, Missouri 63146-3098
www.drugfacts.com
314/216-2100 • 800/223-0554

A Guide to Popular Natural Products

Editor

Ara DerMarderosian, PhD
Professor of Pharmacognosy
Research Professor of Medicinal Chemistry
University of the Sciences in Philadelphia

Advisory Panel

John A. Beutler, PhD
Natural Products Chemist
National Cancer Institute

Michael Cirigliano, MD
Assistant Professor of Medicine
University of Pennsylvania
School of Medicine

Derick DeSilva Jr., MD
President, American Nutraceutical
    Association

Constance Grauds, RPh
President, Association of Natural
    Medicine Pharmacists

David S. Tatro, PharmD
Drug Information Analyst

Facts and Comparisons® Publishing Group:

President and Publisher	Michael R. Riley
Director, Editorial/Production	Steven K. Hebel, RPh
Managing Editor	Teri H. Burnham
Quality Control Editor	Julie A. Scott
Associate Editor	Renée M. Short
Assistant Editor	Jill A. Snitker
Senior Composition Specialist	Jennifer K. Walsh
Director, Drug Information	Bernie R. Olin, PharmD
Assistant Director, Drug Information	Jeanelle T. Beltran, PharmD
Director, Sales and Marketing	Robert E. Brown
Business Development Managers	Heidi Meredith-Pohlman JoAnn Amore
Cover Design	Mark L. Wickersham

Table of Contents

Publisher's Preface

As part of our continued commitment to providing quality, accurate information on natural products, Facts and Comparisons® is proud to add the *Guide to Popular Natural Products* to its distinguished list of reference sources. Interest in natural products, a segment of complementary medicine, continues to escalate, and one of the largest challenges is finding information on these agents that accurately describes their potential value to patient care. This publication provides such a source.

Adapted from the widely popular and highly regarded monthly updated publication *The Review of Natural Products*, the *Guide to Popular Natural Products* excerpts the most popular products into an easy-to-use, abridged format, keeping all the features that have made the complete reference source so successful. There are 125 monographs on botanicals, herbals, and nutriceuticals (combined under the more general term "natural products") included in this publication. Arranged alphabetically for ease of use, each monograph is comprised of the following sections: Scientific name, common name, botany, history, pharmacology, and toxicology.

Each monograph also contains a Patient Information box, which highlights important factors for the patient such as potential uses, side effects, and drug interactions. Other unique features of the *Guide to Popular Natural Products* include a comprehensive index, a therapeutic use index, drug interaction appendices, and a full color section of botanical images to aid the reader in identification of the source of the natural product.

Developed under the direction of Ara Der Marderosian, PhD, a well known and leading expert in the field of natural products, each monograph is fully referenced to the scientific literature and peer reviewed by a distinctive panel of experts from various areas of the medical community. There is no other publication more thoroughly reviewed and evaluated.

Natural products are interesting, intriguing, and extremely popular agents. Sometimes controversial, they can be beneficial as well as harmful. Therefore, it is essential that the information provided to health care professionals and consumers be unbiased, accurate, and trusted. The *Guide to Popular Natural Products* is a tool that considers these issues and presents quality information in an easy-to-use format. We hope that the reader finds this a valuable guide in the selection and use of natural products. We encourage comments and suggestions to help us improve the publication for future editions.

Steven K. Hebel, RPh
Director, Editorial/Production
Facts and Comparisons

Introduction

The *Guide to Natural Products*, a referenced compendial guide to popular phyto-medicines and dietary supplements, is intended to provide the individual with a referenced guide to the numerous plant and dietary supplements now widely used in medicine. It contains more than 100 monographs on natural products alphabetically arranged categorized by scientific name(s), common name(s), patient information (a synopsis of uses, drug interactions, and side effects), history, pharmacology, toxicology, and pertinent medical and scientific references. Color photographs of the major botanicals are also provided for their natural beauty and reference purposes.

This introduction provides an overview of historical and epidemiological data, the complimentary and alternative medicine (CAM) movement, the Dietary Supplement and Health Education Act (DSHEA) of 1994, and sufficient coverage of botany and pharmacology for the reader to appreciate and understand the details of proper use of natural products as medicinal agents.

Historical and epidemiological data: There is little doubt that herbal medicine or pharmacognosy is one of the oldest forms of health care. History records the fact that almost every culture around the world has noted its individual contributions to pharmacognosy and use of foods as medicine. The oldest "prescriptions," found on Babylonian clay tablets, and the hieretic (priestly) writing of ancient Egypt on papyrus are numerous ancient pharmaceutical and medical uses of hundreds of botanicals and foods (eg, olive oil, wine, turpentine, myrrh, opium, castor oil, garlic). This worldwide botanical cornucopia represents an eclectic collection of the most reliable early medicines that even today serve the ills of the world. The World Health Organization records the fact that 80% of the world's population still relies on botanical medicines. Several phytomedicines have advanced to widespread use in modern times and are familiar to all. These include morphine and related derivatives (from opium), colchicine (from Autumn crocus), cocaine (from Coca), digitoxin (from Foxglove), vincristine and vinblastine (from the Vinca plant), reserpine (from Indian Snakeroot), etoposide (from Mayapple), and taxol (from Yew). Many botanicals remain to be reevaluated as continued folkloric use around the world entices researchers to further scientific study.

History and science have shown repeatedly that almost all things are cyclical. Once again, we find ourselves in an era of resurgent interest in natural products as medicine. Ethnobotany, rain forest depletion of species, and certain limits in advancement using synthetic drugs continuously teach us that nature has and will always provide us with clues on how to develop new medicines. This probably will never cease. We have learned over and over the constant need to identify plants as to correct genus, species, variety, and even chemovar (chemical races) in order to obtain the same chemistry and medicinal properties desired for a particular botanical. Computers have helped us identify and categorize plants using the best of classical morphology and modern chemotaxonomy. Lessons from the complex phytochemistry of biologically active constituents have taught us that each plant is a unique and veritable chemical factory. We are trying to reach back to the old pharmacopoeias to update their early attempts to standardize botanical medicines. Modern chemical procedures using chromatography, infra-red spectroscopy, nuclear magnetic resonance spectroscopy, and mass spectrometry for molecular characterization of individual pharmacologically active principles have greatly facilitated the methodology. We now understand the complexity of standardization because of the innate biological variability of plant biochemistry. This allows us to fully appreciate all the complexities and variables that are introduced in plant collection, storage, transport, processing, and extraction to prepare uniform, stable dosage forms.

Natural product research has led to new physiological and pharmacological concepts, particularly when a new compound is found to have a specific biological effect. These have been referred to as "molecular keys" and include such classical examples as morphine (the chemical basis for natural and synthetic opioid analgesics), cocaine (the chemical basis for synthetic local anesthetics like procaine), and ephedra (the chemical basis for CNS stimulants like the amphetamines and the decongestants such as pseudoephedrine). Another recent resurrected plant drug is capsaicin from hot peppers. Previously used in topical analgesics as a "counter-irritant," it is being reintroduced as a true analgesic because in low doses it depletes newly discovered "substances," which is involved in pain transmission.

Along similar lines, the ongoing competition with our new resistant pathogenic microbes has led us back into the race to find new antibiotics from soil microbes and fungi. New pandemic diseases like AIDS have taught us how much we need to stimulate and protect our immune system to fight such diseases. We are all living longer, and we need to help conquer cancer as well, and many promising agents are being developed from plants. New uses of certain supplements and vitamins have also focused our attention on food as medicine (nutraceuticals) and phytochemicals (eg, flavonoids, betacarbolenes, phytosterols) that may help prevent diseases.

Current epidemiological data and the current complimentary and alternative medicine movement: There are several factors that may be cited for the resurgence of interest in complementary and alternative medicine including the use of botanical medicines. These include consumer interest in perceived "natural" medicines, increased interest in fitness, health, and prevention directed toward longer and healthier lives, the general interest in improving the environment, and the increase in chronic diseases related to aging. Coupled with these factors has been an economic rise in costs of conventional medicines, an increased fear of potential adverse reactions to modern powerful drugs, and a desire to self-medicate to circumvent these difficulties. This has led to the current strong broad movement toward complimentary and alternative medicines (CAM) (eg, acupuncture, biofeedback, chiropractic, diet, homeopathy, hypnosis, massage), particularly herbal medicine. A brief overview of the prevalence, costs, and patterns of use of CAM therapies in the US compiled by Dr. David Eisenberg at Peter Bent Brigham Hospital in Boston is quite revealing. Between 1990 and 1997, the prevalence of CAM use increased by 25%, from 33.8% in 1990 to 42.1% in 1997. The total number of visits to CAM providers increased by 47%, from 427 million in 1990 to 629 million in 1997. The total visits to CAM providers (629 million) exceeded total visits to all primary care physicians (386 million) in 1997. The estimated expenditures for alternative medicine professional services increased by 45% exclusive of inflation and in 1997 were estimated at $21.2 billion. An estimated 15 million adults in 1997 took prescription medications concurrently with herbal remedies or high dose vitamins. It is obvious that this is a high risk for potential adverse drug-herb or drug-supplement interactions. The monographs provided herewith are intended to provide information that can preclude some of these difficulties. There is little doubt that even the current use of CAM services is likely under-represented and that insurance coverage for holistic therapies are likely to increase in the future. All health professionals and laity need reliable data to base decisions on which botanical supplements are possibly useful for all the various medical conditions.

The Dietary Supplement Health and Education Act (DSHEA): While several phyto-medicinal agents have been in use for a long time and thoroughly evaluated for safety and efficacy (eg, cascara, psyllium, digitalis, ipecac, belladonna), the majority of herbs have not been fully evaluated. For the most part, this rests with the problem of not being able to patent natural products in the US and the enormous costs (several hundred million dollars) and time (8 to 12 years) required to fully evaluate them. These reasons, coupled with the strong consumer movement to maintain the freedom of choice in self-medication, lead to the DSHEA Act of 1994. For the first time, this law defined herbal products, vitamins, minerals, and amino acids as "dietary supplements." It also prohibited dietary supplements from being regulated as food additives, which normally require premarket approval. Further, it states that the burden of proof for safety and adulteration falls on the FDA. However, if a supplement poses an imminent health hazard, DSHEA does allow the Secretary of Health and Human Services emergency powers to remove it from the market. The act permits general health claims regarding the activity of herbals but does not permit therapeutic claims. The herbal product manufacturer must be able to substantiate any health claim as being truthful and not misleading. The label must also include the following statement: "This statement has not been evaluated by the Food and Drug Administration. This product is not intended to diagnose, treat, cure, or prevent any disease." Finally, the label must include the designation "dietary supplement" and list each ingredient by name and quantity. Another provision allows for the distribution of information at the time of sale, giving a balanced view from scientific and related literature on the herbal products. The literature must not be misleading or false and cannot promote any specific brand and should be displayed in an area physically separate from the product. It is up to the FDA to prove that any such information is misleading or false. Before this time, such literature was felt to be an extension of the label and any implied therapeutic claims could be considered in judging a product "misbranded."

DSHEA allowed for the establishment of a commission to conduct a two-year study of the regulation of label claims and literature used in the sale of supplements. Finally, the bill also establishes the Office of Dietary Supplements (ODS) at the National Institutes of Health to coordinate research on dietary supplements. In order to keep up with the continuously evolving status, legal, and regulatory issues relating to the botanicals covered by ODS, it is recommended that one refer to its web site at:

http://odp.od.nih.gov/ods

Another important web site for general information on complementary and alternative medicine in general is:

http://nccam.nih.gov

Basic botany, pharmacognosy, and pharmacology basic botany: As it relates to herbals, basic botany, pharmacognosy, and pharmacology basic botany requires the understanding that all plants have Latin binomial names (usually accurate and understood around the world) and numerous common names and synonyms (eg, Cannabis sativa L. or marijuana, pot, ganja). Botanical products therefore should be identified with the proper Latin name and the most common synonym. Secondly, the active principles in a given plant may be found in one or more parts of the plant (eg, seeds, flowers, leaves). This is the reason that the plant part used should be indicated on the label of a commercial herbal product. For example, in ginkgo biloa, the active components are found in the leaves; in ginseng (*Panax* species), it is the roots that contain the active constituents. Third, because the species or variety used may have differing concentrations of active principles, it is important to note this as well as geographic source, local environmental conditions of growth, and the processing procedures. All of these factors may influence the final product. Whatever plant part has shown the most active level of therapeutic effect and accompanying clinical evidence should be standardized and used. The proper extract or solvent should be specified by the manufacturer. Some require water soluble extraction while others may need more non-polar or lipid extraction. Many of the commercial extracts do not follow official procedures, so it may be necessary to contact the manufacturer to determine how they produced the product. This may be difficult for proprietary reasons, and this is why particular extracts by particular manufacturers that have been clinically evaluated must be used for further studies verifying effects.

All solvents used to yield tinctures, extracts, and the like need to be fully defined for comparison studies and proper dosage determination. When advanced, concentrated, or standardized to active ingredients, the herb or dietary supplement comes closer to the definition of a drug. Yet many manufacturers do not bother to carry the quality control of their products to as high a level as traditional medicine dictates. The thinking seems to be, "If a tea of such an herb helps my headache, that's all I need to know." Health professionals need to document this type of epidemiological evidence in their practice, so it can be ascertained whether this particular herb really works even in crude form. It must be noted that pharmacologically active compounds in crude herbs are often present in lower concentrations than in conventional advanced, concentrated, or extracted products (tablets, capsules, tinctures, etc.). This usually means that the toxicological risks associated with crude botanicals are minimal with moderate use. This in fact may be true, particularly if there is data indicating safe use in many countries for centuries. The problem is that the US has always promoted the idea of "more is better," and this is where adverse reaction potential increases.

Another important factor about herbal products is that they often contain a wide variety of different compounds from various classes. Often therapeutic action is due to the combined action of several constituents. Some, like the primary metabolites (cellulose, starches, sugars, and fixed oils), are not particularly active pharmacologically. Others, like the secondary metabolites (alkaloids, cardiac glycosides, and steroids), are quite active pharmacologically. Content varies depending on genetics, environment (sunlight and rainfall), and fertilization. In fact, it is possible to see mixed activity depending on which compounds predominate. Selection at different times of the year also affects herb quality and clinical effectiveness.

Potential toxicity, carcinogenicity, or liver toxicity: One must keep in mind dose levels and duration of use. In addition, there are examples of growing concerns about plants such as comfrey (leaves or roots of *Symphytum officinale*) that contain the externally useful drug allantoin (which promotes tissue regeneration) and rosmarinic acid (which acts as an anti-inflammatory). However, when taken internally, the content of pyrrolizidine alkaloids from comfrey is potentially hepatotoxic, mutagenic, and carcinogenic as seen in test animals. Many countries have banned or restricted its use. Unfortunately, because comfrey is regulated in the US as a dietary supplement and not a drug, it has remained on the market. The same story is seen with borage *(Borago officinalis)* and coltsfoot *(Tussilago farfara)* that also contain pyrrolizidine alkaloids. Fortunately, many products such as these have been withdrawn by reputable manufacturers and suppliers.

On occasion, there have been some unusual toxicities reported with commercial herbal products due to contamination with poisonous plants (e.g., belladonna) or arsenic or mercury (imported products) and purposeful adulteration with synthetic drugs such as analgesics, anti-inflammatory agents, corticosteroids, and tranquilizers. These problems can be precluded by using products from reliable sources where rigorous good manufacturing practices (GMPs) are observed. Be aware that many imported products from underdeveloped countries may not adhere to good manufacturing practices.

While documented and published reports on herb-drug interactions are still minimal, there is the possibliity that these can occur: The relatively few reports of herb-drug interactions probably is due to real safety and a lack of professional surveillance. Because herbs have been classed as dietary supplements, there are no requirements for reporting acute or chronic toxicity. This is why the health professional should carefully monitor the use of herbal products by patients. There is a voluntary system for reporting suspected adverse effects (USP at 800-4USP PRN and Medwatch at 800-FDA-1088.

Basic factors for the patient: The following general guidelines should be considered before advising patients about natural products: All products should be purchased from reliable sources. Even though GMPs are implicit in DSHEA guidelines for identity, cleanliness, and good quality control in manufacturing, there are significant differences in the purity, quality, and potency of products on the market. Further, many structure or function claims have not been evaluated by the FDA or by other independent and objective agencies. Generally, the more ambitious the claims, the more one should be suspicious of the quality of the product. One way to determine reliability of a manufacturer is to simply request professional health information from the company about the products, the nature of the company, testing, quality control standards, and the like. As with all legitimate and reliable pharmaceutical firms, such requests should elicit data on which decisions can be made about quality, return policies, and guarantees of structure and function claims in research and literature. Often, the availability of these data is part of a reliable company's advertisements.

Most botanical products (particularly crude herbals) should be dry and appear fresh and have appropriate colors (eg, bright yellows or reds for flowers, green for leaves, and tan for roots). Moldy appearance or off odors are cause for return. Crude herbs, their extracts, or capsule forms should be stored in a cool, dry environment away from direct sunlight and out of the reach of children. Anyone handling crude botanicals should wear plastic gloves. Botanical dust should be kept at a minimum because of contamination concerns and potential allergy problems (eg, to molds, spores, and pollen). All surfaces where herbs are handled should be wiped clean immediately. Botanicals should be dated. Discard it over one year old.

Excessive dosages of phytomedicines should be avoided. Because many herbs are considered mild, the tendency is to use them for prolonged periods of time or to use too much at one time. Patients can delude themselves into thinking that they can avoid more potent and effective drugs by using "natural" herbs. All patients should be advised of risk/benefit ratios on all medical treatments and that serious illnesses can develop by assuming an herb will solve the problem over time. Also patients should be counseled about abuses seen with "diet teas" containing herbal laxatives that may lead to colonic impairments and excessive loss of potassium. Generally, natural products should not be used for serious health conditions without the advice and supervision of a qualified health practitioner. Most natural products are intended to treat mild, short-term disorders (eg, headaches, insomnia, dyspepsia, and constipation). Any natural products causing undesirable side effects should be discontinued or the mode of administration changed. For example, while feverfew may be useful in preventing migraine headaches, aphthous mouth ulcers can result from chewing the leaves. Thus, capsules should be taken to avoid such local effects. Like many prescription and *otc* drugs, most natural products should be discontinued during pregnancy or lactation and not used in young children. Qualified health professionals should be consulted in these situations. Generally, avoid excessive combination products. Most research with prescription and *otc* medications has shown that more than two or three ingredients in one product is not always justifiable. Fixed combinations of active principles often result in excessive doses of one ingredient or use of an ingredient that may not be needed.

There is a good rationale for well conceived combination products when appropriate, standardized dosages of a few synergistic herbals are coupled with vitamins and minerals. Herbal supplement users often start their nutritional regimen coupled with multivitamins. There is a growing market in higher quality, recognized brand-name products that feature concentrated, standardized botanical extracts in combination with appropriate dosages of vitamins and minerals. These offer convenience and simple once daily dosing for patients. Examples of recent commercial products of this type have combined echinacea, vitamin C, and zinc for colds; echinacea polysaccharides and vitamin C may stimulate and improve the immune system, and zinc is an essential nutrient for immune system function. While not a cure, this combination may decrease the incidence and severity of the cold. Similar ideas have spawned combinations of B-vitamins, chromium, and ginseng for energy support, and combinations of St. John's wort and kava-kava for tension and mood control. Further research is obviously needed to substantiate the efficacy of such combinations, but many companies have started to document the usefulness of such products.

However, excessive use of more than a few botanicals in combination can be a potential problem because each botanical contains numerous active principles. There is no doubt that efficacy becomes very difficult, if not impossible, to prove with excessive mixtures. Polypharmacy, an older pharmacy practice where small amounts of 10 to 15 or more ingredients were used in one combination product, is shunned today. Unfortunately, the practice of using many botanicals (often each in minute dosages) is still common in Asian and even in some American botanical products. It is highly unlikely that any of these are effective because there are often too many ingredients in ineffective amounts. Some patients feel that all of these botanicals work together and such combinations are therefore better, or that if one ingredient doesn't work another will. In reality, there is virtually no good clinical data on the efficacy of such complex mixtures.

Ara DerMarderosian, PhD
Editor
Philadelphia, Pennsylvania
April, 1999

Monographs

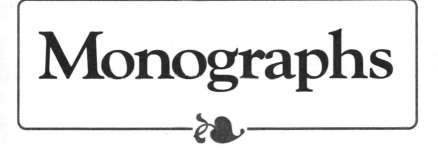

HISTORY: For several decades, health and nutritional benefits have been claimed for products containing *Lactobacillus* cultures. The topical or intravaginal application of yogurt products has been reported to control yeast and bacterial infections. The ingestion of these preparations has been recommended to reduce the symptoms of antibiotic-induced diarrhea or sore mouth as a result of Candida infections.[1] Other reports have indicated that the ingestion of acidophilus-containing products can reduce serum cholesterol levels, improve lactose intolerance, and slow the growth of experimental tumors.[2]

Clinical Uses: Lactobacilli have been shown to inhibit the growth of other vaginal microorganisms including *Escherichia coli*, *Candida albicans*, and *Gardnerella vaginalis*.[3] Several factors may contribute to the possible activity of *Lactobacillus*, including their ability to generate lactic acid, hydrogen peroxide, and exogenous antibacterial compounds, to influence the production of interferon by target cells,[4] and to alter the adherence of bacteria.

The therapeutic benefits of *Lactobacillus* products have been investigated in women with vaginal and urinary tract infections. Women who used either acetic acid jelly, an estrogen cream, a fermented lactobacillus-containing milk product, or metronidazole (eg, *Flagyl*), were evaluated to determine the effects of intravaginal therapy on bacterial vaginosis. Clinical cures were obtained for 13 of 14 women receiving metronidazole but for only 1 of 14 using the fermented milk product.

This latter intervention did not influence the predominance of lactobacilli in the vagina.[5] An evaluation of 16 commercially available products containing *Lactobacillus* in the form of capsules, powders and tablets (in addition to yogurt and milk) found that all 16 products contained lactobacilli, of which 10 strains produced hydrogen peroxide. At least one contaminant was detected in 11 of the products, including *Enterococcus faecium*, *Clostridium sporogenes*, and *Pseudomonas* species. Only 4 of the products contained *L. acidophilus*, and therefore, the authors concluded that most commercially available products may not be appropriate for recolonization of the vagina.[3] The weekly instillation of *Lactobacillus* has been shown to reduce the recurrence rate of uncomplicated lower urinary tract infections in women. The use of a strain that is resistant to nonoxynol-9, a spermicide that kills protective vaginal flora, may have potential for use in women with recurrent cystitis using this contraceptive agent.[6]

L. acidophilus is normally found in the human alimentary tract. Being acid-resistant, it persists in the stomach much longer than other bacteria do. Consequently, the oral administration of products containing *L. acidophilus* may be useful in the management of a variety of conditions associated with altered GI flora. Their beneficial effects may be related to the ability to suppress the growth of pathogens.

When *Lactinex* granules, a combination of *L. acidophilus* and *L. bulgaricus*, were given 4 times daily for 10 days to children concomitantly with amoxicillin (eg, *Amoxil*) therapy under double-blind conditions, 70% of the patients receiving placebo and 66% of those taking *Lactinex* experienced diarrhea. Closer analysis suggested that the incidence of diarrhea diminished during the last 4 days of therapy for the *Lactinex* patients, while it remained constant for those given placebo.[7] However, in a study of 40 children who received amoxicillin concomitantly with fermented lactobacillus milk products, the treated group showed a lower frequency of stool passages and more fully formed feces compared with no treatment.[8]

The ingestion of these products has been associated with decreases in the concentration of several fecal enzymes that have the capacity to convert procarcinogens to carcinogens in the colon. This suggests that consumption of lactobacillus-containing products may have beneficial health effects, although no epidemiological data are available to support this hypothesis.[9]

Effect on cholesterol levels: A mutant strain of *L. acidophilus* with unique metabolic characteristics, led to the isolation of mevalonic acid, an important intermediate of the isoprenoid compound pathway[10] and a precursor to cholesterol synthesis. It has been suggested that appropriately selected strains of *Lactobacillus* may be useful adjuncts for the control of hypercholesterolemia in humans, by virtue of the bacteria's ability to assimilate cholesterol and to grow well in the presence of bile.[11]

TOXICOLOGY: No significant toxicity has been reported among users of *Lactobacillus* products.

[1] Lewis WH. *Medical Botany.* New York, NY: J. Wiley and Sons, 1977.
[2] Gorbach SL. *Ann Med* 1990;22(1):37.
[3] Hughes VL, Hillier SL. *Obstet Gynecol* 1990;75(2):244.
[4] Mihal V, et al. *Cesk Pediatr* 1990;45(10):587.
[5] Fredricsson B, et al. *Gynecol Obstet Invest* 1989;28(3):156.
[6] Reid G, et al. *Clin Microbiol Rev* 1990;3(4):335.
[7] Tankanow RM, et al. *DICP Ann Pharmacother* 1990;24(4):382.
[8] Contardi I. *Clin Ter* 1991;136(6):409.
[9] Marteau P, et al. *Am J Clin Nutr* 1990;52(4):685.
[10] Evans WC. *Trease and Evans' Pharmacognosy,* 13th ed. London, England: Baillíere Tindall, 1989.
[11] Gilliland SE, Walker DK. *J Dairy Sci* 1990;73(4):905.

SCIENTIFIC NAME(S): *Medicago sativa* (L. Common cultivars include Weevelchek, Saranac, Team, Arc, Classic and Buffalo.) Family: Leguminosae

COMMON NAME(S): Alfalfa

⟨⟨⟨⟩⟩⟩ PATIENT INFORMATION ⟨⟨⟨⟩⟩⟩

Uses: The plant appears to reduce cholesterol. No study evidence currently supports use of various parts of the alfalfa plant for diuretic, anti-inflammatory, antidiabetic, or antiulcer purposes.

Side Effects: Alfalfa ingestion has been associated in some instances with pancytopenia and hypocomplementenemia, but alfalfa preparations are generally without side effects.

BOTANY: This legume grows throughout the world under widely varying conditions. The perennial herb has trifoliate dentate leaves with an underground, often woody, stem. Alfalfa grows to ≈ 90 cm. Its blue-violet flowers bloom from July to September.

HISTORY: Alfalfa has played an important role as a livestock forage. It was probably domesticated in southeast Asia. The Arabs fed alfalfa to their horses claiming it made the animals swift and strong, naming the legume "Al-fal-fa" meaning "father of all foods." The medicinal uses of alfalfa stem from anecdotal reports that the leaves cause diuresis, and are useful in the treatment of kidney, bladder, and prostate disorders. Leaf preparations have been touted for their antiarthritic and antidiabetic activity, treatment of dyspepsia, and as an antiasthmatic. Alfalfa extracts are used in baked goods, beverages, and prepared foods. The plant serves as a commercial source of chlorophyll and carotene.[1]

PHARMACOLOGY: There are no studies to provide evidence that alfalfa leaves or sprouts possess effective diuretic, anti-inflammatory, antidiabetic, or antiulcer activity. Alfalfa saponins are hemolytic in vitro.[2]

Alfalfa plant saponins and fiber[3] bind quantities of cholesterol in vitro; sprout saponins interact to a lesser degree. In vitro bile acid adsorption is greatest for the whole alfalfa plant, and this activity is not reduced by the removal of saponins from the plant material. In one study, the ability of alfalfa to reduce liver cholesterol accumulation in cholesterol-fed rats was enhanced by the removal of saponins. Therefore, alfalfa plant saponins appear to play an important role in neutral steroid excretion, but are not essential for increasing bile acid excretion.[4] There is no evidence that canavanine or its metabolites affect cholesterol levels.

TOXICOLOGY: Alfalfa ingestion has provoked pancytopenia and hypocomplementenemia in healthy subjects.[5] L-canavanine has been implicated as the possible causative agent. The toxicity of L-canavanine is due in large part to its structural similarity to arginine. Canavanine binds to arginine-dependent enzymes interfering in their action. Arginine reduces the toxic effects of canavanine in vitro.[6] Further, canavanine may be metabolized to canaline, an analog of ornithine. Canaline may inhibit pyridoxal phosphate and enzymes that require the B_6 cofactor.[7] L-canavanine has also been shown to alter intercellular calcium levels[8] and the ability of certain B- or T-cell populations to regulate antibody synthesis.[9,10] Alfalfa tablets have been associated with the reactivation of systemic lupus erythematosus (SLE) in ≥ 2 patients.[11]

A case of reversible asymptomatic pancytopenia with splenomegaly has been reported in a man who ingested up to 160 g of ground alfalfa seeds daily as part of a cholesterol-reducing diet. His plasma cholesterol fell from 218 mg/dl to 130 to 160 mg/dl.[5] Pancytopenia was believed to be due to canavanine.

A popular self-treatment for asthma and hay fever suggests the ingestion of alfalfa tablets. There is no scientific evidence that this treatment is effective.[12] Fortunately, the occurrence of cross-sensitization between alfalfa (a legume) and grass pollens appears unlikely, assuming the tablets are not contaminated with materials from grasses.[13] One patient died of listeriosis following the ingestion of contaminated alfalfa tablets.[14]

[1] Duke JA. *Handbook of Medicinal Herbs*. Boca Raton, FL: CRC Press, 1985.

[2] Small E, et al. *Economic Botany* 1990;44:226.

[3] Story JA, et al. *J Food Sci* 1982;47:1276.

[4] Story JA, et al. *Am J Clin Nutr* 1984;39:917.

[5] Malinow MR, et al. *Lancet* 1981;i:615.

[6] Natelson S. *J Ag Food Chem* 1985;33:413.

[7] Malinow MR, et al. *Science* 1982;216:415.

[8] Morimoto I. *Kobe J Med Sci* 1989;35:287.

[9] Prete PE. *Arthritis Rheum* 1985;28:1198.

[10] Morimoto I, et al. *Clin Immunol Immunopathol* 1990;55:97.

[11] Roberts JL, et al. *N Engl J Med* 1983;308:1361.

[12] Polk IJ. *JAMA* 1982;247:1493.

[13] Brandenburg DM. *JAMA* 1983;249:3303.

[14] Farber JM, et al. *N Engl J Med* 1990;322:338.

SCIENTIFIC NAME(S): *Aloe vera* L., *A. perryi* Baker (Zanzibar or Socotrine aloe), *A. barbadensis* Miller (also called *A. vera* Tournefort ex Linne or *A. vulgaris* Lamarck; Curacao or Barbados aloe), or *A. ferox* Miller (Cape aloe). *A. vera* Miller and *A. vera* L. may or may not be the same species. Family: Liliaceae

COMMON NAME(S): Cape, Zanzibar, Socotrine, Curacao, Barbados aloes, aloe vera

---

❧❧❧ PATIENT INFORMATION ❧❧❧

Uses: Aloe appears to inhibit infection and promote healing of minor burns and wounds, and possibly of skin affected by diseases such as psoriasis. Dried aloe latex is used, with caution, as a drastic cathartic.

Side Effects: There has been one report that using the gel as standard wound therapy delayed healing. The gel may cause burning sensations in dermabraded skin.

BOTANY: Aloes, of which there are some 500 species, belong to the family Liliaceae.[1] The name, meaning bitter and shiny substance, derives from the Arabic "alloeh." Indigenous to the Cape of Good Hope, these perennial succulents grow throughout most of Africa, southern Arabia, and Madagascar. Although they do not grow in rain forests or arid deserts, they are cultivated in the Caribbean, Mediterranean, Japan, and America. Often attractive ornamental plants, their fleshy leaves are stiff and spiny along the edges and grow in a rosette. Each plant has 15 to 30 tapering leaves, each up to 0.5 m long and 8 to 10 cm wide. Beneath the thick cuticle of the epidermis lies the chlorenchyma. Between this layer and the colorless mucilaginous pulp containing the aloe gel are numerous vascular bundles and inner bundle sheath cells from which a bitter yellow sap exudes when the leaves are cut.[2]

HISTORY: In the 4th millennium B.C., aloe wall carvings were found in Egyptian temples. Called the "Plant of Immortality," it was a traditional funerary gift for the pharaohs. The Egyptian Book of Remedies (ca. 1500 B.C.) notes aloe use in curing infections, treating the skin, and preparing drugs that were chiefly used as laxatives. The Gospel of John (19:39-40) says that Nicodemus brought a mixture of myrrh and aloes for the preparation of Christ's body. Alexander reportedly conquered the Socotra island to obtain control of its aloe resources. In A.D. 74, the Greek physician Dioscorides recorded aloe's use in healing wounds, stopping hair loss, treating genital ulcers, and eliminating hemorrhoids. In the 6th century A.D., Arab traders carried aloe to Asia, and in the 16th century, it was carried to the New World by the Spaniards. Its clinical use began in the 1930s as a treatment for roentgen dermatitis.[2]

PHARMACOLOGY: Aloe latex has been used for centuries as a drastic cathartic. The aloinosides exert strong purgative effects by irritating the large intestine. These should be used with caution in children.

The most common use of the gel remains the treatment of minor burns and skin irritations. The activity of aloe in treating burns may stem from its moisturizing effect, which prevents air from drying the wound.[3] Current theory suggests healing is stimulated by the mucopolysaccharides contained in aloe in combination with sulfur derivatives and nitrogen compounds. Topical aloe treatment for burns has not been adequately documented. Two FDA advisory panels found insufficient evidence to show that *A. vera* is useful in the treatment of minor burns and cuts or vaginal irritations.

More recent studies have found preparations containing aloe to accelerate wound healing, even in frostbitten patients.[5] In patients undergoing dermabrasion, aloe accelerated skin healing by $\approx$ 72 hours compared to polyethylene oxide gel dressing.[4] However, at least one study found that aloe delayed wound healing (83 days vs 53 days).[6]

One study using *A. vera* gel[7] found no activity against *S. aureus* and *E. coli*. Other tests[8] found that *A. chinensis* inhibited growth of *S. aureus*, *E. coli*, and *M. tuberculosis*, but that *A. vera* was inactive. Further, these extracts lost their in vitro activity when mixed with blood. The latex has shown some activity against pathogenic strains.[9] Two commercial preparations (*Aloe gel* and *Dermaide Aloe*) exerted antimicrobial activity against gram-negative and -positive bacteria as well as *Candida albicans* when used in concentrations greater than 90%.[10] Aloe has been found to be more effective than sulfadiazine and salicylic acid creams in promoting wound healing and as effective as sulfadiazine in reducing wound bacterial counts.[11]

Aloe-emodin is antileukemic in vitro;[12] other studies showed *A. vera* gel to be less cytotoxic[13] than indomethacin or prednisolone in tissue cultures.

An emulsion of the gel was reported to cure 17 of 18 patients with peptic ulcers, but no control agent was used in the study.[14]

A Chinese study found that parenteral administration of aloe extract protects the liver from chemical injury and ameliorates ALT levels dramatically in patients with chronic hepatitis.[15]

Only the dried latex is approved for internal use as a cathartic. In some cases, *A. vera* is sold as a food supplement. The FDA has only approved *A. perryi*, *A. vera*, *A. ferox*, and certain hybrids for use as natural food flavorings.[16]

TOXICOLOGY: Since aloe is used extensively as a folk medicine, its adverse effects have been well documented. Except for the dried latex, aloe is not approved as an internal medication. Aloe-emodin and other anthraquinones may cause severe gastric cramping and are contraindicated in children and pregnant women.[17] The external use of aloe usually has not been associated with severe adverse reactions. Reports of burning skin following topical application of aloe gel to dermabraded skin have been described.[18] Contact dermatitis from the related *A. arborescens* has been reported.[1]

[1] Nakamura T, et al. *Contact Dermatitis* 1984;11(1):50.
[2] Grindlay D, et al. *J Ethnopharmacol* 1986;16:117.
[3] Ship AG. *JAMA* 1977;238(16):1770.
[4] Fulton JE, Jr. *J Dermatol Surg Oncol* 1990;16(5):460.
[5] McCauley RL, et al. *Postgrad Med* 1990;88(8):67.
[6] Schmidt JM, et al. *Obstet Gynecol* 1991;78(1):115.
[7] Fly, K. *Economic Bot* 1963;14:46.
[8] Gottshall, et al. *J Clin Invest* 1949;28:920.
[9] Lorenzetti LJ, et al. *J Pharm Sci* 1964;53:1287.

[10] Haggers JP, et al. *J Am Med Technol* 1979;41:293.
[11] Rodriguez-Bigasm, et al. *Plast Reconstr Surg* 1988;81(3):386.
[12] Kupchan, K. *J Nat Prod* 1976;39:223.
[13] Fischer JM. *US Pharmacist* 1982;7(8):37.
[14] Blitz JJ, et al. *J Am Osteopath Assoc* 1963;62:731.
[15] Fan YJ, et al. *Chung Kuo Chung Yao Tsa Chih* 1989;14(12):746.
[16] Hecht A. *FDA Consumer* 1981(July-Aug):27.
[17] Spoerke DG, et al. *Vet Hum Toxicol* 1980;222:418.
[18] Hunter D, et al. *Cutis* 1991;47(3):193.

Angelica

Angelica

SCIENTIFIC NAME(S): *Angelica* sp. Family: Umbelliferae

COMMON NAME(S): Angelica, wild angelica, garden angelica

PATIENT INFORMATION

Uses: Angelica species are used as flavorings, scents, and as a vegetable. It has been a folk remedy for respiratory illnesses and a range of other ailments, including arthritis. Evidence suggests it has immunostimulant, antimutagenic (but also possibly mutagenic), and antitumor effects.

Side Effects: Generally recognized as safe, angelica may be photocarcinogenic. Applied extract produces photosensitivity in some individuals.

BOTANY: Angelica is a tall, aromatic biennial plant of the parsley family with deeply indented, large leaves and strong stems. The plant is commonly used as an attractive border for herb gardens and to shield other herbs from the wind. The stems, leaves, and flowers are light green. The species *A. archangelica*, also referred to as *A. officinalis* (Moench) Hoffm., is native to shady places in Iceland, Lapland, and other northern regions. The species *A. atropurpurea* is found in North America, and *A. sylvestris* L. is a small European species. Other species include *A. curtisi* and *A. rosaefolia*.[1] *A. atropurpurea* also is known in the US by the common name alexanders, which also is used to identify another related plant, *Smyrnium olusatrum*. *A. pubescens* roots are used in Chinese herbal medicine for the treatment of arthritis, headaches, and as a carminative. (See Dong quai monograph).

HISTORY: According to legend, angelica was revealed to humans by an angel as a cure for the plague, hence its name. It was introduced to England during the 16th century. Angelica is best known today in the form of candied or crystallized stems. Dried leaves have been used to make tisanes, which resemble Chinese tea, and as a scent in potpourri. Angelica has been used as a flavoring in gin because of its resemblance to the flavor of juniper berries. The candied leaves and stalks are used as decoration on cakes and pastries. Angelica reduces rhubarb's tartness when cooked together. According to one source, angelica is responsible for the muscatel flavor of Rhine wines.[1] Teas made from the roots and leaves of *A. archangelica* have been used as expectorant, diuretic, diaphoretic, antiflatulent, and externally to treat rheumatic and skin disorders. Angelica has been used as a remedy for respiratory ailments, and in the Faeroe Islands the plant is used as a vegetable.[2]

PHARMACOLOGY: Angelica contains alpha-angelica lactone, which has been shown to augment calcium binding in canine cardiac microsomes in the presence of adenosine triphosphate (ATP). With or without ATP, the compound also augments calcium turnover. Its action may involve increasing the contraction-dependent calcium pool to be released upon systolic depolarization.[3]

An attempt to identify non-viral inducers of interferon failed to find any active extracts of angelica.[4] Experimental confirmation has shown that osthole, a component of *A. pubescens*, has a non-specific relaxing effect on the trachaelis of guinea pigs.[5] Volatile oil from angelica has been shown to inhibit phasic contraction of ileal muscle fibers. In contrast to some other plant extracts, angelica oil has a greater effect on tracheal tissue than on ileal tissue.[6]

A mitogen consisting of 90% sugar and 10% protein has been found in *A. actiloba* (Kitagawa); the activity of this compound is reduced by ≥ 50% in the presence of acid or base.[7] An aqueous extract of *A. koreana* (radix) has shown wormicidal activity against *Clonorchis sinensis*.[8] Alpha-angelica lactone inhibits the formation of metabolites of the carcinogen benzo(α)pyrene in the mouse forestomach and liver, but not in lung tissue.[9] Volatile emissions of *A. archangelica* have demonstrated fungistatic activity against species of *Aspergillus, Rhizopus, Mucor,* and *Alternaria*.[10]

A. archangelica L. has shown some antimutagenic properties in murine bone marrow cells.[11] Antitumor effects on mice with Ehrlich Ascites tumors have been demonstrated by *A. sinensis. In vitro* and *in vivo* immunostimulating effects were also produced.[12] *A. sinensis* given to healthy mice promoted clone-stimulating factors (CSF) in spleen-conditioned medium (SCM).[13] Sodium ferolate, an active component of *A. sinensis* Diels, exhibited hepatoprotective action in mice.[14] Ferulic acid, a phenolic compound in *A. sinesis* Diels, has inhibited uterine contractions in rats.[15]

TOXICOLOGY: Angelica is generally recognized as safe for consumption as a natural seasoning and flavoring. The coumarins and furocoumarins may induce photosensitivity if applied topically.[16] These compounds may also be photocarcinogenic and may be mutagenic in laboratory animals. It is possible to confuse this plant with water hemlock (*Cicuta maculata* L.), which is extremely toxic.

[1] Lowenfeld C, Back P. *The Complete Book of Herbs and Spices*. London: David E. Charles, 1974.
[2] *The New Encyclopedia Britannica*, vol. 1. Chicago: Encyclopedia Britannica, Inc., 1985.
[3] Entman ML, et al. *J Cin Invest* 1969;48(2):229.
[4] Zielinska-Jenczylik J, et al. *Arch Immunol Ther Exp (Warsz)* 1984;32(5):577.
[5] Teng CM, et al. *Naunyn-Schmiedebergs Arch Pharmacol* 1994;349(2):202.
[6] Reiter M, et al. *Arzneimittelforschung* 1985;35(1A):408.
[7] Ohno N, et al. *J Pharmacobiodyn* 1983;6(12):903.
[8] Rhee JK, et al. *Am J Chin Med* 1981;9(4):227.
[9] Ioannou YM, et al. *Cancer Res* 1982;42(4):1199.
[10] Saksena N, et al. *Fitoterapia* 1985;56/4:243.
[11] Salikhova RA, et al. *Vestn Akad Med Nauk SSSR* 1995;(1):58.
[12] Choy YM, et al. *Am J Chin Med* 1994;22(2):137.
[13] Chen YC, Gao YQ *Chung-Kuo Chung Yao Tsa Chih - China J of Chin Materia Med* 1994;19(1):43.
[14] Wang H, Peng RX. *Chung-Kuo Yao Li Hsueh Pao - Acta Pharamacologica Sinica* 1994;15(1):81.
[15] Ozaki Y, Ma JP. *Chem Pharm Bull* 1990;38(6):1620.
[16] Opdyke DL. *Food Cosmet Toxicol* 1975;13(Suppl):683.

SCIENTIFIC NAME(S): *Pimpinella anisum* L. Family: Umbelliferae (Apiaceae). In some texts, anise is referred to as *Anisum vulgare* Gartner or *A. officinarum* Moench. Do not confuse with the "Chinese star anise" (*Illicium verum* Hook. filius. Family: Magnoliaceae).

COMMON NAME(S): Anise, aniseed, sweet cumin

ﮔﮔﮔ PATIENT INFORMATION ﮔﮔﮔ

Uses: Anise has been used as a flavoring in alcohols, liqueurs, dairy products, gelatins, puddings, meats, and candies and as a scent in perfumes, soaps, and sachets. The oil has been used for lice, scabies, and psoriasis. Anise is frequently used as a carminative and expectorant. Anise is also used to decrease bloating and settle the digestive tract in children. In high doses, it is used as an antispasmodic and antiseptic, and for the treatment of cough, asthma, and bronchitis.

Drug Interactions: Anise may interfere with anticoagulant, MAOI, and hormone therapy.

Side Effects: Anise may cause allergic reactions of the skin, respiratory system, and GI tract. Ingestion of the oil may result in pulmonary edema, vomiting, and seizures. It is not recommended for use in pregnancy.

BOTANY: Anise is an annual herb that grows 30 to 60 cm and is cultivated widely throughout the world.[1] The flowers are yellow, compound umbels. Its leaves are feather shaped. The 2 mm long, greenish brown, ridged seeds are used for the food or the drug. They are harvested when ripe in autumn.[2] Aniseed has an anethole-like odor and a sweet, aromatic taste,[3] described as "licorice-like," which has led to traditional use of anise oils in licorice candy.[1]

HISTORY: Anise has a history of use as a spice and fragrance. It has been cultivated in Egypt for ≥ 4000 years. Records of its use as a diuretic and for treatment of digestive problems and toothache are seen in medical texts from this era. In ancient Greek history, it was documented that anise helped breathing, relieved pain, provoked urine, and eased thirst.[2] The oil has been used commercially since the 1800s. The fragrance is used in food, soaps, creams, and perfumes. Anise is often added to licorice candy or used as a "licorice" flavor substitute; it is a fragrant component of anisette.

PHARMACOLOGY: Anise is widely used as a flavoring in all food categories including alcohols, liqueurs, dairy products, gelatins, puddings, meats, and candies.[1] It is sold as a spice, and the seeds are used as a breath freshener.[4] The essential oil is used medicinally as well as in perfumes, soaps, and sachets.[1,5] The oil, when mixed with sassafras oil, is used against insects.[5] Applied externally, the oil has been used for lice and scabies.[2] As a skin penetration enhancer, anise oil has little activity compared with eucalyptus oil and others,[6] but topical application of the constituent bergapten, in combination with ultraviolet light, has been used in psoriasis treatment.[7]

Anise is well known as a carminative and an expectorant. Its ability to decrease bloating and settle the digestive tract is still used today, especially in pediatrics. In higher doses, anise is used as an antispasmodic and an antiseptic for cough, asthma, and bronchitis.[2,3,5,7]

Anise also has been evaluated for its antimicrobial action against gram-negative and gram-positive organisms.[8] Constituent anethole also inhibits growth of mycotoxin-producing *Aspergillus* in culture.[1] Anise is used in dentifrices as an antiseptic and in lozenges and cough preparations for its weak antibacterial effects.[1,4]

TOXICOLOGY: Anise oil has GRAS status and is approved for food use. The acute oral LD-50 of the oil in rats is 2.25 g/kg. No percutaneous absorption of the oil occurred through mouse skin within 2 hours.[9] The oral LD-50 of anethole is 2090 mg/kg in rats; rats fed a diet containing 0.25% anethole for one year showed no ill effects, while those receiving 1% anethole for 15 weeks had microscopic changes in hepatocytes.[4]

The German Commission E monograph lists side effects of anise as "occasional allergic reactions of the skin, respiratory tract, and GI tract."[3] When applied to human skin in a 2% concentration in petrolatum base, anise oil produced no topical reactions. The oil is not considered to be a primary irritant. However, anethole has been associated with sensitization and skin irritation and may cause erythema, scaling, and vesiculation.[10] Anise oil in toothpaste has been reported to cause contact sensitivity, cheilitis, and stomatitis.[5] The constituent bergapten may cause photosensitivity.[9] As mentioned, the cis-isomer of anethole is 15 to 38 times more toxic to animals than the trans-isomer, their relative content being dependent on plant species.[1,5] Ingestion of the oil in doses as small as 1 ml may result in pulmonary edema, vomiting, and seizures.[11] Large doses may interfere with anticoagulant and MAOI therapy. Anethole's estrogenic activity may alter hormone therapy (eg, contraceptive pills). Aniseed is a reputed abortifacient. Excessive use is not recommended in pregnancy.[2,7]

[1] Leung AY. *Encyclopedia of Common Natural Ingredients*, 2nd ed. New York: John Wiley and Sons, 1996;36-38.

[2] Chevallier A. *Encyclopedia of Medicinal Plants*. New York: DK Publishing, 1996:246-47.

[3] Bisset N. *Herbal Drugs and Phytopharmaceuticals*. Stuttgart, Germany: CRC Press, 1994;73-75.

[4] Duke J. *CRC Handbook of Medicinal Herbs*. Boca Raton, FL: CRC Press, 1989;374-75.

[5] Chandler R, et al. *Can Pharm J* 1984 Jan;117:28-29.

[6] Williams, A. et al. *Int J Pharmaceutics* 1989 Dec 22;57:R7-R9.

[7] Newall C, et al. Herbal Medicines. London, England: Pharmaceutical Press, 1996;30-31.

[8] Narasimha B, et al. *Flavor Ind* 1970 Oct;1:725-29.

[9] Meyer F, et al. *Arzneimittelforschung* 1959;9:516.

[10] *Food Cosmet Toxicol* 1973;11:865.

[11] Spoerke DG. *Herbal Medications*. Santa Barbara, CA: Woodbridge Press, 1980.

SCIENTIFIC NAME(S): *Prunus armeniaca* L. (Rosaceae)

COMMON NAME(S): Apricot, Chinese almond

‪PATIENT INFORMATION‬

Uses: Apricots are usually eaten as fruit. Apricot kernel oil is used in cosmetics. In Chinese medicine, it has been used for asthma, cough, and constipation.

Side Effects: Excess ingestion of apricot fruit may cause bone and muscle damage, blindness, hair loss, and reduction in mental capacity. Ingestion of apricot kernels causes cyanide poisoning.

BOTANY: Apricots grow on trees up to 900 cm in height. The plant's leaves are oval and finely serrated. The 5-petaled, white flowers grow together in clusters. Fruits vary in color from yellows and oranges to deep purples. They ripen in late summer.

The apricot is native to China and Japan but is also cultivated in warmer temperate areas of the world, mainly the regions including Turkey through Iran, southern Europe, South Africa, Australia, and California. There are many varieties and species of apricot, differing in flavor, color, and size.[1-4]

HISTORY: In India and China, the apricot has been used for more than 2000 years. During the second century A.D., a physician, Dong Feng, is said to have received his payment in apricot trees. There are also biblical references to the plant.[1,2]

The Greeks wrongly assumed the apricot to have originated in Armenia, hence its botanical name "*Prunus armeniaca.*" The Romans termed the fruit "praecocium" meaning "precocious," referring to the fruit's early ripening. From this, the name "apricot" evolved.[4]

PHARMACOLOGY: Apricots are usually eaten as a fruit, either fresh or dried, made into jams, jellies, or alcoholic beverages. The seeds are used like almonds by Chinese and Afghan cultures. The oil (apricot kernel oil) is also used. Its use in food, flavorings, confection, juices, and jams is common. Some cultures use certain varieties of apricot kernels as almonds.[1,3]

In very small amounts, the toxic prussic acid (hydrogen cyanide) present in apricot kernels is prescribed in Chinese medicine for asthma treatment, cough, and constipation.[2] Decoction of the plant's bark serves as an astringent to soothe irritated skin.[2] The oil is used in cosmetics or as a pharmaceutical vehicle.[1,2] Other folk medicine uses of apricot include treatment of hemorrhage, infertility, eye inflammation, and spasm.[1] Apricot kernel paste may help eliminate vaginal infections.[2]

Laetrile, a semi-synthetic derivative of the naturally occurring "amygdalin," has been used (during late 70s, early 80s) in a highly controversial treatment for cancer.[2,3] A theory claimed that laetrile, when metabolized by the enzyme beta-glucosidase, released toxic cyanide. The enzyme was said to be most prevalent in tumor tissue (as opposed to normal tissue). As a result, this reaction was believed to destroy mainly cancer cells. It was later proven that both cancerous and normal cells contained only trace amounts of this enzyme. Although the treatment may have had slight activity in some cases, it was not as valuable as once thought.[5] A report in 1980 concluded laetrile to be ineffective in cancer treatment. Other proposed theories of laetrile in cancer treatment have not been substantiated by scientific evidence.[1-3]

TOXICOLOGY: Excess ingestion of apricot fruit may cause bone and muscle harm, blindness, hair loss, and reduction in mental capacity.[1] Contact dermatitis has been reported from apricot kernels. Kernel ingestion may be teratogenic as well.[3]

Apricot kernel ingestion is a common source of cyanide poisoning, with > 20 deaths reported.[3] Deaths are reported from ingesting as few as 2 kernels.[1] Amygdalin content in apricot pits varies and can be up to 8%. Wild varieties may contain 20 times the amount of cultivated apricot varieties.[1] Hydrolysis of amygdalin yielding the toxic hydrogen cyanide (HCN) is more rapid in alkaline pH (than acidic in the GI tract), which can delay symptoms of poisoning. Symptoms of cyanide toxicity include dizziness, headache, nausea and vomiting, and quickly progresses to palpitations, hypotension, convulsion, paralysis, coma, and death, from 1 to 15 minutes after ingestion. Antidotes to cyanide poisoning include nitrite, thiosulfate, hydroxocobalamin, and aminophenol.[3]

[1] Duke J. *CRC Handbook of Medicinal Herbs* Boca Raton, FL: CRC Press 1989;394-95.
[2] Chevallier A. *Encyclopedia of Medicinal Plants* New York, NY: DK Publishing 1996;254-55.
[3] Newall C, et al. *Herbal Medicines* London: Pharmaceutical Press 1996;32–33.
[4] Davidson A, et al. *Fruit, a Connoisseur's Guide and Cookbook* London: Mitchell Beazley Publishers 1991;26-27.
[5] Moertel, et al. *N Eng J Med* 306(4):201-6.

SCIENTIFIC NAME(S): *Arnica montana* L. In addition, other related species have been used medicinally including *A. sororia* Greene, *A. fulgens* Pursh., *A. cordifolia* Hook., *A. chamissonis* Less. subsp. *foliosa* (Nutt.) Family: Compositae or Asteraceae

COMMON NAME(S): Leopard's bane, mountain tobacco, mountain snuff, wolf's bane

---

ᶺᶺᶺᶺ PATIENT INFORMATION ᶺᶺᶺᶺ

Uses: Arnica and its extracts have been widely used in folk medicine. It is used externally as a treatment for acne, boils, bruises, rashes, sprains, pains, and other wounds. It has also been used for heart and circulation problems, to reduce cholesterol, and to stimulate the CNS.

Side Effects: The plant is poisonous and ingestion can cause stomach pain, diarrhea, vomiting, dyspnea, cardiac arrest, and death. Contact dermatitis also has occurred.

BOTANY: Arnica is a perennial that grows from 30 to 60 cm.[1,2] Its oval, opposite leaves, with bright yellow, daisy-like flowers, form a basal rosette close to the soil surface.[1-3] The dried flower heads and rhizome are used.[2,4] Arnica is native to the mountainous regions of Europe to southern Russia.[3,4]

HISTORY: Alcoholic tinctures were used by early settlers to treat sore throats, as a febrifuge, and to improve circulation. Homeopathic uses included the treatment of surgical or accidental trauma, as an analgesic, and in the treatment of postoperative thrombophlebitis and pulmonary emboli.[5] It has been used externally for acne, bruises, sprains, and muscle aches, and as a general topical counterirritant.[6] Arnica has been used extensively in European folk medicine. Arnica's bactericidal properties were employed for abrasions and gunshot wounds.[7]

PHARMACOLOGY: Not only is arnica employed in hair tonics, antidandruff preparations, perfumery, and cosmetics, it is used in herbal and homeopathic medicines as well.[4,7] The plant has a slight anti-inflammatory and mild analgesic effect, most likely because of the sesquiterpene lactones it contains. Helenalin and dihydrohelenalin, compounds contained in arnica, exert mild anti-inflammatory and antibacterial activity.[6,8] Arnica improved feelings of stiffness associated with hard physical exertion (vs placebo) when tested in 36 marathon participants in a double-blinded, randomized trial.[9]

Metronidazole was more effective than arnica in controlling postoperative pain, inflammation, and healing in patients who had their wisdom teeth removed. Patients receiving arnica had greater pain and inflammation than those receiving placebo.[10]

Arnica contains a group of polysaccharides with 65% to 100% galacturonic acid that can inhibit the complement system, thereby modifying the immune system reponse.[11] This polysaccharide displays marked phagocytosis enhancement in vivo,[12] yet another compound stimulates macrophages to excrete tumor necrosis factor.[13] Arnica has immunostimulatory activity.[14,15]

Extracts of arnica blossoms have been used in traditional medicine to improve blood flow. The sesquiterpene lactones helenalin and 11-alpha, 13-dihydrohelenalin have been shown to inhibit platelet aggregation by interacting with platelet sulfhydryl groups, suggesting therapeutic potential for these compounds.[16] Arnica increases the rate of reabsorption of internal bleeding.[2]

Arnica has been used traditionally as a topical agent to improve wound healing and externally for acne, boils, bruises, rashes, sprains, pains, and other wounds.[3,7] Constituent helenalin and related esters have strong antimicrobial activity.[3] It has bactericidal[8] and fungicidal activity,[4,7] as well as counterirritant properties[8] as a result of the constituents arnidiol and foradiol.[17] Arnica also has been used for heart problems,[2,3,7] to improve circulation,[3] reduce cholesterol,[3,7] and stimulate the CNS.[7]

TOXICOLOGY: The internal use of arnica and its extracts cannot be recommended. The plant is considered poisonous, and oral use should be avoided or strictly controlled.[2,3,8] Arnica irritates mucous membranes, and causes stomach pain, diarrhea, and vomiting.[4,8] Gastroenteritis has occurred with high oral dosages; dyspnea and cardiac arrest may occur resulting in death.[3] The flowers and roots of the plant have caused vomiting, drowsiness, and coma when eaten by children. Gastric lavage or emesis followed by supportive treatment is recommended.[18] A 1 oz tincture reportedly produced serious, but not fatal effects.[4] In animal experimentation, the helenolide constituents of arnica were cardiotoxic.[3,8]

The plant's sesquiterpene lactones are responsible for its oxytocic activity. In folk medicine, arnica was used as an abortifacient because of these actions.[3]

Numerous cases of contact dermatitis have been reported. Chemical and animal experimentation have proven the high sensitizing capacity of the plant. Sesquiterpene lactones helenalin, helenalin acetate, and methacrylate are the primary culprits in this type of allergy.[19] Another report is available identifying the allergans in arnica.[20] Three cases of patients with occupational contact dermatitis to arnica have been reported.[21] A case report of a 65-year-old male suffered from chronic eczema on his face and hands related to arnica's sesquiterpene lactones.[22]

[1] Schauenberg P, et al. *Guide to Medicinal Plants.* New Canaan, CT: Keats Pub., 1977.

[2] Chevallier A. *Encyclopedia of Medicinal Plants.* New York, NY: DK Publishing, 1996;170.

[3] Bisset N. *Herbal Drugs and Phytopharmaceuticals.* Stuttgart, Germany: CRC Press, 1994:83–87.

[4] Leung A. *Encyclopedia of Common Natural Ingredients,* 2nd ed. New York: John Wiley & Sons, 1996;40–41.

[5] Ghosh A. *Lancet* 1983;8319:304.

[6] DerMarderosian A. *Natural Product Medicine.* Philadelphia, PA: George F. Stickley Co, 1988;253–54.

[7] Duke J. CRC *Handbook of Medicinal Herbs.* Boca Raton, FL: CRC Press, 1989;64.

[8] Newall C, et al. *Herbal Medicines.* London, England: Pharmaceutical Press, 1996;34–35.

[9] Tveiten D, et al. *Tidsskr Nor Laegeforen* 1991;111(30):3630–31.

[10] Kaziro G. *Br J Oral Maxillofac Surg* 1984;22(1):42–49.

[11] Knaus U, et al. *Planta Med* 1988;54:565.

[12] Puhlmann J. *Phytochemistry* 1991;30(4):1141–45.

[13] Puhlmann J, et al. *Planta Medica* 1989;55:99.

[14] Wagner H, et al. *Arzneimittelforschung* 1984;34(6):659–61.

[15] Wagner H, et al. *Arzneimittelforschung* 1985;35(7):1069–75.

[16] Schroder H, et al. *Thromb Res* 1990;57:839.

[17] Tyler V. *Herbs of Choice.* New York: Pharmaceutical Products Press, Haworth Press, Inc. 1994:157.

[18] Hardin JW, et al. *Human Poisoning from Native and Cultivated Plants.* Duke University Press, 1974.

[19] Hausen B. *Hautarzt* 1980;31(1):10–17.

[20] Hausen B. *Contact Dermatitis* 1978;4(5):308.

[21] Hausen B. *Contact Dermatitis* 1978;4(1):3–10.

[22] Spettoli E, et al. *Am J Contact Dermat* 1998;9(1):49–50.

SCIENTIFIC NAME(S): *Persea americana* Mill. Synonymous with *P. gratissima* Gaertn. Also referred to as *Laurus persea* L. Family: Lauraceae

COMMON NAME(S): Avocado, alligator pear, ahuacate, avocato

ᕶᕶᕶ PATIENT INFORMATION ᕶᕶᕶ

Uses: The fruit is commonly eaten and the fruit oil used for cosmetics. Studies indicate avocado reduces cholesterol and improves lipid profile. Seed derivatives reportedly have antitumor activity in rodents.

Side Effects: Large quantities of seeds or leaves appear to be toxic.

BOTANY: The avocado grows to 1500 cm to 1800 cm in height. It bears a large fleshy fruit that is oval or spherical in shape; the skin of the fruit can be thick and woody. The plant is native to Mexico and Central America.[1]

HISTORY: The pulp has been used as a pomade to stimulate hair growth and hasten the healing of wounds. The fruit also has been purported as an aphrodisiac and emmenagogue. American Indians have used the seeds to treat dysentery and diarrhea. Today, the fruit is eaten and the oil is a component of numerous cosmetic formulations.

PHARMACOLOGY: Avocado oil has been used extensively for its ability to heal and soothe the skin. This use is based on the high hydrocarbon content of the pulp and oil, which may help dry skin.

Avocados are frequently included in health diets, and recent evidence suggests they are effective in modifying lipid profiles. In a randomized study, women chose either a diet high in monounsaturated fatty acids enriched with avocado or a high complex-carbohydrate diet. After 3 weeks, the avocado diet resulted in a reduction in total cholesterol level from baseline (8.2%);

a decrease (4.9%) occurred with the comparison diet. Low-density lipoprotein cholesterol and apolipoprotein B levels decreased in the avocado group.[2]

TOXICOLOGY: The poisoning of grazing animals that have ingested avocado has been observed in species as diverse as fish and birds.[1] One review reported that feeding dried avocado seed in a 1:1 ratio with normal food rations killed all mice tested.[3] The amount of avocado ingested ranged from 10 to 14 g. Signs of toxicity became apparent after 2 to 3 days and the animals generally died within the next 24 hours. Gross findings included hemorrhage into the brain, lungs, and liver.

In cattle and goats, acute toxicity has been characterized by a cessation of milk flow and nonbacterial mastitis. Fish have been killed as a result of avocado leaves falling into a backyard pond.[3] Although the specific mechanism of toxicity is not clear, leaves fed to goats reproducibly decreased milk production and increased AST and LDH enzyme levels. A published case report suggests that the anticoagulant effects of warfarin may be antagonized by the avocado.[4]

---

[1] Leung AY. *Encyclopedia of Common Natural Ingredients Used in Food, Drugs, and Cosmetics.* New York, NY: John Wiley and Sons, 1980.

[2] Colquhoun DM, et al. *Am J Clin Nutr* 1992;56:671.

[3] Craigmill AL, et al. *Vet Hum Toxicol* 1984;26:381.

[4] Blickstein D, et al. *Lancet* 1991;337:914.

SCIENTIFIC NAME(S): *Berberis vulgaris* L. and *B. aquifolium* Pursh. However, more appropriately designated *Mahonia aquifolium* Nutt. Family: Berberidaceae

COMMON NAME(S): Barberry, Oregon grape, trailing mahonia, berberis, jaundice berry, woodsour, sowberry, pepperidge bush, sour-spine[1,2]

⁂ PATIENT INFORMATION ⁂

Uses: The fruits have been used in jams and jellies. Plant alkaloids have been found to be bactericidal, antidiarrheal, anticonvulsant, hypotensive, and sedative. Berberine is a uterine stimulant.

Side Effects: Barberry can produce stupor, daze, diarrhea, and nephritis.

BOTANY: The barberry *B. vulgaris* grows wild throughout Europe but has been naturalized to many regions of the eastern US. *B. aquifolium* is an evergreen shrub native to the Rocky Mountains. Barberry grows to > 300 cm with branched, spiny holly-like leaves. Its yellow flowers bloom from May to June and develop into red to blue-black oblong berries.[3]

HISTORY: The plant has a long history of use, dating back to the Middle Ages. The extracts of the plant are used today in homeopathy for treatment of intestinal disorders and sciatica. A decoction of the plant has been used to treat GI ailments and coughs.[3] The plant has been used as a bitter tonic and antipyretic. More than three dozen traditional uses for barberry have been cited,[4] including cancer,[5] cholera, and hypertension. The alkaloid berberine was included as an astringent in eye drops, but its use has become rare. The fruits have been used to prepare jams and jellies. The medicinal use of the plant has been limited by the bitter taste of the bark and root.

PHARMACOLOGY: Berberine (100 mg 4 times a day), given either alone or together with tetracycline (eg, *Achromycin V*), was found to significantly improve acute watery diarrhea and excretion of vibrios after 24 hours, compared with placebo in patients with cholera-induced diarrhea. Berberine had no benefit over placebo in patients with non-cholera diarrhea.[6] Berberine does not appear to exert its antidiarrheal effect by astringency, and the mechanism of action has not been defined.[7]

Berberine has anticonvulsant, sedative, and uterine-stimulant properties. Local anesthesia can occur following SC injection of berberine.[4] Berbamine produces a hypotensive effect.[8]

TOXICOLOGY: Symptoms of poisoning are characterized by stupor and daze, diarrhea, and nephritis.

[1] Windholz M ed. *The Merck Index*, 10th ed. Rahway, NJ: Merck and Co., 1983.
[2] Leung AY. *Encyclopedia of Common Natural Ingredients Used in Food, Drugs and Cosmetics.* New York, NY: John Wiley and Sons, 1980.
[3] Schauenberg P, Paris F. *Guide to Medicinal Plants.* New Canaan, CT: Keats Publishing, Inc., 1977.
[4] Duke JA. *Handbook of Medicinal Herbs.* Boca Raton, FL: CRC Press, 1985.
[5] Hartwell JL. *Lloydia* 1968;31(2):71.
[6] Maung KU, et al. *BMJ* 1985;291:1601.
[7] Akhter MH, et al. *Indian J Med Res* 1979;70:233.
[8] Tyler VE. *The New Honest Herbal.* Philadelphia, PA: G.F. Stickley Co, 1987.

Bayberry

SCIENTIFIC NAME(S): *Myrica cerifera* L. Family: Myricaceae

COMMON NAME(S): Bayberry, wax myrtle plant

༄༅༄ PATIENT INFORMATION ༄༅༄

Uses: Bayberry tea has been used as a tonic, stimulant, and diarrhea treatment. Plant parts are also used to heal wounds. Bayberry wax is used to make fragrant candles.

Side Effects: Bayberry should not be taken internally. Ingestion may cause GI distress. Long-term injection produced malignancies in rats.

BOTANY: The bayberry grows as a large evergreen shrub or small tree that is widely distributed throughout the southern and eastern US. It is known for its small bluish white berries.[1]

HISTORY: The bayberry is best known for its berries, from which a wax is derived to make fragrant bayberry candles. In folk medicine, it has been used internally as a tea for its tonic and stimulant properties in the treatment of diarrhea. The dried root bark is often used medicinally.[2] The plant is astringent, which may account for this latter use along with its use for topical wound healing.[1]

PHARMACOLOGY: Myricadiol has been reported to have mineralocorticoid activity. Myricitrin has choleretic activity, stimulating the flow of bile.[1] The dried root is reported to have antipyretic properties.[2]

TOXICOLOGY: The elevated tannin concentration of the plant precludes its general internal use. The percutaneous injection of bark extracts in rats produced a significant number of malignant tumors following long-term (78-week) administration.[1,2] Ingestion of the plant may cause gastric irritation and vomiting.[3] The plant is said to be an irritant and sensitizer.[4]

---

[1] Tyler VE. *The New Honest Herbal.* Philadephia, PA: G.F. Stickley Co., 1987.

[2] Leung AY. *Encyclopedia of Common Natural Ingredients Used in Food, Drugs, and Cosmetics.* New York, NY: John Wiley and Sons, 1980.

[3] Spoerke DG Jr. *Herbal Medications.* Santa Barbara, CA: Woodbridge Press, 1980.

[4] Duke JA. *Handbook of Medicinal Herbs.* Boca Raton, FL: CRC Press, 1985.

PATIENT INFORMATION

Uses: Although bee pollen is nutritionally rich, claims that it enhances athletic performance have not been reliably verified. Some evidence indicates it may benefit a range of conditions, from constipation to aging.

Side Effects: Ingestion produces allergic reactions in sensitive individuals. Attempts to hyposensitize by administering bee pollen may produce severe anaphylaxis and other acute or chronic responses.

SOURCE: Bee pollen consists of plant pollens collected by worker bees, combined with plant nectar and bee saliva. Packed by the insects into small pellets, it is used as a food source for the male drones. Commercially, the pollen is gathered at the entrance of the hive by forcing the bees to enter through a portal partially obstructed with wire mesh, thus brushing the material off the hind legs into a collection vessel. Because of the increasing popularity of this health food, this means of pollen collection has been supplemented by the direct collection of the material from within the hives. Alternately, pollen is collected directly from the wind-pollinated plants by automated means, and the pollen is compressed into tablets, with or without added nutritional supplements.[1]

HISTORY: The use of bee pollen increased during the late 1970s following testimonials by athletes that supplementation with this product increased stamina and improved athletic ability.

PHARMACOLOGY: Articles in the lay press reported that athletes could enhance their performance by ingesting bee pollen; however, an investigation conducted by the National Athletic Trainer Association with Louisiana State University swim team members found no beneficial effect.[2] The results of a study conducted in track runners suggested that athletes who took bee pollen recovered faster after exercise; therefore, it would help relieve common tiredness and lack of energy. Critics of the study found the test group to be small, the blinding to be inadequate, and the conclusions to be premature.[3]

Bee pollen has been recommended to immunologically strengthen multiple sclerosis patients being treated with prednisolone and *Proper-Myl*.[4] Bee pollen may relieve or cure cerebral hemorrhage, bodily weakness, anemia, weight loss, enteritis, colitis, and constipation.[5] However, all of these require clinical verification.

TOXICOLOGY: Reports of adverse reactions to bee pollen have been related to allergic reactions after ingestion by sensitive persons. There is a popular, but unadvisable, home practice of using bee pollen to treat allergic disorders. Despite the usually limited response to oral hyposensitization techniques and the potential for severe allergic reactions, this practice has spread considerably.

In one anaphylaxis report, a 46-year-old man with a history of seasonal allergic rhinitis took a teaspoonful of bee pollen to treat his hay fever symptoms. Fifteen minutes later he developed paroxysm of sneezing, and by 30 minutes, experienced generalized angioedema, itching, dyspnea, and lightheadedness. He recovered following treatment with epinephrine, corticosteroids, and diphenhydramine.[1]

Other investigators have reported similar allergic reactions after single doses among patients with a history of allergic rhinitis. The dose required to precipitate an acute allergic reaction was

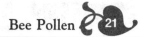

less than 1 tablespoonful of bee pollen.[6] By contrast, the development of hypereosinophilia, neurologic, and GI symptoms in a woman who ingested bee pollen for > 3 weeks also was reported.[7] These chronic allergic symptoms resolved upon discontinuation of the preparation. Although infrequent, some reports of severe allergic reactions to bee pollen have been observed. A 33-year-old man with no prior allergies had an acute anaphylactic reaction 15 minutes after ingesting bee pollen. He recovered fully after emergency medical treatment with epinephrine, Lactated Ringer's solution, and methylprednisolone sodium succinate.[8]

[1] Mansfield LE, Goldstein GB. *Ann Allergy* 1981;47:154.

[2] Montgomery PL. *New York Times* 1977(Feb 6).

[3] Blustein P. *Wall Street Journal* 1981(Feb 12).

[4] Iarosh AA, et al. *Vrach Delo* 1990;(2):83.

[5] Tyler VE. *The Honest Herbal: A Sensible Guide to the Use of Herbs and Related Remedies*, 3rd ed. New York: Haworth Press, 1993.

[6] Cohen, SH, et al. *J Allergy Clin Immunol* 1979;64(4):270.

[7] Lin FL, et al. *J Allergy Clin Immunol* 1989;83(4):793.

[8] Geyman JP. *J Am Board Fam Pract* 1994;7(3):250.

Betel Nut

SCIENTIFIC NAME(S): *Areca catechu* L. Family: Palmae

COMMON NAME(S): Betel nut, areca nut, pinlang, pinang

❧❧❧ PATIENT INFORMATION ❧❧❧

Uses: Many Asians chew betel nut, usually along with other components in a quid. Betel nut is a CNS and salivary stimulant. The leaves may act as an antitussive and topically as a counterirritant.

Side Effects: Oral cancer and precancerous conditions are common among users. Betel may exacerbate asthma and contribute to periodontitis.

BOTANY: The areca tree is a feathery palm that grows to ≈ 15 m in height. It is cultivated in tropical India, Sri Lanka, south China, the East Indies, the Philippines, and parts of Africa. The hard nut is about 2.5 cm in length.[1]

HISTORY: The chewing of betel nut quids dates to antiquity. Betel nut is used in India and the Far East as a mild stimulant and digestive aid. The quid is generally composed of a mixture of tobacco, powdered or sliced areca nut, and slaked lime often obtained from powdered snail shells. This mixture is wrapped in the leaf of the "betel" vine (*Piper betel* L. Family: Piperaceae). Users may chew from 4 to 15 quids a day with each quid being chewed for about 15 minutes.[2] Because of its CNS-stimulating effects, betel nut is used in a manner similar to the Western use of tobacco or caffeine.[3] Chewing the nut stimulates salivary flow, thereby aiding digestion. The leaves have been used externally as a counterirritant and internally as an antitussive.

PHARMACOLOGY: Arecoline is an alkaloid, contained in betel nut, that has been used in veterinary medicine as a cathartic for horses and as a worm killer. The alkaloids of betel nut cause pupil dilation, vomiting, diarrhea, and in high doses, convulsions and death. Extracts of the nut have been used for the management of glaucoma in traditional medicine.[4] Betel nut chewing induces a number of physiologic changes including an increase in saliva-tion,[5] gradual resorption of oral calcium induced by the lime, gingivitis, periodontitis, and chronic osteomyelitis.[6]

TOXICOLOGY: As with chewing or smoking tobacco, the long-term use of betel nut has serious adverse health effects. Leukoplakia, which is considered to be a precancerous lesion, and squamous cell carcinoma of the oral mucosa have been found with unusually high frequency in long-term users of betel nut. Studies in New Guinea also have shown that chewing a betel nut-slaked lime mixture has been associated with oral leukoplakia that is precancerous in up to 10% of the cases.[7] By contrast, in persons chewing betel nut alone, such lesions are infrequent.

Experimental evidence indicates that arecaidine and arecoline have the greatest carcinogenic potential. When tested by an in vitro cell transformation assay, both alkaloids gave a positive response, implicating both as suspected human carcinogens.[8] Other compounds are also highly active in decreasing mucosal cell viability, colony-forming efficiency, and in causing DNA strand breaks and cross-links in buccal cells in vitro. These effects indicate that these compounds may contribute to the oral carcinogenicity associated with chewing betel nut quid.[9]

The incidence of oral cancers increases among heavy long-term chewers of betel quids; whether this is caused by the

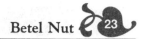
alkaloids, to the associated tannin (which accounts for 15% of the nut weight), or to carcinogens in the tobacco that is often added to the quid, is unknown. The protective value of chewing betel leaf is also unknown.

The results of one study of Filipino betel chewers found that dietary supplementation with retinol (100,000 IU/week) and beta-carotene (300,000 IU/week) for 3 months was associated with a 3-fold decrease (from 4.2% to 1.4%) in the mean proportion of oral cells with nuclear alterations suggestive of precancerous lesions.[2]

Arecaine is poisonous and affects respiration and heart rate, increases intestinal peristalsis, and can cause tetanic convulsions. Although doses of the seed in the range of 8 to 10 g have been reported to be fatal, others have suggested that doses up to 30 g may have a low toxicity potential.[10]

Betel nut chewing has been associated with an aggravation of asthma, and a dose-response relationship may exist between the use of this drug and the development of asthmatic symptoms.[11]

[1] Evans WC. *Trease and Evans' Pharmacognosy*, 13th ed. London, England: Bailliere Tindall, 1989.

[2] Stich HF, et al. *Lancet* 1984;8388(i):1204.

[3] Boyland E. *Planta Med* 1968(Suppl):13.

[4] Morton JF. *Major Medicinal Plants*. Springfield, IL: CC Thomas, 1977.

[5] Reddy MS, et al. *Am J Clin Nutr* 1980;33:77.

[6] Westermeyer J. *JAMA* 1982;248:1835.

[7] McCallum CA. *JAMA* 1982;247(19):2715.

[8] Ashby J, et al. *Lancet* 1979;1(8107):112.

[9] Sundqvist K, et al. *IARC Sci Publ* 1991;105:281.

[10] Duke JA. *Handbook of Medicinal Herbs*. Boca Raton, FL: CRC Press, 1985.

[11] Kiyingi KS. *PNG Med J* 1991;34(2):117.

SCIENTIFIC NAME(S): *Stachys officinalis* (L.) Trevisan, also referred to as *Betonica officinalis* L. in some older texts. Family: Labiatae

COMMON NAME(S): Betony, wood betony, and bishop wort. The genus is often collectively referred to as hedge-nettles.

⋙⋙ PATIENT INFORMATION ⋙⋙

Uses: Betony is used as an astringent to treat diarrhea and as a gargle or tea for mouth and throat irritations. It has been used to treat anxiety and headaches.

Side Effects: Betony overdosage can cause stomach irritation. Do not take during pregnancy.

BOTANY: Betony is a square-stemmed, mat-forming perennial of the mint family. It is distributed widely throughout western and southern Europe. It has a rosette of hairy leaves and a dense terminal spike of pink, white, or purple flowers that bloom from June to September. The plant reaches a height of 1 m. The above-ground parts are dried and used medicinally.[1,2]

HISTORY: Betony's use has been known since the Roman Empire, where it was considered a panacea for practically every disease. During the Middle Ages, the plant was ascribed magical powers.[3]

The plant is still used in traditional medicine. A weak infusion is sometimes taken as a tea. It is used as an astringent to treat diarrhea and as a gargle or tea for irritations of the mouth and throat. It has been given to treat anxiety, as a tincture, or smoked for the treatment of headaches.[4]

PHARMACOLOGY: The high tannin content of the plant most likely contributes to the antidiarrheal effect. In large doses, the plant may have purgative and emetic action. A powder of the dried pulverized leaves has been used to induce sneezing.[5] Betony possesses sedative properties, relieving nervous stress and tension. It is still used as a remedy for headache and facial pain. In combination with herbs such as comfrey or linden, betony is effective for sinus headache and congestion.[2] Other uses for betony include treatment of diarrhea and nosebleeds, a gargle for gums, mouth, and throat, and irritations of mucous membranes. Folk remedies of betony include treatment of tumors, spleen and liver sclerosis, colds, convulsions, kidney stones, palpitations, stomachache, and toothaches.[4] Betony is known to stimulate the digestive system and the liver.[2]

TOXICOLOGY: There is little evidence of betony toxicity; however, overdosage may cause GI irritation because of the tannin content.[4] Betony polyphenols were found to be toxic in animals.[6] Betony should not be taken during pregnancy.[2]

[1] Bremness L. *The Complete Book of Herbs.* London, England: Dorling Kindersley Ltd., 1988;278.

[2] Chevallier A. *Encyclopedia of Medicinal Plants.* New York, NY: DK Publishing, 1996:270.

[3] Tyler VE. *The New Honest Herbal.* Philadelphia, PA: G.F. Stickley Co., 1987.

[4] Duke J. *CRC Handbook of Medicinal Herbs.* Boca Raton, FL: CRC Press Inc., 1989;457.

[5] Schauenberg P, et al. *Guide to Medicinal Plants.* New Canaan, CT: Keats Publishing Inc., 1977.

[6] Lipkan G, et al. *Farmatsevtychnyi Zhurnal* 1974;29(1):78–81.

SCIENTIFIC NAME(S): *Vaccinium myrtillus,* Myrtilli fructus. Family: Ericaeae

COMMON NAME(S): Bilberries, bog bilberries,[1] whortleberries

---

🌿🌿 PATIENT INFORMATION 🌿🌿

Uses: Tea prepared from dried bilberries are used internally to treat nonspecific diarrhea and topically for inflamed mouth and throat mucosa. Bilberry extracts improve visual acuity and ability to adjust to changing light. Derivatives demonstrate vasoprotective, antiedema, and gastroprotective effects.

Side Effects: None known.

BOTANY: Bilberry fruit originates from northern and central Europe and has been imported from parts of southeastern Europe. These black, coarsely wrinkled berries contain many small, shiny brownish red seeds. They have a somewhat caustic and sweet taste.[1]

HISTORY: The historical uses of dried bilberry fruit include a supportive treatment of acute, non-specific diarrhea when administered as a tea and serving as a topical decoction for the inflammation of the mucous membranes of the mouth and throat.[1]

During World War II, British Royal Air Force pilots ate bilberry preserves before night missions in order to improve their vision. After the war, studies confirmed the folk beliefs that bilberry extracts could improve visual acuity and lead to faster visual adjustments between light and darkness.[2]

PHARMACOLOGY: Dried bilberry fruit is used as an antidiarrhetic, especially in mild cases of enteritis. It is also used as a topical treatment for mild inflammation of the mucous membranes of the mouth and throat.[1]

Most clinical studies have concentrated on the fruit's anthocyanoside content.

Anthocyanosides present in bilberry are also effective in promoting and intensifying arteriolar rhythmic diameter changes which aid in the redistribution of microvascular blood flow and interstitial fluid formation.[3]

An investigation using an anthocyanidin pigment (IdB 1027) found in bilberries showed protective gastric effects without influencing acid secretion. The pigment was administered orally using 600 mg twice daily for 10 days in 10 laboratory animals. The results showed an increase in the gastric mucosal release of prostaglandin E2, which may explain the antiulcer and gastroprotective effects of IdB 1027.[4]

Anthocyans and vitamin E are natural antioxidants which produce a protective effect on liver cells damaged by injury.[5]

TOXICOLOGY: The effects of ingesting large doses of bilberry are not known. There are no known side effects or interactions with other drugs.

It is important that the fruit has not been attacked by insects and is free of mold. The berries should be as soft as possible or the long-stored drug will become hard and brittle.[1]

[1] Bissett NG, ed. *Herbal Drugs and Phytopharmaceuticals.* Stuttgart: Medpharm Scientific Publishers, 1994.

[2] Murray MT. *The Healing Power of Foods.* Rocklin, CA: Prima Publishing, 1993.

[3] Colantuoni A, et al. *Arzneimittelforshung* 1991;41(9):905.

[4] Mertz-Nielsen A, et al. *Ital J Gastroenterol* 1990;22(5):288.

[5] Mitcheva M, et al. *Cell Microbiol* 1993;39(4):443.

Bitter Melon

SCIENTIFIC NAME(S): *Momordica charantia L.* Family: Cucurbitaceae

COMMON NAME(S): Bitter melon, balsam pear, bitter cucumber, balsam apple, "art pumpkin," cerasee, carilla cundeamor

---

⟩⟩⟩⟩ PATIENT INFORMATION ⟨⟨⟨⟨

Uses: Bitter melon has hypoglycemic, antimicrobial, and antifertility effects.

Drug Interactions: Increased hypoglycemic effect when *M. charantia* and chlorpropamide are coadministered.

Side Effects: Use with caution in hypoglycemic patients. The red arils around bitter melon seeds are toxic to children. The plant is not recommended in pregnant women because it may cause uterine bleeding and contractions or may induce abortion.

BOTANY: Bitter melon, an annual plant $\approx$ 180 cm tall, is cultivated in Asia, Africa, South America, and India. The plant has lobed leaves, yellow flowers, and bitter-tasting, orange-yellow fruit. The unripe fruit is green and cucumber-shaped with bumps on its surface. The parts used include the fruit, leaves, seeds, and seed oil.[1-3]

HISTORY: Bitter melon has been used for tumors, asthma, skin infections, GI problems, and hypertension.[4] The plant has been used as a traditional medicine in China, India, Africa, and the southeastern US, and for the treatment of diabetes symptoms.[3]

PHARMACOLOGY: Beneficial effects of bitter melon have been studied and reviewed.[3,5-7] These effects include hypoglycemic, antimicrobial, antifertility, and others.

The hypoglycemic effects of bitter melon have been clearly established in several studies.[8,9] Constituents of the plant contributing to its hypoglycemic properties include charantin, polypeptide P, and vicine.[2,10-12] Reduction of blood glucose and improvement of glucose tolerance are the mechanisms by which the plant exerts its actions.

Other mechanisms for hypoglycemic effects include extrapancreatic actions, such as increased glucose uptake by tissues, glycogen synthesis in liver and muscles, triglyceride production in adipose tissue, and gluconeogenesis.[13] One report suggests the mechanism to be partly attributed to increased glucose use in the liver, rather than an insulin secretory effect.[14] Hepatic enzyme studies demonstrate hypoglycemic activity by depression of blood glucose synthesis through depression of enzymes glucose-6-phosphatase and fructose-1,6-bisphosphatase, along with enhancement of glucose oxidation by enzyme G6PDH pathway.[15]

Bitter melon improves glucose tolerance.[16] One study reported improved glucose tolerance in 18 type 2 diabetes patients with 73% success from a bitter melon juice preparation.[17] An additional report observed a 54% decrease in postprandial blood sugar, as well as a 17% reduction in glycosylated hemoglobin in 6 patients taking 15 g of aqueous bitter melon extract.[2] One trial studied patients taking a powder preparation of the plant.[18] Bitter melon did not promote insulin secretion but did increase carbohydrate use.[4]

Roots and leaf extracts have shown antibiotic activity.[3,4] One study reports 33.4% cytostatic activity from bitter melon aqueous extract,[19] as constituents momorcharins have antitumor properties and can inhibit protein synthesis.[20] Similarly, the plant also inhibits replication of viruses, including polio, herpes simplex 1, and HIV.[3,10] A study on antipseudomonal activity reports bitter melon to be effective, but not promising.[21]

Bitter melon exhibits genotoxic effects in *Aspergillus nidulans*.[22] It is cytotoxic in leukemia cells as a guanylate cyclase inhibitor. The ripe fruit has been said to induce menstruation.[1]

Other effects of bitter melon include anti-inflammatory actions,[10] treatment for GI ailments[1,4] and hemorrhoids.[23] The plant has also been used for skin diseases,[4] for its lipid effects, and hypotensive actions.[4,10] The plant has also been used as an insecticide.[3,4]

TOXICOLOGY: Bitter melon extract is said to be nontoxic.[3] The plant is relatively safe at low doses and for a duration of ≤ 4 weeks.[1] There are no published reports of serious effects in adults given the "normal" oral dose of 50 ml. Bitter melon has low clinical toxicity, with some possible adverse GI effects.[10]

Because of the plant's ability to reduce blood sugar, take caution in susceptible patients who may experience hypoglycemia.[1] Two small children experienced hypoglycemic coma resulting from the intake of a tea made from the plant. Both recovered upon medical treatment.[10] Another report concerning increased hypoglycemic effect noted an interaction in a 40-year-old diabetic woman between *M. charantia* and chlorpropamide, which she was taking concurrently for her condition.[24]

The red arils around bitter melon seeds are toxic to children. The juice given to a child in one report caused vomiting, diarrhea, and death.[4]

The seed constituent, vicine, is a toxin said to induce "favism," an acute condition characterized by headache, fever, abdominal pain, and coma.[3,10]

Bitter melon is not recommended in pregnant women because of its reproductive system toxicities, induction of uterine bleeding and contractions or abortion induction.[3,23,10]

[1] Chevallier A. *Encyclopedia of Medicinal Plants.* New York, NY: DK Publishing, 1996:234.
[2] Murray M. *The Healing Power of Herbs*, 2nd ed. Rocklin, CA: Prima Publishing, 1995;357-58.
[3] Cunnick J, et al. *J Nat Med* 1993;4(1):16-21.
[4] Duke J. *CRC Handbook of Medicinal Herbs.* Boca Raton, FL: CRC Press Inc., 1989;315-16.
[5] Sankaranaravanan J, et al. *Indian J Pharm Sci* 1993;55(1):6-13.
[6] Platel K, et al. *Nahrung* 1997;41(2):68-74.
[7] Avedikian J. *California Pharmacist* 1994 Aug;42:15.
[8] Lei Q, et al. *J Tradit Chin Med* 1985 Jun;5(2)99-106.
[9] Aslam M, et al. *Internat Pharm J* 1989 Nov-Dec;3:226-29.
[10] Raman A, et al. *Phytomedicine* 1996;2(4):349-62.
[11] Wong C, et al. *J Ethnopharmacology* 1985 Jul;13:313-21.
[12] Handa G, et al. *Indian J Nat Prod* 1990;6(1):16-19.
[13] Welihinda J, et al. *J Ethnopharmacology* 1986 Sep;17:247-55.
[14] Sarkar S, et al. *Pharmacol Res* 1996 Jan;33(1):1-4.
[15] Shibib B, et al. *Biochem J* 1993 May 15;292(Pt. 1):267-70.
[16] Leatherdale B, et al. *BMJ (Clin Res Ed)* 1981 Jun 6;282(6279):1823-24.
[17] Welihinda J, et al. *J Ethnopharmacology* 1986 Sep;17:277-82.
[18] Akhtar M. *JPMA J Pak Med Assoc* 1982 Apr;32(4):106-7.
[19] Rojas N, et al. *Revista Cubana de Farmacia* 1980 May-Aug;14:219-25.
[20] Bruneton J. *Pharmacognosy, PhytoChemistry, Medicinal Plants.* Paris, France: Lavoisier, 1995;192.
[21] Saraya A, et al. *Mahidol Univ J Pharm Sci* 1985 Jul-Sep;12:69-73.
[22] Ramos R, et al. *J Ethnopharm* 1996;52(3):123-27.
[23] Hocking G. *A Dictionary of Natural Products.* Medford, NJ: Plexus Publishing Inc., 1997;504-5.
[24] Aslam M, et al. *Lancet* 1979 Mar 17;1:607.

SCIENTIFIC NAME(S): *Cimicifuga racemosa* (L.) Nutt. Family: Ranunculaceae. Plants associated with cohosh (although white cohosh and blue cohosh are quite distinct) include other *Cimicifuga* species, *Macrotys actaeoides* and *Actaea racemosa* L.

COMMON NAME(S): Black cohosh, baneberry, black snakeroot, bugbane, squawroot, rattle root[1]

ꙮꙮꙮ PATIENT INFORMATION ꙮꙮꙮ

Uses: Black cohosh has been used to help manage some symptoms of menopause and as an alternative to HRT therapy. It may be useful for hypercholesterolemia treatment or peripheral arterial disease.

Side Effects: Overdose causes nausea, dizziness, nervous system and visual disturbances, reduced pulse rate, and increased perspiration.

BOTANY: Black cohosh grows in open woods at the edges of dense forests from Ontario to Tennessee and west to Missouri. This perennial grows to 240 cm and is topped by a long plume of white flowers that bloom from June to September. Its leaflets are shaped irregularly with toothed edges. The term "black" refers to the dark color of the rhizome. The name "cohosh" comes from an Algonquian word meaning "rough," referring to the feel of the rhizome.[2]

HISTORY: The roots and rhizomes of this herb are used medicinally. Traditional uses include the treatment of dysmenorrhea, dyspepsia, and rheumatisms. A tea from the root has been recommended for sore throat. The Latin name cimicifuga means "bug-repellent" for which the plant has been used. American Indians used the plant to treat snakebites.

The old-time remedy "Lydia Pinkham's Vegetable Compound" from the early 1900s contained many natural ingredients, one of which was black cohosh.[3]

PHARMACOLOGY: *Remifemin*, the brand-name of the standardized extract of the plant, has been used in Germany for menopausal management since the mid-1950s.[4]

In women treated for 8 weeks with *Remifemin* and luteinizing hormone, but not follicle-stimulating hormone, levels were reduced significantly. This product is used for the management of menopausal hot flashes. Analysis of the commercial product identified ≥ 3 fractions that contribute synergistically to the suppression of LH and bind to estrogen receptors. These data suggest that black cohosh has a measurable effect on certain reproductive hormones.[5] The product may offer an alternative to conventional hormone replacement therapy (HRT). In patient populations with a history of estrogen-dependent cancer (although it possesses some estrogenic activity), *Remifemin* shows no stimulatory effects on established breast tumor cell lines dependent on estrogen's presence. Instead, inhibitory actions were seen. In addition, the product exerts no effect on endometrium, so there is no need to oppose therapy with progesterone as with conventional HRT. The plant extract's action proves to be more like estriol than estradiol. Estradiol is associated with a higher risk for breast, ovarian, and endometrial cancers. Estriol mainly exerts its effects on the vaginal lining rather than the uterine lining as estradiol does. However, more studies are

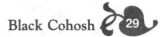

needed to address osteoporosis and bone health with use of the product.[4]

One report finds no signs of uterine growth and vaginal cornification in ovariectomized rats given black cohosh extract. This helps to confirm that the plant's beneficial effects on menopausal discomfort cannot be explained as estrogenic's typical effects.[6]

A clinical and endocrinologic study has been performed in 60 patients < 40 years old who had undergone hysterectomies. Four randomized treatment groups included estriol, conjugated estrogens, estrogen-gestagen sequential therapy, or black cohosh extract. Results of this report showed no significant differences between groups in success of therapy.[7]

Other actions of black cohosh include the following: Constituent actein that has been shown to have a hypotensive effect in rabbits and cats and causes peripheral vasodilation in dogs;[8,9] anti-microbial activity both by black cohosh[10] and related species *Cimicifuga dahurica*;[11] in vivo hypocholesterolemic activity; and therapy for patients with peripheral arterial disease by causing peripheral vasodilation and increase in blood flow from constituent actein.[11]

TOXICOLOGY: Overdose of black cohosh may cause nausea, vomiting, dizziness, nervous system and visual disturbances, reduced pulse rate, and increased perspiration. The constituent actein does not possess toxicity in animal studies.[11]

Large doses of the plant may induce miscarriage.[2] Black cohosh is contraindicated in pregnancy and may cause premature birth in large doses.[11]

A case report describes a 45-year-old woman who experienced seizures, possibly related to consumption of an herbal preparation containing black cohosh.[12]

[1] Meyer JE. *The Herbalist.* Hammond, IN. Hammond Book Co., 1934.
[2] Dobelis IN, ed. *Magic and Medicine of Plants.* Pleasantville, NY: Reader's Digest Association, 1986.
[3] Tyler V. *Pharmacy in History* 1995;37(1):24-28.
[4] Murray M. *Am J Nat Med* 1997;4(3):3-5.
[5] Duker E, et al. *Planta Medica* 1991;57(5):420-24.
[6] Einer-Jensen N, et al. *Maturitas* 1996;25(2):149-53.
[7] Lehmann Willenbrook E, et al. *Zentralbl Gynakol* 1988;110(10):611-18.
[8] Genazzani E, et al. *Nature* 1962;194:544.
[9] Corsano S, et al. *Gazz Chimica Ital* 1969;99:915.
[10] Bukowiecki H, et al. *Acta Pol Pharm* 1972;29:432.
[11] Newall C, et al. *Black Cohosh Herbal Medicines.* London, England: Pharmaceutical Press, 1996;80-81.
[12] Shuster J. *Hosp Pharm* 1996 Dec;31:1553-54.

Bloodroot

SCIENTIFIC NAME(S): *Sanguinaria canadensis* L. Family: Papaveraceae

COMMON NAME(S): Bloodroot, red root, red puccoon, tetterwort, Indian red plant, Indian plant, sanguinaria

---

٭٭٭ PATIENT INFORMATION ٭٭٭

Uses: Used externally in folk remedies to treat rheumatism, warts, polyps, and cancers. Evidence indicates derived compounds are antineoplastic. Derivatives in mouthwash and toothpaste limit dental plaque.

Side Effects: Ingestion is not recommended because of its low oral toxicity.

BOTANY: This perennial grows in rich woods from Ontario to Manitoba, Florida, and Oklahoma. It grows close to the ground and produces a large white flower in April. The stout rhizome contains a red juice that oozes following damage to the root; hence the name, bloodroot. The root and rhizome are collected and dried for use.

HISTORY: Bloodroot has a long history of use, especially in Russia and North America. A root tea was used externally by American Indian tribes for the treatment of rheumatisms. Other folk uses included the treatment of warts, nasal polyps, and skin cancers. During the mid-1800s, topical preparations containing bloodroot extracts were used as part of the "Fell Technique" for the treatment of breast tumors. Solutions of the root were also used as a dental analgesic. Extract of the root has been used as an emetic, expectorant,[1] and in combination products as a cough remedy.[2] A number of these folk uses have spurred research into the pharmacology of this plant.

PHARMACOLOGY: Sanguinarine, the pharmacologically active compound in bloodroot, can induce slight CNS depression and narcosis if ingested. These compounds have papaverine-like action on smooth and heart muscle. It inhibits sodium/potassium ATPase in the guinea pig brain and can react with nucleophiles in particular sulfhydryl enzymes, thereby inhibiting oxidative decarboxylation of pyruvate.[3]

Because of its long folk history in the treatment of cancers, the root has been investigated in detail for its antineoplastic activity. Carcinomas of the human nose and ear have responded to topical treatment with a preparation containing bloodroot extract.[4]

Bloodroot toothpastes are commercially available for use in the reduction of plaque. A large body of well-designed studies has found that toothpastes and oral rinses containing sanguinarine help reduce and limit the deposition of dental plaque in as little as 8 days.[5] Sanguinarine contains a negatively charged iminiun ion that permits it to bind to dental plaque.[6] Sanguinarine is effective in vitro against a number of common oral bacteria, some of which are considered to play an important role in plaque formation.[7,8] Bloodroot extracts have also been shown to reduce glycolysis activity in saliva.[9]

TOXICOLOGY: Despite the general opinion that bloodroot is considered to have a low oral toxicity potential,[10] its ingestion has been discouraged because of safety concerns. Sanguinarine appears to be poorly absorbed from the GI tract.[3]

When ingested in large doses, extracts of the root produced nausea and vomiting. Sanguinarine may cause slight CNS depression.[11]

Sanguinarine is a mild irritant to the eye and dust of the root irritates mucous

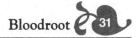

membranes.[12] Sanguinarine rinses in concentrations ranging from 0.03% to 0.045% generally did not induce mucosal irritation. No dermal sensitization or irritation has been noted in humans. Although the oral toxicity is low, it is suggested that reasonable precautions be used during processing of the crude drug to protect against inhalation exposure.[13] It is not mutagenic in the Ames mutagen assay.[3]

If ingested in large quantities, gastric lavage or emesis followed by symptomatic treatment has been suggested if tolerated by the patient.[14]

[1] Morton JF. *Major Medicinal Plants*. Springfield, IL: C.C. Thomas, 1977.

[2] Leung AY. *Encyclopedia of Common Natural Ingredients Used in Food, Drugs, and Cosmetics*. New York, NY: J. Wiley and Sons, 1990.

[3] Becci PJ, et al. *J Toxicol Environ Health* 1987;20:199.

[4] Phelan JT, et al. *Surgery* 1963;53:310.

[5] Southgard GL, et al. *J Am Dent Assoc* 1984;108:338.

[6] Bonesvoll P, et al. *Arch Oral Biol* 1978;23:289.

[7] Dzink JL, et al. *Antimicrob Agents Chemother* 1985;27:663.

[8] Eisenberg AD, et al. *J Dent Res* 1985;64:341.

[9] Boulware RT, et al. *J Dent Res* 1984;63:1274.

[10] Lewis WH, et al. *Medical Botany*. New York, NY: John Wiley and Sons, 1977.

[11] Hakim, et al. *Nature* 1961;189:198.

[12] Duke JA. *Handbook of Medicinal Herbs*. Boca Raton, FL: CRC Press, 1985.

[13] Schwarts H, et al. *Toxicologist* 1985;5:702.

[14] Hardin JW, et al. *Human Poisoning from Native and Cultivated Plants*, 2nd ed. Durham, NC: Duke University, 1974.

Blue Cohosh

SCIENTIFIC NAME(S): *Caulophyllum thalictroides* (L.) Michx. Family: Berberidaceae

COMMON NAME(S): Blue cohosh, blue ginseng, squaw root, papoose root, yellow ginseng

---

PATIENT INFORMATION

Uses: Folk use as an antispasmodic, uterine stimulant, and treatment for rheumatism. It is a general stimulant, possibly antimicrobial and contraceptive.

Side Effects: Raw seeds are reportedly poisonous; leaves are toxic.

BOTANY: Blue cohosh is a perennial herb that grows to 60 to 90 cm. It has yellow-green or green-purple flowers that can be found in rich moist woods from Canada to South Carolina. The flowers develop into dark blue seeds.[1]

HISTORY: Early uses of blue cohosh include the treatment of rheumatism, cramps, epilepsy, and uterus inflammation. In the 1800s, blue cohosh gained a reputation as an antispasmodic, menstrual flow stimulant, and labor inducer.[2] The plant has reportedly normalized the menstrual cycle when given with pennyroyal.[3] In addition, it continues to find use in black ethnic medicine.[4]

PHARMACOLOGY: Methylcytisine and caulophylline, compounds in blue cohosh, are pharmacologically similar to nicotine, resulting in increased blood pressure, small intestine stimulation, and hyperglycemia. In animal tests, it was 10 to 40 times less active than nicotine, and convulsions produced by the drug were less severe than those resulting from nicotine.[5]

Caulophyllosaponin, another blue cohosh compound, and caulosaponin are uterine stimulants which also have a toxic effect on cardiac muscle, probably caused by vasoconstrictor activity on the coronary blood vessels.[6] Investigators in India found low-dose extracts of blue cohosh given to rats inhibit ovulation and result in uterine changes that will inhibit nidation, suggesting the plant may have contraceptive potential.[7] There is some indication that extracts of related blue cohosh species exert antimicrobial activity.[8]

TOXICOLOGY: The leaves and seeds of the plant contain alkaloids and glycosides and can cause severe stomach pain when ingested. The seeds are bitter, and poisonings have been reported following their ingestion.[3] Strong heat denatures the toxicity of the seeds, and roasted seeds are used as a coffee substitute. Poisoning is usually treated by gastric lavage or emesis followed by supportive treatment.[9] Powdered dried blue cohosh is said to be irritating to mucous membranes.[1,3]

[1] Dobelis IN, ed. *Magic and Medicine of Plants.* Pleasantville, NY: Reader's Digest Association, Inc., 1986.

[2] Tyler VA. *The New Honest Herbal. Philadelphia,* PA: G.F. Stickley Co., 1987.

[3] Duke JA. *Handbook of Medicinal Herbs.* Boca Raton, FL: CRC Press, 1985.

[4] Boyd EL, et al. *Home Remedies and the Black Elderly.* Levittown, PA: Pharmaceutical Information Associates, Ltd., 1991.

[5] Scott CC, et al. *Therapeutics* 1943;79:334.

[6] Ferguson HC, et al. *J Am Pharm Assoc* 1954;43:16.

[7] Chandrasekhar K, et al. *J Reprod Fertil* 1974;38:236.

[8] Anisimov MM, et al. *Antibio Khimioter* 1972;17:834.

[9] Hardin JW, et al. *Human Poisoning from Native and Cultivated Plants.* Durham, NC: Duke University Press, 1974.

SCIENTIFIC NAME(S): *Eupatorium perfoliatum* L. Family: Asteraceae

COMMON NAME(S): Boneset, thoroughwort, vegetable antimony, feverwort, agueweed, Indian sage, sweating plant, eupatorium, crosswort

---

⟐⟐⟐ PATIENT INFORMATION ⟐⟐⟐

Uses: Boneset has chiefly been used to treat fevers.

Side Effects: Large amounts of teas or extracts can cause severe diarrhea. Because of liver damage and other toxic effects of its alkaloids, the use of boneset is discouraged.

BOTANY: Boneset is an ubiquitous plant found growing in swamps, marshes, and shores from Canada to Florida and west to Texas and Nebraska. The plant is easily recognized by its long, narrow, tapering leaves that oppose each other around a single stout stem, giving the impression of one long leaf pierced at the center by the stem. Hence, its name "perfolia," meaning through the leaves. The plant grows from July to October to a height of 90 to 120 cm, flowering in late summer with white blossoms. The entire plant is hairy and light green in color.

HISTORY: Boneset has been used as a charm and medicinal remedy for centuries by the American Indians. As a charm, the root fibers were applied to hunting whistles, since they were believed to increase the whistle's ability to call deer.[1] As an herbal remedy, Indians used boneset as an antipyretic. The early settlers used the plant to treat rheumatisms, dropsy, dengue fever, pneumonia, and influenza. The name "boneset" was derived from the plant's use in the treatment of break-bone fever, a term describing the high fever that often accompanies influenza.[2]

PHARMACOLOGY: Based on data from early medical compendia, boneset is believed to have diuretic and laxative properties in small doses; large doses may result in emesis and catharsis.[3] The "usual" dose of boneset was the equivalent of 2 to 4 grams of plant administered as a fluid extract. When used as a household remedy, the plant has been taken as a tea ranging in concentration from 2 teaspoonsful to 2 tablespoonsful of crushed dried leaves and flowering tops steeped in a cup to a pint of boiling water. Boneset had been used by physicians to treat fever, but its use was supplanted by safer and more effective antipyretics. It is not known which components of boneset reduce fever, or what the relative degree of effectiveness is of these compounds.

A number of the sesquiterpene lactones isolated from the plant and related species (ie, eupatilin, eupafolin), and flavones (eupatorin) have been shown to possess cytotoxic or antineoplastic activity.[3,4]

An extract of *E. perfoliatum* combined with other herbs has been shown to stimulate phagocyte activity in vitro.[5] Compounds isolated from the related species *E. odoratum* have been found to enhance blood coagulation by accelerating clotting time through the activation of certain clotting factors.[6]

TOXICOLOGY: Although few reports of adverse effects have been reported with the use of boneset, the FDA has classified this plant as an "Herb of Undefined Safety."[7] Large amounts of teas or extracts result in severe diarrhea. The identification of pyrrolizidine alkaloids in *Eupatorium* species is disconcerting. This class of alkaloids is known to cause hepatic impairment after long-term ingestion. While direct evidence for a hepatotoxic effect from boneset does not exist, there is sufficient evidence to indicate that any plant containing pyrrolizidine alkaloids should not be ingested.

The sesquiterpene lactones of the related species *E. cannabinum* L. have been reported to induce contact dermatitis, although no documented cross-allergenicity to *E. perfoliatum* has been reported.[8]

Symptoms of toxicity are often observed in grazing animals and include weakness, nausea, loss of appetite, thirst, and constipation. Animals may show muscle trembling and drooling progressing to muscle paralysis and death. Milk sickness in humans has been attributed to boneset poisoning from animals.[9] These symptoms also are seen after ingestion of the related *E. rugosum* (white snakeroot), and the activation of a toxic component by the cytochrome P450 system appears to be required for the toxic effect to occur.[10]

[1] Densmore F. *How Indians Used Wild Plants.* NY: Dover Publications, 1974.

[2] Dobelis IN, ed. *Magic and Medicine of Plants.* Pleasantville, NY: Reader's Digest Association, Inc., 1986.

[3] Leung AY. *Encyclopedia of Common Natural Ingredients Used in Food, Drugs and Cosmetics.* New York, NY: John Wiley and Sons, 1980.

[4] Woerdenbag HJ, et al. *Br J Cancer* 1989;59:68.

[5] Wagner H, et al. *Arzneimittelforschung* 1991;41:1072.

[6] Triratana T, et al. *J Med Assoc Thai* 1991;74:283.

[7] Duke JA. *Handbook of Medicinal Herbs.* Boca Raton, FL: CRC Press, 1985.

[8] Evans FJ, et al. *Planta Medica* 1980;38:289.

[9] Spoerke DG Jr. *Herbal Medications.* Santa Barbara, CA: Woodbridge Press, 1980.

[10] Beier RC, et al. *Vet Hum Toxicol* 1990;32:81.

Borage

SCIENTIFIC NAME(S): *Borago officinalis* L. Family: Boraginaceae

COMMON NAME(S): Borage, common borage, bee bread, common bugloss, starflower, ox's tongue, cool tankard[1,2,3]

⟐⟐⟐ PATIENT INFORMATION ⟐⟐⟐

Uses: Leaves and flowers may be eaten, used for tea, or steeped in wine. Although credited with increasing lactation, dispelling melancholy, and relieving cold symptoms, borage exhibits little pharmacological significance.

Side Effects: None known.

BOTANY: A hardy annual that grows to about 60 cm, the entire plant is covered with coarse hairs. Borage has oval leaves and star-shaped bright blue flowers with black anthers. The flowers bloom from May to September. Borage is found throughout Europe and North America. The fresh plant has a salty flavor and a cucumber-like odor.[3]

HISTORY: Borage leaves have been a part of European herbal medicine for centuries. In the Middle Ages, the leaves and flowers were steeped in wine to dispel melancholy. It has been suggested for the relief of rheumatisms, colds, bronchitis, and to increase breast milk production.[3] Infusions of the leaves and stems were once used to induce sweating and diuresis. Although it is now only sold as an herbal remedy, borage has been an official drug in Germany, Spain, Portugal, Romania, Venezuela, and Mexico.[3] The preserved leaves, soaked in vinegar, have been used as hors d'oeuvres and are eaten like spinach.[4] An infusion of borage flowers and dried stems is valued for its refreshing effect. It is often used to accent salads, pickles, and vegetables.[3]

PHARMACOLOGY: In small amounts, borage may have a slight constipating effect most likely because of the tannin content.[5] The mucilage may contribute to the purported expectorant action. The mild diuretic effect has been attributed to the presence of malic acid and potassium nitrate.[6] Borage is often found in *otc* herbal preparations designed for the relief of cold symptoms. While there is no direct evidence for its beneficial action, at least one of its components has the ability to act as an expectorant.

TOXICOLOGY: Borage has been used without significant adverse effects for hundreds of years. It can be eaten raw or cooked like spinach or in jams, jellies, and teas. The presence of toxic pyrrolizidine alkaloids in borage has not been demonstrated in contrast to other Boraginaceae. The toxicologic importance of its chemotaxonomic association with toxic members of the family Boraginaceae is not known. However, current research suggests that it may be harmful in large doses.[2]

---

[1] Tyler VE, et al. *Pharmacognosy*, 9th ed. Philadelphia, PA: Lea and Febiger, 1988.

[2] Dobelis IN, ed. *Magic and Medicine of Plants*. Pleasantville, NY: Reader's Digest Association, 1986.

[3] Awang DVC. *Can Pharm J* 1990;123:121.

[4] Schauenberg P, et al. *Guide to Medicinal Plants*. New Canaan, CT: Keats Publishing, 1977.

[5] Hannig E. *Die Pharmazie* 1950;5:35.

[6] Tyler VE. *The New Honest Herbal*. Philadelphia, PA: G.F. Stickley Co., 1987.

SCIENTIFIC NAME(S): *Arctium lappa* L. (Synonymous with *A. majus* Bernh, great burdock as well as *A. minus* Bernh., lesser burdock.) Family: Asteraceae or Compositae

COMMON NAME(S): Bardana, beggar's buttons, clotbur, edible burdock, great bur, great burdocks, lappa

---

᪥᪥᪥ PATIENT INFORMATION ᪥᪥᪥

Uses: Treatment of fever, infection, cancer, fluid retention, and kidney stones. Safety and effectiveness for these have not been adequately evaluated. In addition, burdock has been used topically to cleanse the skin and treat dandruff.

Side Effects: Oral: Root tea poisoning caused by atropine (eg, blurred vision, headache, drowsiness, slurred speech, loss of coordination, incoherent speech, restlessness, hallucinations, hyperactivity, seizures, disorientation, flushing). Topical: Allergic skin irritation.

BOTANY: Burdock is native to Europe and northern Asia and naturalized in the US. The plant is a perennial or biennial herb, growing to 3 m tall. Burdock has large, ovate, acuminate leaves with broad pinkish flowers with reddish violet tubular florets surrounded by many involucral bracts ending in a stiff spiny or hooked tip. The root pieces, used in teas, are hard, minimally fibrous, longitudinally wrinkled, and grayish brown to black.[1,2]

HISTORY: In traditional medicine, the fruits (seeds), roots, and leaves of burdock have been used as decoctions or teas for a wide range of ailments including colds, catarrh, gout, rheumatism, stomach ailments, cancers, and as a diuretic, diaphoretic, and laxative. It has been promoted as an aphrodisiac and externally for skin problems.

PHARMACOLOGY: Several reports cover the burdock's antipyretic, antimicrobial, antitumor, diuretic, and diaphoretic properties.[2] Some cosmetic and toiletry products used for skin cleaning, antidandruff, and hair tonic applications are given in recent literature. Among the more recent studies are the uses of burdock in the treatment of urolithiasis,[3] potential inhibition of HIV-1 infection in vitro,[4] platelet activating factor (PAF) antagonism,[5] effects of dietary fiber in digestion,[6] potential antitumor activity of burdock extract,[7] and a desmutagenic factor isolated from burdock.[8]

TOXICOLOGY: While burdock is generally considered a safe and edible food product, a few reports have appeared on burdock root tea poisoning[9] caused by adulteration and allergic contact dermatitis caused by burdock.[10]

[1] Bisset G, ed. *Herbal Drugs and Phytopharmaceuticals.* Stuttgart: Medpharm Scientific Publishers, 1994.

[2] Leung A, et al. *Encyclopedia of Common Natural Ingredients,* 2nd ed. New York: John Wiley and Sons, 1996.

[3] Grases F, et al. *Int Urol Nephrol* 1994;26(5):507.

[4] Yao X, et al. *Virology* 1992;187(1):56.

[5] Iwakami S, et al. *Chem Pharm Bull* 1992;40(5):1196.

[6] Tadeda H, et al. *J Nutr Sc Vit* 1991;37(6):611.

[7] Donbradi C, et al. *Tumori* 1966;53(3):173.

[8] Morita K, et al. *Mut Res* 1984;129(1):25.

[9] Bryson P, et al. *JAMA* 1978(May 19);239:2157.

[10] Rodriguez P, et al. *Contact Dermatitis* 1995;33(3):134.

SCIENTIFIC NAME(S): *Calendula officinalis* L. Family: Compositae

COMMON NAME(S): Calendula, garden marigold, gold bloom, holligold, marygold, pot marigold, marybud[1]

❧❧ PATIENT INFORMATION ❧❧

Uses: Calendula has been used topically in folk medicine to treat wounds and internally to reduce fever, treat cancer, and control dysmenorrhea. Extracts have proved antibacterial, antiviral, and immunostimulating in vitro. Petals are consumed as a seasoning. The plant has been used to repel insects.

Side Effects: Allergic reactions to the botanical family and one case of anaphylaxis have been reported.

BOTANY: Believed to have originated in Egypt, this plant has almost world-wide distribution. There are numerous varieties of this species, each one varying primarily in flower shape and color. Calendula grows to about 60 cm in height, and the wild form has small, bright yellow-orange flowers that bloom from May to October. It is the ligulate florets, mistakenly called the flower petals, that have been used medicinally. This plant should not be confused with several other members of the family that also carry the "marigold" name.

HISTORY: The plant has been grown in European gardens since the 12th century and its folkloric uses are almost as old. Tinctures and extracts of the florets had been used topically to promote wound healing and reduce inflammation. Systemically, they have been used to reduce fever, control dysmenorrhea, and treat cancer. The dried petals have been used like saffron as a seasoning and to adulterate saffron.[2]

The pungent odor of the marigold has been used as an effective pesticide. Marigolds are often interspersed among vegetable plants to repel insects.[3]

PHARMACOLOGY: Despite the historical use of calendula and the detailed studies of its chemistry, there are almost no studies regarding its efficacy in the treatment of human disorders.

Calendula extracts have been used topically to promote wound healing, and experiments in rats have shown this effect is measurable. An ointment containing 5% flower extract in combination with allantoin was found to "markedly stimulate" epithelialization in surgically induced wounds. On the basis of histological examination of the wound tissue, it was concluded that the ointment increased glycoprotein, nucleoprotein, and collagen metabolism at the site.[4]

Russian investigators found that sterile preparations of calendula extracts alleviated signs of chronic conjunctivitis and ocular inflammatory conditions in rats.[5] The extracts also had a systemic anti-inflammatory effect. Other Russian investigators have used plant extract mixtures containing calendula for the treatment of chronic hyposecretory gastritis.

Calendula extracts have in vitro antibacterial, antiviral,[6,7] and immunostimulating properties.[8] Published reports of small clinical trials conducted in Poland and Bulgaria suggest that extracts of the plant may be useful in the management of duodenal ulcers, gastroduodenitis, and gum disease.

TOXICOLOGY: Despite its widespread use, there have been no reports in the Western literature describing serious reactions to the use of calendula preparations. A report of anaphylactic shock in a patient who gargled with a calendula infusion has been reported in Russia.

Allergies to members of the family Compositae (chamomile, feverfew, dandelion) have been attributed to the pollens of these plants. There is a potential for allergic reactions with calendula use.

In animals, doses of ≤ 50 mg/kg of extract had essentially no pharmacologic effect and induced no histopathologic changes following either acute or chronic administration.[9] Saponin extracts of calendula showed antimutagenic activity.[10]

[1] Meyer JE. *The Herbalist.* Hammond, IN: Hammond Book Co, 1934.

[2] Duke JA. *Handbook of Medicinal Herbs.* Boca Raton, FL: CRC Press, 1985.

[3] Lewis WH, et al. *Medical Botany: Plants Affecting Man's Health.* New York: John Wiley & Sons, 1977.

[4] Klouchek-Popava E, et al. *Acta Physiol Pharmacol Bulg* 1982;8:63.

[5] Marinchev VN, et al. *Oftalmol Zh* (USSR) 1971;26:196.

[6] Dumenil G, et al. *Ann Pharm Fr* 1980;38:493.

[7] De Tommasi N, et al. *J Nat Prod* 1990;53(4):830.

[8] Wagner H, et al. *Arzneimittelforschung* 1985;35:1069.

[9] Iatsyno AI, et al. *Farmakol Toksikol* 1978;41:556.

[10] Elias R, et al. *Mutagenesis* 1990;5(4):327.

SCIENTIFIC NAME(S): *Capsicum frutescens* L., *Capsicum annuum* L., or any of a large number of hybrids or varieties of the species. Family: Solanaceae

COMMON NAME(S): *C. frutescens:* capsicum, cayenne pepper, red pepper, African chilies; *C. annuum* var. conoides: tabasco pepper, paprika, pimiento, Mexican chilies; *C. annuum* var. longum: Louisiana long pepper or hybridized to the Louisiana sport pepper.

ꙮꙮ PATIENT INFORMATION ꙮꙮ

Uses: Many varieties are eaten as vegetables and spices. The component capsaicin is both an irritant and analgesic used in self-defense sprays and as pain treatments for post-surgical neuralgia and shingles.

Side Effects: Topical, mucosal, and GI irritation are common.

BOTANY: *C. frutescens* is a small spreading annual shrub that is indigenous to tropical America. It yields an oblong, pungent fruit, while *Capsicum annum* (the common green pepper) yields paprika. It was believed that all peppers derived from *C. frutescens* or *C. annuum* or their hybrids. It is now recognized that ≈ 5 species and their hybrids contribute as sources of "peppers."[1] Capsicum peppers should not be confused with the black and white pepper spices derived from the unripened fruit of *Piper nigrum.*

HISTORY: Capsicum was first described in the mid-1400s by a physician accompanying Columbus to the West Indies. The names come from the Latin "capsa," meaning box, referring to the partially hollow, box-like fruit. Capsicum has been desired as a spice and cultivated in some form in almost every society. Peppers are among the most widely consumed spices in the world with an average daily per capita consumption in some Southeastern Asian countries approaching 5 g of red pepper (≈ 50 mg of capsaicin).[2] Preparations of capsicum have been used as topical rubifacients and extracts have been ingested as a stomachic, carminative, and GI stimulant.

PHARMACOLOGY: Capsicum is a powerful irritant because of the effect of the oleoresin and capsaicin. Solutions applied topically can produce sensations varying from warmth to burning, depending on the concentration. With repeated applications, an apparent desensitization to the burning occurs. This effect has been studied in detail and has resulted in the elucidation of the mechanism of action of capsaicin.

In one study, 4 applications of a 0.1% solution of capsaicin were applied topically to the skin of healthy subjects and compared to untreated skin. Histamine was injected intradermally at the application site to test for chemical responsiveness. As expected, injection at the untreated area evoked a wheal, flare, and itching. Interestingly, the capsaicin-treated areas developed a wheal but no flare. The flare response, also called axon reflex vasodilation, is believed to be mediated by release of the vasoactive compound substance P. This compound is involved in the transmission of painful stimuli from the periphery to the spinal cord. Following an initial application, substance P is released, causing the sensation of pain. However, upon repeated administration, substance P is depleted and a lack of pain sensation ensues. This effect usually occurs within 3 days of regular application. Pretreatment with capsaicin also abolishes airway edema and bronchoconstriction induced by cigarette smoke and other irritants.[3]

Capsaicin has become a valuable "pharmacologic probe" for the evaluation of nociception. Of more practical importance has been the use of capsaicin ointments for the treatment of pain caused by herpes-zoster (shingles). Often in patients affected with shingles, excruciating pain may persist around the infected nerve tracts for months to years after the initial flare. *Zostrix* cream (GenDerm Corp.), containing either 0.025% or 0.075% capsaicin, was effective when applied topically in the management of post-herpetic neuralgia.[4,5] It also has been found to be effective in the management of trigeminal and diabetic neuralgia, causalgia, and post-mastectomy and post-surgical neuralgias.

Inhalation of capsaicin solution can desensitize nasal nerves that cause a runny nose, sneezing, and congestion. In one study, such symptoms were alleviated in 8 volunteers receiving repeated nose sprays of capsaicin.[6]

One product (*WarmFeet,* Divajex Inc, Tustin CA) contains powdered capsicum mixed with several herbs, which is sprinkled into socks or massaged on the feet to stimulate a sensation of warmth during cold weather.

TOXICOLOGY: The most well-known adverse effect of peppers is an intolerable burning sensation that occurs following contact with moist mucous membranes. Thus, it is commonly used in many self-defense sprays. When sprayed into an attacker's eyes, *Pepper Defense* (Security Barn, New Port Richey, FL) causes immediate blindness and irritation for up to 30 minutes, with no permanent damage. If capsicum comes in contact with mucous membranes, it should be flushed with water. Anecdotal reports suggest that flushing the area with milk may be beneficial.

Topical irritation is common with use of commercial creams. One study in patients with post-herpetic lesions was terminated early because about one-third of the patients experienced "unbearable" burning.[7]

In rats, the acute oral LD-50 of *Tabasco* brand red pepper sauce 241 ml/kg.[8] After 90 days of diet supplementation with the sauce, no signs of toxicity were noted. Mild eye irritation was observed when instilled, but vinegar, an ingredient in the sauce, was shown to contribute to this effect.[9]

The intense GI burning that often accompanies the ingestion of peppers may be reduced by removing the seeds from the pepper pods before ingestion[10] or by ingesting bananas along with the peppers.[11] One study found no difference in the healing rate of duodenal ulcers among patients who ingested 3 g of capsicum daily compared to untreated controls.[12]

[1] Leung AY. *Encyclopedia of Common Natural Ingredients Used in Food, Drugs and Cosmetics.* New York, NY: John Wiley and Sons, 1980.

[2] Buck SH, et al. *Tips* 1983;4:84.

[3] Editorial. *Lancet* 1983;B335:1198.

[4] Bernstein JE, et al. *J Am Acad Dermatol* 1987;17:93.

[5] Olin BR, Hebel SK, eds. *Drug Facts and Comparisons.* St. Louis, MO: Facts and Comparisons, 1992(Jul):632.

[6] Snyder M. *USA Today* 1992(Mar 18).

[7] *F-D-C Reports* 1989(Feb 27).

[8] Winek CL, et al. *Drug Chem Toxicol* 1982;5(2):89.

[9] Monsereenusorn Y. *Res Commun Chem Pathol Pharmacol* 1983;41(1):95.

[10] Prevost, RJ. *Lancet* 1982;8277(1):917.

[11] Roberts RM. *Lancet* 1982;8270(1):519.

[12] Kumar N, et al. *BMJ* 1984;288:1803.

Cascara

SCIENTIFIC NAME(S): *Rhamnus pushiana* D.C. (Syn. *Frangula purshiana* [D.C.] A. Gray ex J.C. Cooper) Family: Rhamnaceae

COMMON NAME(S): Buckthorn, cascara sagrada, chittem bark, sacred bark

---

✿✿✿ PATIENT INFORMATION ✿✿✿

Uses: Cascara extracts are used in laxatives.

Drug Interactions: No direct interactions known. Chronic use that leads to potassium deficiency can potentiate the effects of cardiotonic glycosides (eg, digitalis).

Side Effects: Cascara should not be used during pregnancy and lactation. Extended use may cause chronic diarrhea and weakness.

BOTANY: Cascara sagrada is the dried bark of *Rhamnus pushiana* collected from small- to medium-sized wild deciduous trees. They usually range from 600 to 1200 cm high and have thin, elliptic to ovate-oblong, acutely pointed leaves. The greenish flowers are arranged in umbellate cymes, and the fruit is purplish black and broadly obovoid (8 mm long). The commercial bark is flattened or transversely curved and longitudinally ridged with a brownish to red-brown color. It has gray or white lichen patches and occasional moss attachments. Cascara trees are found in North America in California, Oregon, Washington, Idaho, Montana, and as far north as southeast British Columbia.[1,2]

HISTORY: American cascara is a folkloric medicine of relatively recent origin, having been introduced as a laxative by early Mexican and Spanish priests of California (probably *Rhamnus californica*). *R. purshiana* itself was not described officially until 1805, and the bark was not brought into regular medicinal use until 1877. The European counterpart (European buckthorn, *Rhamnus frangula*) was described much earlier by the Anglo-Saxons. The berries were official in the 1650 London Pharmacopoeia.[3]

PHARMACOLOGY: As in other laxatives (eg, aloe, senna), the anthraquinone glycosides are responsible for the cathartic properties in cascara. Cascarosides A and B are the major active principles which act on the large intestine to induce peristalsis and evacuation.[2] More specifically, the anthraquinone glycosides produce an active secretion of water and electrolytes within the lumen of the small intestine and inhibit the absorption of these from the large intestine. This causes an increase in the volume of the bowel contents and strengthens the dilatation pressure in the intestine to stimulate peristalsis. They exert this action with a minimum of side effects.[4] In general, the cascarosides are more active than their hydrolyzed by-products.[2] Furthermore, these cascarosides have a sweet and more pleasant taste than the aloins and, hence, should be extracted separately, if possible.[3] Cascara is largely used in the form of a liquid extract, elixir, or as tablets made from a standardized dry extract.[2]

The daily dose ranges from 20 to 160 mg of the cascara derivatives for the treatment of constipation.[4] The average dose range of total hydroxyanthracene derivatives is 20 to 70 mg daily.[5] The laxative action is seen within 6 to 8 hours after administration. Basically, cascara can be used in most conditions where easy defecation with a soft stool is desired (eg, constipation, hemorrhoids, anal fissures, post rectal-anal surgery). It is contraindicated during pregnancy and lactation.[4]

No major side effects are known; however, chronic use or abuse (eg, for weight loss) can result in electrolyte loss, especially potassium. Chronic use can also lead to pigmentation of the intestinal mucosa (melanosis coli). No direct interactions are known with cascara except where chronic use leads to a potassium deficiency which can potentiate the effects of cardiotonic glycosides (eg, digitalis). The anthraquinone glycosides should not be used for long periods of time because they can cause the above problems or lead to laxative dependence.[4]

Because freshly prepared cascara products contain anthrones, they can lead to severe vomiting and intestinal cramping. Therefore, the bark should be stored for at least a year before use or artificially changed by heating (in air) to reduce the content of anthrones.

Recent studies have shown that aloe-emodin has antileukemic activity against the P-388 lymphocytic leukemia in mice,[2] *Rhamnus* anthraquinones can act as sunscreens in cosmetics,[6] and cascarosides are not readily metabolized in animal model gut microflora.[7] Studies also suggest that a Formosan *Rhamnus* species contains physcion and frangulin B which exhibited a high activity against human hepatoma PLC/PRF/5 and KB cell lines.[8] *R. purshiana* extracts are capable of inactivating herpes simplex virus.[9] In addition, anthranoids are transformed to their corresponding glucuronide and sulfate derivatives and appear in the urine and bile.[10] One study showed that a mixture of *Curcuma amara* and *R. purshiana* roots have choleretic and serum cholesterol lowering effects in rats.[11]

TOXICOLOGY: Extended or habitual use of cascara is to be avoided because it can cause chronic diarrhea and weakness, as a result of excessive potassium loss. Chronic use can cause melanin pigmentation of the mucous membranes of the colon.[4,12] Emodin can produce dermatitis.[12]

[1] Osol A, Farrar GE, eds. *The Dispensatory of the United States of America*, 25th ed. Philadelphia: JB Lippincott, 1955.

[2] Leung AY. *Encyclopedia of Common Natural Ingredients Used in Food, Drugs, and Cosmetics*. New York: J Wiley Interscience, 1980.

[3] Evans WC. *Trease and Evans' Pharmacognosy*, 13th ed. New York: Bailliere Tindall, 1989.

[4] Bisset NG, ed. Herbal Drugs and *Phytopharmaceuticals*. Stuttgart: Medpharm Scientific Publishers, 1994.

[5] Reynolds JEF, ed. *Martindale: The Extra Pharmacopoeia*, 31st ed. London: Royal Pharmaceutical Society, 1996.

[6] Bader S, et al. *Cosmetics and Toiletries* 1981;96:67.

[7] Dreessen M, et al. *Pharm Acta Helv* 1988;63(9–10):287.

[8] Wei BL, et al. *J Nat Prod* 1992;55:967.

[9] Sydiskis RJ, et al. *Antimicrob Agents Chemother* 1991;35(12):2463.

[10] de Witte P, et al. *Hepatogastroenterology* 1990;37(6):601.

[11] Beynen AC. *Artery* 1987;14(4):190.

[12] Duke JA. *Handbook of Medicinal Herbs*. Boca Raton, FL: CRC Press, 1985.

SCIENTIFIC NAME(S): *Uncaria tomentosa* (Willd.) DC and *Uncaria guianensis* (Aubl.) Gmel. Family: Rubiaceae

COMMON NAME(S): Cat's claw, life-giving vine of Peru, samento, uña de gato

---

⚘⚘⚘ PATIENT INFORMATION ⚘⚘⚘

Uses: Various species have been used as an astringent, anti-inflammatory, contraceptive, for gastric ulcers, rheumatism, cancer treatment, and as a general tonic. Studies have verified some anticancer and immunostimulant properties. The major alkaloid is hypotensive.

Side Effects: Data suggest little hazard in ingestion.

BOTANY: Cat's claw, or uña de gato (Spanish), is a tropical vine of the madder family (Rubiaceae). The name describes the small curved-back spines on the stem at the leaf juncture. The genus *Uncaria* is found throughout the tropics, mainly in Southeast Asia, the Asian continent, and South America. The two species of current interest, *Uncaria tomentosa* (Willd.) DC and *Uncaria guianensis* (Aubl.) (Gmel.), are found in South America. These species are lianas or high-climbing, twining, woody vines.[1,2] Both species are known in Peru as uña de gato.

There are 34 reported species of *Uncaria*. One Asian species, known as gambir or pole catechu (*Uncaria gambir* (Hunter) Roxb.), is a widely used tanning agent which has long medicinal use as an astringent and antidiarrheal.[3]

HISTORY: *U. guianensis* has long folkloric use in South America as a wound healer and for treating intestinal ailments.[2] Large amounts of *U. guianensis* are collected in South America for the European market, while American sources prefer *U. tomentosa*.[1]

The bark decoction of *U. guianensis* is used in Peru as an anti-inflammatory, antirheumatic, and contraceptive, as well as in treating gastric ulcers and tumors, gonorrhea (by the Bora tribe), dysentery (by the Indian groups of Columbia and Guiana), and cancers of the urinary tract in women.[2]

The Ashanica Indians believe that samento (also *U. tomentosa*) has "life-giving" properties, and use a cup of the decoction each week or two to ward off disease, treat bone pains, and cleanse the kidneys.[4] Recent interest in uña de gato stems from a reference to the plant in a popular book, *Witch Doctor's Apprentice, Hunting for Medicinal Plants in the Amazonian.*[5]

Reviews and scientific studies by the National Cancer Institute in the last decade have led to verification of some of the anticancer and immunostimulant properties.[2] Some of the demand for the bark has been attributed to European reports on its clinical use with AZT in AIDS treatment. The demand for the bark in the US is based on the purported usefulness of its tea in treating diverticulitis, hemorrhoids, peptic ulcers, colitis, gastritis, parasites, and leaky bowel syndrome.[4]

PHARMACOLOGY: Both species, *U. tomentosa* and *U. guianensis*, have been used folklorically in the form of a bark decoction for a wide range of disorders, including gastric ulcers, inflammation, rheumatism, tumors, and as a contraceptive. Specifically, *U. guianensis* has been employed to treat dysentery, gonorrhea, and cancer of the urinary tract in women.[1]

Recent reports have demonstrated *Uncaria's* role in improving immunity in cancer patients,[4] as well as its antimutagenic properties.[6] All the individual alkaloids of *U. tomentosa,* with the exception of hynchophylline and mitraphyllin, have immunostimulant properties[7] and the ability to enhance phagocytosis in vitro. Other researchers have shown pteropodine and isopteropodine to have immune-stimulating effects.[4]

The major alkaloid rhynchophylline has been shown to be antihypertensive, to relax the blood vessels of endothelial cells, dilate peripheral blood vessels, inhibit sympathetic nervous system activities, lower the heart rate, and lower blood cholesterol.[4,8] The alkaloid mytraphylline has diuretic properties,[4] while the alkaloid hirsutine inhibits urinary bladder contractions and possesses local anesthetic properties.[4,9] At higher dosages, hirsutine showed a "curare-like" ability on neuromuscular transmission.[4,10] The Oriental crude drug "chotoko" (the dried climbing hooks of *Uncaria* species) has hypotensive properties.[11] Six quinovic acid glycosides in *U. tomentosa* have antiviral activity *in vitro.*[12,13] The alkaloid gambirine isolated from *U. callophylla* has cardiovascular properties.[14]

TOXICOLOGY: Plant extracts and fractions of *U. tomentosa* exhibit no mutagenic effects, but show a protective antimutagenic property in vitro and decreased the mutagenicity in a smoker who had ingested a decoction of the plant for 15 days.[6] While there is little published data on the toxicology of uña de gato, there is an international patent (1982) and a German dissertation (1984) which indicate low toxicity for this material.[4] The scattered pharmacological studies also seem to indicate little hazard in ingesting the plant decoction.

[1] Duke J, et al. *Amazonian Ethobotanical Dictionary.* Boca Raton, FL: CRC Press, 1994.
[2] Foster S. *Health Food Bus* 1995(Jun);24.
[3] Duke JA. *Handbook of Medicinal Herbs.* Boca Raton, FL: CRC Press, 1985.
[4] Jones K. *Am Herb Assoc* 1994;10(3):4.
[5] Maxwell, N. *Witch Doctor's Apprentice, Hunting for Medicinal Plants in the Amazonian,* 3rd ed. New York: Citadel Press, 1990.
[6] Wagner H, et al. *Planta Med* 1985:419.
[7] Hemingway SR, et al. *J Pharm Pharmacol* 1974;26(Suppl):113P.
[8] Harada M, et al. *Chem Pharm Bull* 1979;27(5):1069.
[9] Harada M, Ozaki Y. *Chem Pharm Bull* 1976;24(2):211.
[10] Anonymous. *Peruvian Cat's Claw: A Gift from Nature.* Gilroy, CA: Bour-Man Medical.
[11] Endo K, et al. *Planta Med* 1983;49:188.
[12] Aquino R, et al. *J Nat Prod* 1989;52(4):679.
[13] Aquino R, et al. *J Nat Prod* 1990;53(3);559.
[14] Rizzi R, et al. *J Ethnopharmacol* 1993;38(1):63.

SCIENTIFIC NAME(S): *Matricaria chamomilla* L. and *Anthemis nobilis*. Sometimes referred to as *Chamaemelum nobile* (L.) All. Family: Compositae (Asteraceae)

COMMON NAME(S): *M. chamomilla* is known as German, Hungarian, or genuine chamomile, and *A. nobilis* is called English or Roman chamomile (common chamomile).

❧❧❧ PATIENT INFORMATION ❧❧❧

Uses: Teas and extracts of the flower heads have been used as anti-inflammatories, GI antispasmodics, and sedatives. Research has found chamomile components with these effects and antiallergic activity.

Side Effects: Although toxicity appears to be low, sensitive individuals have experienced contact dermatitis, anaphylaxis, and other reactions. Inhibition of GI activity may slow drug absorption.

BOTANY: *M. chamomilla* grows as an erect annual and *A. nobilis* is a slow-growing perennial. The fragrant flowering heads of both plants are collected and dried for use as teas and extracts.

HISTORY: Known since Roman times for their medicinal properties, the plants have been used as antispasmodics and sedatives in the folk treatment of digestive and rheumatic disorders. Teas have been used to treat parasitic worm infections and as a hair tint and conditioner. The volatile oil has been used to flavor cigarette tobacco.

PHARMACOLOGY: Bisabolol, a chamomile comound, exerts numerous pharmacologic effects that may account for the many traditional uses of chamomile. The compound effectively reduces inflammation, and is antipyretic in yeast-induced fever in rats.[1] It shortens the healing time of cutaneous burns in guinea pigs.[2] The compound also inhibits the development of gastric ulcers in rats, induced by indomethacin, stress, and ethanol, and shortens the healing time of acetic acid-induced ulcers.[3]

Chamomile infusions have been used traditionally as GI antispasmodics. Alcohol extracts of *M. chamomilla* showed antispasmodic effects in vitro.[4] Bisabolol and the lipophilic compounds bisabolol oxides A and B, as well as the essential oil, have a papaverine-like antispasmodic effect. Bisabolol is about as potent as papaverine and twice as potent as the oxides.[5] The chamomile flavones apigenin, luteolin, patuletin, and quercitin also have marked antispasmodic effects as do the coumarins umbelliferone and herniarine.

The hydrophilic components of chamomile, principally the flavonoids, also contribute to the anti-inflammatory process. The most active flavonoids are apigenin and luteolin, with potencies similar to that of indomethacin.[6]

Because of the low water solubility of the essential oil, teas prepared from chamomile flowers contain only ≈ 10% to 15% of the oil present in the plant. Despite the relatively low concentration of lipophilic components in water infusions, chamomile teas are generally used over long periods of time, during which a cumulative therapeutic effect may result.[7]

TOXICOLOGY: The toxicity of bisabolol is low following oral administration in animals. The acute LD-50 is ≈ 15 ml/kg in rats and mice. In a 4-week subacute toxicity study, the administration of bisabolol (1 to 2 ml/kg body weight) to rats caused no significant toxicity. No teratogenicity or developmental abnormalities were noted in rats and rabbits after chronic administration of 1 ml/kg bisabolol.[8]

The tea, prepared from the pollen-laden flower heads, has resulted in contact dermatitis,[9] anaphylaxis,[10] and other severe hypersensitivity reactions in persons allergic to ragweed, asters, chrysanthemums, and other members of the family Compositae.[11] Although some experts suggest that persons with allergies to ragweed pollens should refrain from ingesting chamomile, good evidence for this cross-sensitivity remains to be established.

The dried flowering heads are emetic when ingested in large quantities.[12]

[1] Jakovlev V, et al. *Planta Medica* 1979;35:125.

[2] Isaac O. *Planta Medica* 1979;35:118.

[3] Szelenyi I, et al. *Planta Medica* 1979;35:218.

[4] Forster HB, et al. Antispasmodic effects of some medicinal plants. *Planta Medica* 1980;40:309.

[5] Achterrath-Tuckerman U, et al. *Planta Medica* 1980;39:38.

[6] Hamon NW. *Can Pharm J* 1989(Nov):612.

[7] Farnsworth NR. *JAMA* 1972;221:410.

[8] Habersang S, et al. *Planta Medica* 1979;37:115.

[9] Rowe AH. *J Allergy* 1934;5:383.

[10] Benner MH, et al. *J Allergy Clin Immunol* 1973;52:307.

[11] *Med Lett Drugs Ther* 1979;21:29.

[12] Lewis WH, et al. *Medical Botany.* New York, NY: John Wiley and Sons, 1977.

SCIENTIFIC NAME(S): *Larrea divaricata* Cav. [synon. with L. *tridentata* (DC) Coville], also referred to as *L. glutinosa* Engelm. Family: Zygophyllacea

COMMON NAME(S): Chaparral, creosote bush, greasewood, hediondilla[1]

❧❧❧ PATIENT INFORMATION ❧❧❧

Uses: Chaparral tea has been widely used in folk medicine to treat conditions ranging from the common cold to snakebite pain. A derivative was formerly used as a food preservative. Anecdotal and in vitro evidence suggests antineoplastic effects.

Side Effects: No longer classified safe. Chaparral may cause liver damage, contact dermatitis, and stimulate most malignancies.

BOTANY: The chaparrals are a group of closely-related wild shrubs found in the arid regions of the southwestern US and Mexico. Chaparral found in health food stores usually consists of leaflets and twigs. This branched bush grows to 270 cm. Its leaves are bilobed and have a resinous feel and strong smell.

HISTORY: Chaparral tea was used as a remedy by Native Americans and has been suggested for the treatment of bronchitis and the common cold, to alleviate rheumatic pain, stomach pain, chicken pox, and snakebite pain. A strong tea from the leaves has been mixed with oil as a burn salve.[2] It is an ingredient in some *otc* weight loss teas.

In 1959, the National Cancer Institute (NCI) was informed through lay correspondence that several cancer patients claimed beneficial effects on their cancers from drinking chaparral tea. Years later, a similar treatment was brought to the attention of physicians at the University of Utah, when an 85-year-old man with a proven malignant melanoma of the right cheek with a large cervical metastasis refused surgery and treated himself with chaparral tea. Eight months later he returned with marked regression of the tumor.[3] Additional cases observed by the physicians at the University of Utah included four patients who responded to some degree to treatment with the tea, including two with melanoma, one with metastatic choriocarcinoma, and one with widespread lymphosarcoma. After 2 days of treatment, the patient with lymphosarcoma discontinued chaparral treatment, despite the disappearance of 75% of his disease. The choriocarcinoma patient who had not responded well to other therapies, responded well to chaparral tea for 2 months after which the disease became progressive. Of the melanoma patients, one experienced a 95% regression and the remaining disease was excised; the other, after remaining in remission for 4 months, subsequently developed a new lesion.[4]

Reports subsequently appeared in the lay literature describing the virtues of chaparral tea as an antineoplastic treatment.

PHARMACOLOGY: Nordihydroguaiaretic acid (NDGA) is believed to be responsible for the biological activity of chaparral. Up until 1967, when more effective antioxidants were introduced, NDGA was used in the food industry as a food additive to prevent fermentation and decomposition. It is theorized that any anticancer effect of chaparral tea is caused by the ability of NDGA to block cellular respiration. NDGA and its related compounds inhibit the beef heart mitochondrial nicotinuamide adenine dinucleotide (NADH) oxidase system and succinoxidase system, and therefore, exert some antioxidant activity at the cellular level.[5] NDGA also inhibits collagen- and ADP-induced platelet aggregation and platelet adhesiveness in aspirin-treated patients.[6]

Studies conducted by the NCI found that in vitro, NDGA was an effective anticancer agent, being described as "the penicillin of the hydroquinones and the most potent antimetabolite in vitro."[7] However, this activity is almost completely abolished in vivo. Chaparral failed to show any significant anticancer activity in two separate NCI chemotherapy screening tests in mice.[4] There is some evidence that when combined with ascorbic acid, NDGA shows some inhibitory effect against small Ehrlich ascites tumors in mice.

Other disconcerting data from 34 cancer patients treated for varying periods of time with chaparral suggest that a majority of malignancies are stimulated by NDGA, while some go on to regress.[4]

TOXICOLOGY: The creosote bush can induce contact dermatitis.[8] NDGA has been found to induce mesenteric lymph node and renal lesions in rats;[9] because of these problems, it was removed from the Generally Recognized as Safe (GRAS) list in 1970.[10]

Several recent reports have linked the ingestion of chaparral tea with the development of liver damage.[9,11] In all 3 cases, the patients took chaparral tablets or capsules for 6 weeks to 3 months. They developed signs of hepatic damage as evidenced by liver enzyme abnormalities; these resolved following discontinuation of the plant material. These reports indicate that chronic ingestion of chaparral may be associated with liver damage.

[1] Dobelis IN, ed. *Magic and Medicine of Plants.* Pleasantville, NY: Reader's Digest Association, Inc., 1986.
[2] Sweet M. *Common Edible and Useful Plants of the West.* Healdsburg, CA: Naturegraph Publications, 1976.
[3] Smart CR, et al. *Cancer Chemother Rep* 1969;53:147.
[4] *Unproven Methods of Cancer Management.* American Cancer Society, 1970.
[5] Gisvold O, Thaker E. *J Pharm Sci* 1974;63:1905.
[6] Gimeno MF, et al. *Prostaglandin Leukotrein Med* 1983;111:109.
[7] Burk D, Woods M. *Radiat Res Suppl* 1963;3:212.
[8] Lampe KF, McCann MA. *AMA Handbook of Poisonous and Injurious Plants.* Chicago, IL: AMA, 1985.
[9] MMWR. 1992;43:812.
[10] Tyler VE. *The Honest Herbal.* Philadelphia, PA: G.F. Stickley Co., 1981.
[11] Katz M, et al. *J Clin Gastroenterol* 1990;12:203.

SCIENTIFIC NAME(S): *Vitex agnus-castus* L. Family: Verbenaceae

COMMON NAME(S): Chaste tree, chasteberry, monk's pepper

❧❧❧ PATIENT INFORMATION ❧❧❧

Uses: Chaste tree has been used by women to balance progesterone and estrogen production and regulate menstruation. It has been used for breast pain, ovarian insufficiency, uterine bleeding, and to increase breast milk production.

Side Effects: Minor side effects include GI reactions, itching, rash, headaches, and increased menstrual flow.

BOTANY: The chaste tree is a shrub that grows in moist river banks in southern Europe and the Mediterranean region.[1] It can grow to 660 cm in height and blooms in summer, developing light purple flowers and palm-shaped leaves. The dark brown-to-black fruits are the size of a peppercorn. Collected in autumn, the fruits have a pepperish aroma and flavor.[2,3]

HISTORY: The dried, ripe fruit is used in traditional medicine. The plant has been recognized since antiquity and described in works by Hippocrates, Dioscorides, and Theophrastus.[2] In Homer's epic, *The Iliad*, the plant was featured as a "symbol of chastity, capable of warding off evil."[3] Early physicians recognized its effect on the female reproductive system, suggesting its use in controlling hemorrhages and expelling the placenta after birth. The English name "chaste tree" derives from the belief that the plant reduces unwanted libido. Monks have chewed its parts to decrease sexual desire.[2,3] At least one report is available discussing the chaste tree's use in ancient medicine to the present.[4]

PHARMACOLOGY: Chaste tree berries are thought to be antiandrogenic, inhibiting male hormonal actions. In females, the berries exert progesterogenic effects, balancing progesterone and estrogen production from the ovaries and regulating menstrual cycles.[3] A preparation of chaste tree (0.2% w/w) has been available in Germany since the 1950s and is used in treatment of breast pain, ovarian insufficiency (some cases resulting in pregnancy), and uterine bleeding.[5] Crude herb, alcoholic, or aqueous extracts of pulverized fruit are used in commercial preparations.[6]

When studied in 52 women with luteal phase defects caused by latent hyperprolactinemia, a chaste tree preparation reduced prolactin release, normalized luteal phases, and eliminated deficits in luteal progesterone without side effects.[7] Chaste tree extract contains an active principle that binds to dopamine (D_2) receptor sites, inhibiting prolactin release. This suggests therapeutic usefulness of the plant for treatment of premenstrual breast pain associated with prolactin hypersecretion.[8]

A case report in a female patient evaluated chaste tree therapy in multiple follicular development. Hormone levels after administration of the herb became "disordered;" thus, the authors concluded that chaste tree should not be used to promote normal ovarian function.[9]

Chaste tree is reportedly effective in treating endocrine abnormalities such as menstrual neuroses and dermatoses. It has also been used to treat acne.[5]

In lactating women, extracts of the plant have also been used to increase milk production.[2] When analyzed chemically, the breast milk revealed no compositional changes after chaste tree use.[5]

TOXICOLOGY: Chaste tree administration has not been associated with significant adverse events. In one large German market surveillance study, 17 of 1542 women discontinued treatment because of an adverse event.[2] Minor side effects include GI reactions, allergic reactions (eg, itching and rash), headaches, and menstrual flow increase.[2,5] The safety of the plant has not been determined in children.

[1] Mabberley DJ. *The Plant-Book: A Portable Dictionary of the Higher Plants*. Cambridge: Cambridge University Press, 1987.

[2] Brown DJ. *Quarterly Rev Nat Med* 1994;Summer:111.

[3] Chevallier A. *Encyclopedia of Medicinal Plants*. New York, NY: DK Publishing 1996;149.

[4] Newall C, et al. *Herbal Medicines*. London, England: Pharmaceutical Press 1996;19-20.

[5] Houghton P. *Pharm J* 1994 Nov 19;253:720-21.

[6] Leung, AY. *Encyclopedia of Common Natural Ingredients*. New York, NY: John J. Wiley and Sons 1996;151.

[7] Milewicz A, et al. *Arzneimittelforschung* 1993;43(7):752-56.

[8] Jarry H, et al. *Exp Clin Endocrinol* 1994;102(6):448-54.

[9] Cahill D, et al. *Hum Reprod* 1994;9(8):1469-70.

SCIENTIFIC NAME(S): Chondroitin sulfate, chondroitin sulfuric acid, chonsurid, structum

COMMON NAME(S): Chondroitin

༺༘ PATIENT INFORMATION ༺༘

Uses: Chondroitin has been used to treat arthritis. It has also been studied for use in drug delivery and antithrombotic and extravasation therapy.

Side Effects: There is little information on chondroitin's long-term effects. Most reports conclude that it is not harmful.

SOURCE: Chondroitin is a biological polymer that acts as the flexible connecting matrix between the protein filaments in cartilage.[1] Chondroitin can come from natural sources (eg, shark or bovine cartilage) or can be manufactured in the lab using different methods.[2] Danaparoid sodium, a mixture of heparin sulfate, dermatan sulfate, and chondroitin sulfate (21:3:1), is derived from porcine intestinal mucosa.[3]

HISTORY: Chondroitin sulfates were first extracted and purified in 1960. Studies suggested that if enough chondroitin sulfate was available to cells manufacturing proteoglycan, stimulation of matrix synthesis could occur, leading to an accelerated healing process.[4]

PHARMACOLOGY: One report evaluated half-lives of distribution and elimination, volumes of distribution, excretion values, urine and blood levels, and bioavailablity.[5] Another report concludes oral chondroitin sulfate B (dermatan sulfate) to reach significant plasma levels, with 7% bioavailability.[6] In 22 patients with renal failure, chondroitin sulfate half-life was prolonged, but it could be administered for clot prevention during hemodialysis in this population.[7]

There is considerable controversy regarding absorption of chondroitin. Absorption of glucosamine is 90% to 98%, but chondroitin absorption is only 0% to 13% because of molecule size.

Chondroitin is 50 to 300 times larger than glucosamine. Chondroitin may be too large to be delivered to cartilage cells. In addition, there also may be purification and identification problems with some chondroitin products, some of which have tested subpotent.[4]

Chondroitin's role in treating arthritis has gained popularity. Articular cartilage is found between joints (eg, finger, knee, hip) allowing for easy, painless movement. It contains 65% to 80% water, collagen, and proteoglycans. Chondrocytes are also found within this matrix to produce new collagen and proteoglycans from building blocks, including chondroitin sulfate, a glycosaminoglycan (GAG). Glucosamine, another of the beneficial substances in this area, stimulates chondrocyte activity. It is also the critical building block of proteoglycans and other matrix components.[4] Both chondroitin and glucosamine play vital roles in joint maintenance, which is the reason the combination of the two are found in many arthritic nutritional supplements.

In inflammation and repeated wear of the joint, chondrocyte function is disturbed, altering the matrix and causing breakdown.[8] Proper supplementation with glycosaminoglycans (eg, chondroitin sulfate) may enable chondrocytes to replace proteoglycans, offering "chondroprotection."[9] Cartilage contains the biological resources to enhance repair of degenerative injuries and inflammation. It has been proposed that a certain chondroitin sulfate sequence, released from cartilage proteoglycans, can inhibit elastase, regulating the matrix.[10]

Several studies in finger, knee, and hip joint therapy indicate beneficial results in osteoarthritis treatment.[11] An overview of chondroitin sulfate in another report concluded the product has no clear value in osteoarthritis treatment.[12]

Chondroitin sulfate has been used as a drug delivery system for diclofenac and flurbiprofen.[13] The polymer also has been used as a stabilization agent for iron injection hyperalimentation.[14]

Chondroitin sulfate B (dermatan sulfate) has potential as an antithrombolytic agent, as it inhibits venous thrombi, with less effect upon bleeding than heparin. It is an effective anticoagulant in hemodialysis.[15] Dermatan sulfate's efficacy, compared with heparin, has been determined in acute leukemia patients.[16]

Chondroitin sulfate has been used to treat extravasation after ifosfamide therapy, decreasing pain and inflammation.[17] It has also been used to treat extravasation from vindesine,[18] doxorubicin, and vincristine[19] and an etoposide needlestick injury in a health care worker.[20] Levels of chondroitin sulfate increase 10 to 100 times in tumors compared with normal tissue. In one report, all 44 cancer patients analyzed showed the structural anomaly of the urinary chondroitin sulfate. This may provide a potential new marker for diagnosis and follow-up of cancer therapy.[21] General reviews are available on chondroitin sulfate and chondroitin sulfate B.[22,23]

TOXICOLOGY: Little information about long-term toxic effects of chondroitin sulfate is available. Because the drug is concentrated in cartilage, the theory is that it produces no toxic or teratogenic effects.[11] Long-term clinical trials with larger populations are needed to fully determine toxicity.[24]

[1] Budavari S, et al, eds. The Merck Index, 11th ed. Rahway: Merck and Co., 1989.
[2] Ma S, et al. Chin Pharm J 1993 Dec 28;741-43.
[3] Reynolds J, ed. Martindale, the Extra Pharmacopoeia, 13th ed. London: Royal Pharmaceutial Society, 1996.
[4] Benedikt H. Nat Pharm 1997;1(8):1,22.
[5] Conte A, et al. Arzneimittelforschung 1991;41(7):768-72.
[6] Dawes J, et al. Br J Clin Pharm 1991 Sep;32:361-66.
[7] Gianese F, et al. Br J Clin Pharm 1993 Mar;35:335-39.
[8] Krane S, et al. Eur J Rheumatol Inflamm 1990;10(1):4-9.
[9] Pipitone V. Drugs Exp Clin Res 1991;17(1):3-7.
[10] Paroli E. Int J Clin Pharmacol Res 1993;13 Suppl:1-9.
[11] Leeb B, et al. Wien Med Wochenschr 1996;146(24):609-14.
[12] Anonymous. Prescrire Int 1995;4(20):165-67.
[13] Murata Y, et al. J Controlled Release 1996 Feb;38:101-8.
[14] Yamaji A, et al. J Nippon Hosp Pharm Assoc 1979 Jan;5:30-35.
[15] Lane D, et al. Lancet 1992 Feb 8;339:334-35.
[16] Cofrancesco E. Lancet 1992 May 9;339:1177-78.
[17] Mateu J, et al. Ann Pharmacother 1994 Nov;28:1243-44.
[18] Mateu J, et al. Ann Pharmacother 1994 Jul-Aug;28:967-68.
[19] Comas D, et al. Ann Pharmacother 1996 Mar;30:244-46.
[20] Mateu J, et al. Am J Health Syst Pharm 1996 May 1;53:1068,1071.
[21] Dietrich C, et al. Lab Invest 1993;68(4):439-45.
[22] Dosa E, et al. Acta Pharm Hungarica 1977 May;47:102-12.
[23] Tamagnone G, et al. Drugs of the Future 1994 Jul;19:638-40.
[24] American College of Rheumatology Patient Information WEB page (60 Executive Park S. Ste. 150, Atlanta, GA 30329), 1997. http://www.rheumatology.org/patient/970127.htm.

SOURCE: Chromium is abundant in the earth's crust and found in concentrations ranging from 100 to 300 ppm.[1] Commercially, it is obtained from chrome ore among other sources. The organic form of chromium exists in a dinicotino-glutathionine complex in natural foods, and appears to be absorbed better than the inorganic form. Good dietary sources of chromium include brewer's yeast, liver, potatoes with skin, beef, fresh vegetables, and cheese.[2]

HISTORY: Chromium is important as an additive in the manufacture of steel alloys (chrome-steel, chrome-nickel-steel, stainless steel) and greatly increases the durability and resistance of these metals. Synthetically produced $_{51}$Cr is used as a tracer in various hematologic disorders and in the determination of blood volume.[3] Because chromium is a recognized element required for normal glucose metabolism, a number of *otc* products promote the use of chromium, alone or in combination with glucose tolerance factor (GTF) to improve carbohydrate utilization. The effectiveness of these products has not been established, although they represent nutritionally sound sources of chromium.

PHARMACOLOGY: The recommended daily allowance for chromium in healthy adults is 50 to 200 mcg.[4]

Trivalent chromium plays a role in a cofactor complex for insulin, and is involved in normal glucose utilization.[5] Chromium forms part of the GTF that may facilitate binding of insulin to insulin receptors, thereby amplifying its effects on lipid and carbohydrate metabolism.[6]

Chromium deficiency is rare in the general population but may play a role in the development of adult diabetes mellitus and atherosclerosis.[6] Persons who have a high intake of highly refined foods may be at risk for developing chromium deficiency, as are patients receiving total parenteral nutrition. Trace metal solution for IV administration are available containing chromium alone or in combination with other metals.[7] These patients may experience peripheral neuropathy or encephalopathy that can be alleviated by administration of chromium. Marginal levels of chromium have been associated with decreased glucose utilization during pregnancy and in the elderly. Administration of chromium has improved glucose tolerance in these patients. It should be noted that supplemental amounts of dietary chromium do not have a hypoglycemic effect in healthy individuals.[5] Most absorbed chromium is eliminated through the kidneys (3 to 50 mcg/day).[6,7]

TOXICOLOGY: Acute oral ingestion of chromate salts may lead to irritation of the GI tract (nausea, vomiting, ulcers), circulatory shock, or hepatitis.[7] Renal damage (including acute tubular necrosis) has been observed following occupational exposure to chromium.[8] Trivalent chromium compounds (the kind found in foods) show little or no toxicity.

Exposure to occupational dust contaminated with hexavalent chromium and CrO_3 or CrF_2 (which are used as corrosion inhibitor pigments, and in metallurgy and electroplating) has been associated with the development of mucous hypersecretion and respiratory (lung) cancers.[9] The incidence of lung cancer is increased up to 15 times the normal rate in workers exposed to chromite, chromic oxide, or chromium ores.[10] The hexavalent species of chromium appears to be most highly associated with the development of cancers.[11]

Topical effects following exposure to chromium and chromates may lead to incapacitating eczematous dermatitis and ulceration. Ulceration and perforation of the nasal septum have also occurred.[10] About 1% to 4% of a topically applied dose of hexavalent and trivalent chromium penetrates guinea pig skin in 24 hours. Only 2 mcg of hexavalent chromium are required to induce a topical reaction in sensitive individuals.[12] Chromium may be chelated by the systemic administration of dimercaprol.[10]

[1] Windholz M, ed. The Merck Index, 10th ed. Rahway, NJ: Merck & Co., 1983.

[2] Faelten S. The Complete Book of Minerals for Health. Emmaus, PA: Rodale Press, Inc., 1981.

[3] Davey RJ. Transfus Med Rev 1988;2(3):151.

[4] The National Research Council: Recommended Dietary Allowances, 10th ed. Washington, DC: National Academy of Sciences, 1989.

[5] AMA Drug Evaluations Annual 1991. American Medical Association, 1990.

[6] Dubois F, et al. Pathol Biol (Paris) 1991;39(8):801.

[7] Olin BR, Hebel SK, eds. Drug Facts and Comparisons. St. Louis, MO: Facts and Comparisons, 1992.

[8] Wedeen RP, et al. Environ Health Perspect 1991;92:71.

[9] Wilson JD, et al, eds. Harrison's Principles of Internal Medicine, 12th ed. New York, NY: McGraw-Hill, 1991.

[10] Meyers FH, et al, eds. Review of Medical Pharmacology, 5th ed. Los Altos, CA: Lange Medical Publications, 1976.

[11] Lees PS. Environ Health Perspect 1991;92:93.

[12] Bagdon RE, Hazen RE. Environ Health Perspect 1991;92:111.

SCIENTIFIC NAME(S): *Eugenia caryophyllata* Thunb. also described as *Caryophyllus aromaticus* L. and *Syzygium aromaticum* L. Merr. and Perry. Family: Myrtaceae

COMMON NAME(S): Clove, caryophyllus

༚༚༚༚ PATIENT INFORMATION ༚༚༚༚

Uses: Cloves have been used for their antiseptic and analgesic effects and studied for use in platelet aggregation inhibition, antithrombotic activity, and chemoprotective and antipyretic effects.

Side Effects: Blood-tinged sputum and hemoptysis have been noted in clove cigarette smokers. Clove oil can irritate skin and mucous membranes.

BOTANY: The clove plant grows in warm climates and is cultivated commercially in Tanzania, Sumatra, the Molucca Islands, and South America. The tall evergreen grows to 20 m tall and has leathery leaves. The clove spice is the dried flower bud. Essential oils are obtained from the buds, stems, and leaves. The dark brown buds are 12 to 22 mm in length with 4 projecting calyx lobes. The 4 petals above the lobes fold over to form a hood, which hides numerous stamens. The cloves are strongly aromatic.[1]

HISTORY: Clove oil was used as an expectorant and antiemetic with inconsistent clinical results. Clove tea was used to relieve nausea. The use of the oil in dentistry as an analgesic and local antiseptic continues today. The oil has been used topically as a counterirritant.

PHARMACOLOGY: Clove oil has antihistaminic and spasmolytic properties, most likely because of the presence of eugenyl acetate.[2] Cloves have a positive effect on healing stomach ulcers.[1] A 15% tincture of cloves has been effective in treating topical ringworm infections. As with many other volatile oils, clove oil has inhibited gram-positive and gram-negative bacteria. Its fungistatic action has been documented, suggesting use as an antidermatophytic drug.[3] Clove oil also has anthelmintic and larvicidal properties. Another report suggests clove oil suppresses aflatoxin production.[4] Sesquiterpenes from cloves show potential as anticarcinogenic agents.[5] Similarly, eugenol present in clove oil may ameliorate effects of environmental food mutagens.[6] Whole cloves were chemoprotective against liver and bone marrow toxicity in mice.[7] Eugenol in high concentrations can inhibit reactive oxygen species generated by macrophages during inflammation.[8] Eugenol has also been found to possess marked antipyretic activity in animals, similar to the activity of acetaminophen.[9]

Aqueous extracts of clove increase trypsin activity. Eugenol inhibits prostaglandin biosynthesis, the formation of thromboxane B_2, and arachidonic acid-induced platelet aggregation in vitro. This effect has been postulated to contribute to the antidiarrheal effect of other oils that contain eugenol.[10] Other reports also confirm inhibition of platelet aggregation and antithrombotic activity of clove oil.[11,12]

Clove oil is applied for the symptomatic treatment of toothaches and used for the treatment of dry socket. Recent studies indicate that newer techniques, such as the application of collagen paste, may be more effective than clove oil/zinc oxide preparations in the management of alveolitis.[13]

TOXICOLOGY: Cloves and clove oils are used safely in foods, beverages, and toothpastes. In general, the level of clove used in foods does not exceed 0.236%; the oil is not used in amounts > 0.06%. Toxicity has been observed following ingestion of the oil, but this type of poisoning is rare and poorly documented. In rats, the oral LD-50 of eugenol is 2680 mg/kg; however, the toxicity of the compound increases almost 200-fold when administered by the intratracheal route (LD-50 11 mg/kg).[14] This increase in toxicity by the pulmonary route has become more important in light of the toxicity reported among persons who have smoked clove cigarettes. Clove cigarettes, called kreteks, generally contain ≈ 60% tobacco and 40% ground cloves. More than a dozen brands of kreteks exist and are popular in Asian countries. This popularity is growing in the US and Europe.

More than a dozen cases of pulmonary toxicity have been reported in people who have smoked clove cigarettes.[15,16] There is evidence that clove cigarettes may anesthetize the throat, leading to deeper and more prolonged inhalation of the smoke. Blood-tinged sputum and hemoptysis have been noted in smokers and may be related to eugenol's antiplatelet effects.[10] The American Lung Association has issued a warning against clove cigarette use, noting that they can have a higher tar content than ordinary cigarettes. However, one study did not find any carcinogenic effect of hot aqueous clove extracts in the *Drosophila* mutagenicity assay, although metabolites and pyrolysis products of eugenol are carcinogenic.[17]

Clove oil can be a skin and mucous membrane irritant and sensitizer.[18] A case of a 24-year-old woman reports permanent local anesthesia and anhidrosis following clove oil spillage into the facial area.[19] Other case reports exist, including treatment of a 2-year-old child suffering from disseminated intravascular coagulation and liver failure following clove oil ingestion,[20] and development of depression and electrolyte imbalance in a 7-month-old child after accidental oral ingestion of clove oil.[21] There has been no documentation of toxicity in the bud, leaf, or stem of the plant.[18]

[1] Bisset N. *Herbal Drugs and Phytopharmaceuticals.* Stuttgart, Germany: CRC Press, 1994;130–31.

[2] Leung AY. *Encyclopedia of Common Natural Ingredients Used in Food, Drugs and Cosmetics.* NY: John Wiley and Sons, 1980.

[3] El-Naghy M, et al. *Zentralb Mikrobiol* 1992;147(3-4):214–20.

[4] Hasan H, et al. *Zentralb Mikrobiol* 1993;148(8):543–48.

[5] Zheng G, et al. *J Nat Prod* 1992;55(7):999–1003.

[6] Soudamini K, et al. *Indian J Physiol Pharmacol* 1995;39(4):347–53.

[7] Kumari M. *Cancer Lett* 1991;60(1):67–73.

[8] Joe B, et al. *Biochim Biophys Acta* 1994;1224(2):255–63.

[9] Feng J, et al. *Neuropharmacology* 1987;26(12):1775–78.

[10] Rasheed A, et al. *N Engl J Med* 1984;310:50.

[11] Srivastava K. *Prostaglandins Leukot Essent Fatty Acids* 1993;48(5):363–72.

[12] Saeed S, et al. *J Pakistan Med Assoc* 1994;44(5):112–15.

[13] Mitchell R. *Int J Oral Maxillofac Surg* 1986;15:127.

[14] LaVoie EJ, et al. *Arch Toxicol* 1986;59:78.

[15] *MMWR* 1985;34:297.

[16] Hackett PH, et al. *JAMA* 1985;253:3551.

[17] Abraham SK, et al. *Ind J Exp Biol* 1978;16:518.

[18] Newall C, et al. *Herbal Medicines.* London: The Pharmaceutical Press, 1996;79.

[19] Isaacs G. *Lancet* 1983 Apr 16;1(Apr. 16):882.

[20] Brown S, et al. *Blood Coagul Fibrinolysis* 1992;3(5):665-68.

[21] Lane B, et al. *Hum Exp Toxicol* 1991;10(4):291–94.

SCIENTIFIC NAME(S): *Tussilago farfara* L. Family: Compositae

COMMON NAME(S): Coltsfoot, coughwort, feuilles de tussilage (Fr.), horse-hoof, huflattichblätter (Ger.), kuandong hua

---

❧❧❧❧ PATIENT INFORMATION ❧❧❧❧

Uses: Coltsfoot has been widely used in folk medicine to treat respiratory ills, especially coughs, sore throats, and asthma. Extracts were used to flavor candy.

Side Effects: Some individuals may be allergic. The alkaloids are carcinogenic, hepatotoxic, and genotoxic. Coltsfoot is too dangerous to be used internally.

BOTANY: Coltsfoot is a low-growing perennial (up to 30 cm high) with fleshy, woolly leaves. The plant produces a stem with a single golden-yellow, narrow, ligulate flower head that blooms from April to June. As the stem dies, hoof-shaped leaves appear. The plant is native to Europe, but also grows in sandy places throughout the US and Canada.[1] Coltsfoot is collected from wild plants in the Balkans, Eastern Europe, and Italy.[2] It has been part of Chinese folk medicine for centuries.

HISTORY: The buds, flowers, and leaves of coltsfoot have been used in traditional medicine for dry cough and throat irritation. The plant has been used in Chinese herbal medicine for the treatment of respiratory diseases, including cough, asthma, and acute and chronic bronchitis. It is also a component of numerous European commercial herbal preparations for treating respiratory disorders. A mixture containing coltsfoot has been smoked for the management of coughs and wheezes, but the smoke is potentially irritating. Its silky seeds have been used as a stuffing for mattresses and pillows.[3] Extracts of coltsfoot were used as flavorings for candies. Early references point to the usefulness of coltsfoot's mucilage for soothing throat and mouth irritation.[2]

PHARMACOLOGY: Coltsfoot has been used to soothe sore throats. The mucilage is most likely responsible for the demulcent effect of the plant. The mucilage is destroyed by burning. Smoking the plant or inhaling vapors of the leaves steeped in water would not be expected to provide any degree of symptomatic relief. Instead, the smoke may exacerbate existing respiratory conditions. Coltsfoot, in a mixture of Chinese herbs, has been evaluated in 66 cases of convalescent asthmatics and found useful in lowering airway obstruction.[4]

A compound designated L-652,469, isolated from coltsfoot buds, has been found to be a platelet-activating factor (PAF) inhibitor and a calcium channel blocker. PAF is an integral component of the complex cascade mechanism involved in both acute and chronic asthma. A number of naturally occurring PAF antagonists are being clinically evaluated for the treatment of this and other inflammatory diseases. The isolation of PAF antagonists from coltsfoot indicates that the traditional uses of the plant in the management of certain inflammatory respiratory diseases may be verifiable.[5]

Tussilagone increased the rate of respiration. Cardiovascular effects appear to be peripherally mediated, while the site of respiratory stimulation is central. Aqueous leaf extracts and phenolic components have been found to have in vitro antibacterial activity generally limited to gram-negative bacteria.[6]

TOXICOLOGY: The use of teas prepared from coltsfoot has not generally been associated with acute toxicity. Several members of this plant family (eg, chamomile, ragweeds) cause common allergies,[7] and some people may exhibit cross-sensitivity to coltsfoot. While coltsfoot is a weak topical sensitizer in guinea pigs, other plants of the family are strong sensitizers (blessed thistle, dwarf sunflower) and cross-sensitivity may exist.[8]

Several reports have noted the presence of hepatotoxic pyrrolizidine alkaloids in coltsfoot. In one long-term safety study, the alkaloid senkirkine (0.015% by weight in dried flowers) was incorporated into rat diets in concentrations of up to 8% of the diet for 2 years. Among the rats fed the 8% meal, two-thirds developed cancerous tumors of

the liver characteristic of pyrrolizidine toxicity.[9] This alkaloid is also present in the leaves.[10] The acute IV LD-50 of tussilagone is 28.9 mg/kg.[11]

Of recent interest is a case reported on reversible hepatic veno-occlusive disease in an infant after consumption of what was initally identified as coltsfoot, later found to be *Adenostyles alliariae*.[12] Seneciphylline and related hepatotoxins were identified via thin-layer chromatography, mass spectrometry, and NMR spectroscopy.

Coltsfoot has been classified by the FDA as an herb of "undefined safety."[13] The pyrrolizidine alkaloids of coltsfoot are hepatotoxic, genotoxic, and cancerogenic.[2]

[1] Tyler, VE. *The New Honest Herbal*. Philadelphia: GF Stickley Co., 1987.
[2] Bisset NG. *Herbal Drugs and Phytopharmaceuticals*. Stuttgart: Medpharm Scientific Publishers, 1994.
[3] Duke JA. *Handbook of Medicinal Herbs*. Boca Raton, FL: CRC Press, 1985.
[4] Fu JX. *Chung Hsi I Chieh Ho Tsa Chih* 1989;9(11):658.
[5] Hwang SB, et al. *Eur J Pharmacol* 1987;141(2):269.
[6] Didry N, et al. *Ann Pharm Fr* 1982;40(1):75.
[7] Anonymous. *Med Lett* 1979;21(7):29.
[8] Zeller W, et al. *Arch Dermatol Rec* 1985;227(1):28.
[9] Roder E, et al. *Planta Med* 1981;43:99.
[10] Smith LW, et al. *J Nat Prod* 1981;44:129.
[11] Li YP, et al. *Gen Pharm* 1988;19(2):261.
[12] Sperl W, et al. *Eur J Pediatr* 1995;154(2):112.
[13] DerMarderosian AH, et al. *Natural Products Medicine*. Philadelphia: GF Stickley Co., 1988.

Comfrey

SCIENTIFIC NAME(S): *Symphytum officinale* L., *S. asperum* Lepechin, *S. tuberosum, Symphytum × uplandicum* Nyman (Russian comfrey) is a hybrid of *S. officinale* and *S. asperum.* Family: Boraginaceae

COMMON NAME(S): Comfrey, Russian comfrey, knitbone, bruisewort, blackwort, slippery root

---

❧❧❧ PATIENT INFORMATION ❧❧❧

Uses: Comfrey has been used as a vegetable, as topical treatment for bruises, burns and sprains, and as internal medicine.

Side Effects: Evidence indicates that comfrey is unsafe in any form and potentially fatal.

BOTANY: A perennial that grows to about 90 cm in moist grasslands, comfrey has lanceolate leaves and bell-shaped purple or yellow-white flowers.

HISTORY: Comfrey has been cultivated in Japan as a green vegetable and used in American herbal medicine.[1] Its old name, knitbone, derives from the external use of poultices of the leaves and roots to heal burns, sprains, swelling, and bruises. Comfrey has been claimed to heal gastric ulcers, hemorrhoids, and to suppress bronchial congestion and inflammation.[1] Its use has spanned over 2000 years.[2]

PHARMACOLOGY: Ointments containing comfrey have been found to possess anti-inflammatory activity, which appears to be related to the presence of allantoin and rosmarinic acid[3] or to another hydrocolloid polysaccharide.[4] Lithospermic acid, isolated from the root, appears to have antigonadotropic activity.[5]

TOXICOLOGY: Despite its common use, the long-term ingestion of comfrey may pose a health hazard. Several members of the family Boraginaceae contain related alkaloids reported to cause liver toxicity in animals and humans. Some of these compounds predispose hepatic tumor development.

Similarly, the alkaloids of Russian comfrey caused chronic liver damage and pancreatic islet cell tumors after 2 years of use in animal models. Eight alkaloids have been isolated from *Symphytum × uplandicum*.[6] Alkaloid levels range from 0.003% to 0.115% with highest concentrations in small young leaves.[7] An indirect estimate of alkaloid ingestion determined the consumption of toxic alkaloids to be 2 mg/700 g of flour. Based on this value, Roitman's calculation of 8 to 26 mg of toxic alkaloids per cup of comfrey root tea (4 to 13 times as great as the episode above) suggests that comfrey ingestion poses a significant health risk.[8] Herbal teas and similar preparations of *Symphytum* contain the pyrrolizidine alkaloid that has been shown to cause blockage of hepatic veins and lead to hepatonecrosis.[9] Veno-occlusive disease has been reported in a woman who ingested a comfrey-pepsin preparation for 4 months;[8] one woman died following the ingestion of large quantities of yerba mate tea.[10] A woman who consumed large amounts of comfrey preparations developed ascites-caused veno-occlusive disease,[11] and 4 Chinese women who self-medicated with an herbal preparation that contained pyrrolizidine alkaloids from an unknown plant source also developed the disease.[12] One man presented portal hypertension with hepatic veno-occlusive disease and later died of liver failure. It was discovered that he used comfrey in his vegetarian diet.[13] Oral ingestion of pyrrolizidine-containing plants, such as comfrey, poses the greatest risk since the alkaloids are converted to toxic pyrrole-like derivatives following ingestion;[14] however, the alkaloids of comfrey applied to the skin of rats were detected in the urine, and lactating rats excrete pyrrolizidine alkaloids into breast milk.[15] If animals consume plants containing pyrrolizidine alkaloids, they could pass these alkaloids on to humans via milk.[16]

[1] Bianchi F, Corbetta F. *Health Plants of the World.* New York: Newsweek Books 1975.
[2] Castlemen M. *Herb Quarterly* 1989;44:18.
[3] Andres R, et al. *Planta Med* 1989;55:643.
[4] Franz G. *Planta Med* 1989;55:493.
[5] Wagner H, et al. *Arzneimittelforschung* 1970;20(5):705.
[6] Culvenor CCJ, et al. *Experientia* 1980;36:377.
[7] Mattocks, AR. *Lancet* 1980;2:1136.
[8] Ridker PM, et al. *Gastroenterology* 1985;88:1050.
[9] Larrey D. *Presse Med* 1994;23(15):691.
[10] McGee J, et al. *J Clin Pathol* 1976;29:799.
[11] Bach N, et al. *JAMA* 1989;87:97.
[12] Kumana CR, et al. *Lancet* 1983;ii:1360.
[13] Yeong ML, et al. *J Gastroenterol Hepatol* 1990;5(2):211.
[14] Mattocks AR. *Nature* 1986;217:724.
[15] Schoenta R. *Toxicol Lett* 1982;10:323.
[16] Panter KE, James LF. *J Animal Sci* 1990;68(3):892.

SCIENTIFIC NAME(S): *Vaccinium macrocarpon* Ait. (cranberry, trailing swamp cranberry), *V. oxycoccos* L. (small cranberry), *V. erythrocarpum* Michx. (Southern mountain cranberry), *V. vitis* (lowbush cranberry), *V. edule* (highbush cranberry). Family: Ericaceae.[1]

COMMON NAME(S): See above.

❧❧❧ PATIENT INFORMATION ❧❧❧

Uses: Cranberries and cranberry juice appear to combat urinary tract infections. The acids lower urine pH levels enough to slow urine degradation and odor in incontinent patients.

Side Effects: Extremely large doses can produce GI symptoms such as diarrhea.

BOTANY: A number of related cranberries are found in areas ranging from damp bogs to mountain forests from Alaska to Tennessee. Cranberry plants grow as small trailing evergreen shrubs. Their flowers vary from pink to purple and bloom from May to August depending on the species. The *Vaccinium* genus also includes the blueberry (*V. angustifolium* Ait.) and bilberry (*V. myrtillus*).

HISTORY: During the mid-1800s, German physicians observed that the urinary excretion of hippuric acid increased after the ingestion of cranberries. It was believed that cranberries, prunes, and plums contained benzoic acid or another compound that the body metabolized and excreted as hippuric acid (a bacteriostatic agent in high concentrations). This hypothesis has been disputed because the amounts of benzoic acid present in these fruits ($\approx$ 0.1% by weight) could not account for the excretion of the larger amounts of hippuric acid.

Despite a general lack of scientific evidence to indicate that cranberries or their juice were effective urinary acidifiers, interest persists among the public in the medical use of cranberries. Cranberries are used in eastern European cultures because of their folkloric role in the treatment of cancers and in reducing fever. Cranberries make flavorful jams and preserves.

PHARMACOLOGY: The ability of cranberries to acidify urine was based on an experiment with two healthy subjects.[2] Following a basal diet, one subject was given 305 g of cooked cranberries and the other an unspecified amount of prunes. In the first subject, urinary pH decreased from 6.4 to 5.3 with a concomitant increase in the excretion of total acids. Hippuric acid excretion increased from 0.77 g to 4.74 g. Presumably, urinary hippurate came from the slow biotransformation of quinic and benzoic acids or from a glucoside that hydrolyzes to quinic acid. Since mammalian tissues cannot convert quinic to hippuric acid, intestinal bacteria may play a role in this conversion.[3]

Despite these observations, the value of cranberries in treating urinary tract infections continues to be controversial. In one study, 3 of 4 subjects given 1.5 to 4 L per day of cranberry cocktail (1/3 juice mixed with water and sugar) showed only transient changes in urinary pH.[4] The maximum tolerated amounts of cranberry juice (about 4 L per day) rarely result in enough hippuric acid excretion to achieve urinary concentrations that are bacteriostatic at the optimum activity level of pH 5. The antibiotic activity of hippuric acid decreases about 5-fold at pH 5.6.[5] When 5 subjects were given 1.2 to 4 L per day of cranberry juice, urinary pH decreased only 0.2 to 0.5 units after 4 days of treatment; no urinary pH was ever lowered to pH 5.[5] A recent placebo controlled study assessed the value of drinking 300 ml/day of cranberry juice on bacteria and white blood cell counts in the urine of 153 elderly women.[6] The odds of having bacteria or white blood cells in the urine were lower in the group of women that ingested the real cranberry juice and their odds of remaining bacteria-free from one month to the next were only 27% of the controls (p = 0.006). This is one of the largest and best designed studies of its kind and suggests that there may be a microbiologic basis for cranberry's activity.

Therefore, it is likely that the juice does not exert a direct antibacterial effect via a compound such as hippuric acid, but that an alternate mechanism accounts for the anti-infective activity.[7] This is supported by the observation that cranberry and blueberry juices contain a high molecular weight compound that inhibits the common urinary pathogen *Escherichia coli* from adhering to infection sites within the urinary tract, thereby limiting the ability of the bacteria to initiate and spread infections.[8]

One promising use for the juice is as a "urinary deodorant." The malodor of fermenting urine from incontinent patients is a persistent, demoralizing problem in hospitals and long-term care facilities. Cranberry juice appears to lower urinary pH sufficiently to retard the degradation of urine by *E. coli*, limiting the generation of the pungent ammoniacal odor.[9-11]

Using the juice in combination with antibiotics has been suggested for the long-term suppressive therapy of urinary tract infections.[12,13] Anecdotal reports have described the benefits of drinking 6 oz of juice twice daily to relieve symptoms of chronic pyelonephritis and to decrease the recurrence of urinary stones.[12] The juice shows slight antiviral activity in vitro.[14]

TOXICOLOGY: There have been no reports of significant toxicity with the use of cranberries or their juice. The ingestion of large amounts (> 3 to 4 L per day) of the juice often results in diarrhea and other GI symptoms.

[1] Dobelis IN. *Magic and Medicine of Plants*. Pleasantville, NY: Reader's Digest Association, 1986.

[2] Blatherwick NR, Long ML. *J Biol Chem* 1923;57:815.

[3] DerMarderosian AH. *Drug Therapy* 1977;7:151.

[4] Kahn DH, et al. *J Am Dietetic Assn* 1967;51:251.

[5] Bodel PT, et al. *J Lab Clin Med* 1959;54:881.

[6] Avorn J, et al. *JAMA* 1994;271:751.

[7] Tyler V. *The Honest Herbal: A Sensible Guide to the Use of Herbs and Related Remedies*. Binghamtom, NY: The Haworth Press, 1993.

[8] Ofek I, et al. *N Engl J Med* 1991;324:1599.

[9] Kraemer RJ. *Southwestern Med* 1964;45:211.

[10] Dugan C, Cardaciotto PS. *J Psychiatric Nurs* 1966;8:467.

[11] Walsh BA. *J ET Nurs* 1992;19:110.

[12] Zinsser HH, et al. *NY State J Med* 1968;68:3001.

[13] Papas PN, et al. Cranberry juice in the treatment of urinary tract infections. *Southwestern Med* 1966;47:17.

[14] Konowalchuk J, Speirs JI. *Appl Envir Microbiol* 1978;35:1219.

SCIENTIFIC NAME(S): *Taraxacum officinale* Weber, also referred to as *Leontodon taraxacum* L. Family: Compositae

COMMON NAME(S): Dandelion, lion's tooth

ꮪꮪꮪ PATIENT INFORMATION ꮪꮪꮪ

Uses: Dandelion has been used for its nutritional value in addition to other uses including diuresis, regulation of blood glucose, liver and gall bladder disorders, as an appetite stimulant, and for dyspeptic complaints.

Side effects: Contact dermatitis and gastric discomfort have been reported.

BOTANY: The dandelion is a weedy compositae plant with a rosette of leaves radiating from its base. The stem is smooth, hollow, and bears a solitary yellow head consisting solely of ray flowers, which produces a cluster of numerous tiny, tufted, single-seed fruits. The plant has a deep taproot. The leaves may be nearly smooth-edged, toothed, or deeply cut; the toothed appearance gives rise to the plant's name.[1] This perennial plant can reach 50 cm in height. It grows wild in most parts of the world and is cultivated in France and Germany.[2]

HISTORY: The dandelion was used in the 10th century by Arab physicians for medicinal purposes.[3] The plant was also recommended in an herbal written in the 13th century by the physicians of Myddfai in Wales.[2] It is native to Europe and Asia, but was naturalized in North America and now grows as a weed in nearly all temperate climates. It is cultivated by some European growers and more than 100 specialized varieties have been developed. The bitter greens are used raw in salads, in wine-making, or cooked like spinach. The root is roasted and used to brew a coffee-like beverage said to lack the stimulant properties of coffee. Dandelions have long been used in herbal remedies for diabetes and disorders of the liver and as a laxative and tonic. The juice of the leaves has been used to treat skin diseases, loss of appetite, and stimulate the flow of bile.[3]

PHARMACOLOGY: Dandelion has been classified as a hepatic, mild laxative, cholegogue, diaphoretic, analgesic, stimulant, tonic, and a regulator of blood glucose.[4-10] The roots have been used as a laxative, diuretic, tonic, hepatic, and for spleen ailments.[5,7,9] Root and leaves have been used for heartburn, bruises, chronic rheumatism, gout, diabetes, eczema, and other skin problems, as well as for cancers.[7,9]

Its diuretic effect, likely a result of sesquiterpene lactone activity and high potassium content,[6] has been used to treat high blood pressure.[2,6] A later report observed no significant diuretic activity from the plant.[11] These same sesquiterpene lactones may contribute to dandelion's mild anti-inflammatory activity.[4,7]

It is effective as a detoxifying herb, working primarily on the liver and gallbladder to remove waste. It may aid in gallbladder ailments and help dissolve gallstones.[2] However, dandelion should only be used for gallstones under a physician's direction; it is generally contraindicated in bile duct obstruction, empyema, or ileus.[4,6,7,8] Increases of bile secretion in rats ($\geq 40\%$) have been attributed to activity of bitter sesquiterpene lactones in the root.[7] These lactones also increase gastric secretions that can cause gastric discomfort.[6-7] Use for dyspeptic disorders may be attributed to the anti-ulcer and gastric antisecretory activity of taraxerol, one of the terpenoid alcohols also found in the root.[12] Dandelion is also considered an appetite-stimulating bitter.[6,12] The bitter principles, previously known as taraxacin, that have recently been identified as eudesmanolides, are contained in the leaves and appear to be unique to dandelion.[6]

Hypoglycemic effects have been demonstrated in healthy, non-diabetic rabbits with a maximum decrease in blood glucose achieved at a dose of 2 g/kg.[4] The maximum effect of dandelion was reported to be 65% of the effect produced by tolbutamide 500 mg/kg.[4] Another report found no effect on glucose homeostasis in mice.[13] Inulin, reported to have antidiabetic activity, may contribute to dandelion's glucose regulating properties.[9,14]

In vitro antitumor activity with a mechanism similar to that of lentinan (a tumor polysaccharide) has been reported.[4]

TOXICOLOGY: Like many plants in this family, dandelions are known to cause contact dermatitis in sensitive individuals.[15,16] A case report of a 9-year-old boy describes positive patch test reactions to dandelion and other compositae-plant oleo resins.[17] Two out of 7 patients, each with histories of dandelion dermatitis, reacted not only to dandelion extracts, but to a sesquiterpene mix.[18] These sesquiterpene lactones are believed to be the allergenic principles in dandelion.[2] Taraxinic acid 1'-O-beta-D-glucopyranoside has also been identified as an allergenic component.[19]

Acute toxicity of dandelion is low. LD_{50} values in mice for the root are 36.8 g/kg and for herb are 28.8 g/kg.[2] A case report describes toxicity in a patient taking an herbal combination tablet that included dandelion. It was unclear as to which constituents were responsible.[20] Dandelion may be potentially toxic because of the high content of potassium, magnesium, and other minerals.[21]

[1] Seymour ELD. *The Garden Encyclopedia.* 1936.
[2] Chevallier A. *Encyclopedia of Medicinal Plants.* New York, NY: DK Publishing, 1996;140.
[3] Loewenfeld C, Back P. *The Complete Book of Herbs and Spices.* David E. Charles. London: Seymour, 1974.
[4] Newall C, et al. *Herbal Medicines.* London, England: Pharmaceutical Press, 1996;96-97.
[5] Duke J. *CRC Handbook of Medicinal Herbs.* Boca Raton, FL: CRC Press Inc., 1989;476-77.
[6] Bisset Ng, ed. Max Wichtl. *Herbal Drugs and Phytopharmaceuticals.* Boca Raton, FL: CRC Press Inc., 1994;486-89.
[7] Leung AY; Fosters. *Encyclopedia of Common Natural Ingredients.* New York: John Wiley and Sons, Inc., 1996;205-7.
[8] Brooks S. *Prot J Bot Med* 1998;2(3):268.
[9] Brooks S. *Prot J Bot Med* 1996;1(3):163.
[10] Brooks S. *Prot J Bot Med* 1995:1(1):70.
[11] Hook I, et al. *Int J Pharmacognosy* 1993;31(1):29-34.
[12] Brooks S. *Prot J Bot Med* 1996;1(4):231.
[13] Swanston-Flatt S, et al. *Diabetes Res* 1989;10(2):69-73.
[14] Duke JA. *Handbook of Biologically Active Phytochemicals and Their Activities.* Boca Raton, FL: CRC Press, Inc., 1992;86.
[15] Larregue M, et al. *Ann Dermatol Venerol* 1978;105:547.
[16] Hausen BM, et al. *Derm Beruf Umwelt* 1978;26:198.
[17] Guin J, et al. *Arch Dermatol* 1987;123(4):500-2.
[18] Lovell C, et al. *Contact Dermatitis* 1991;25(3):135-88.
[19] Hausen BM. *Derm Beruf Umwelt* 1982;30:51.
[20] DeSmet P, et al. *BMJ* 1996 Jul 13;313:92.
[21] Hamlin T. *Can J Hosp Pharm* 1991;44(1):39-40.

SCIENTIFIC NAME(S): *Salvia miltiorrhiza* Bunge, Family: Labiatae

COMMON NAME(S): Danshen, Tan-Shen, Tzu Tan-Ken (roots of purple sage), Hung Ken (red roots), Shu-Wei Ts'ao (rat-tail grass), Ch'ih Shen (scarlet sage), Pin-Ma Ts'ao (horse-racing grass)

≈≈≈ PATIENT INFORMATION ≈≈≈

Uses: Danshen has been used for circulation improvement. Danshen has also been used to alleviate menstrual irregularity, abdominal pains, and insomnia.

Drug Interactions: Adverse effects of warfarin are exaggerated when danshen and warfarin are coadministered.

Side Effects: Severe clotting abnormalities and an interaction between danshen and methylsalicylate medicated oil have been reported.

BOTANY: Danshen is a perennial herb found mainly on sunny hillsides and stream edges. Violet-blue flowers bloom in the summer. The leaves are oval, with finely serrated edges. The fruit is an oval brown nut. Danshen's roots, from which many of the common names are derived, are a vivid scarlet red.[1] Danshen is related to common sage, the culinary herb.

HISTORY: The herb has been used for menstrual irregularity, to "invigorate" the blood, and for other ailments such as abdominal pain and insomnia.[1]

PHARMACOLOGY: Danshen has been used in improving circulation. Its ability to "invigorate" the blood is proven in many Chinese studies. Danshen has been used for menstrual problems and to relieve bruising.[1]

In animal studies, a combination of danshen with chuanxiong excelled in preventing capillary contraction, thus improving circulation in a hypoxic, high-altitude environment.[3] However, this same combination was not satisfactory to prevent cardiopulmonary changes caused by high altitudes in humans.[4]

Another danshen combination, this time with foshousan, may offer protection to erythrocytes, improving blood flow to the placenta and increasing fetal birth weight in pregnant rats exposed to cigarette smoke.[5]

Danshen use in ischemic stroke has been reported.[6]

Antithrombotic actions of danshen have also been reported.[7] Acetylsalvionolic acid A was found to exert suppressive effects on collagen-induced platelet 5-HT release while inhibiting aggregation in vitro.[8] The rosmarinic acid isolated from danshen also displayed antithrombotic effects when injected into rats. This was because of platelet aggregation and promotion of fibrinolytic activity as well.[9]

Danshen use results in possible dilation of blood vessels, increase in portal blood flow, and prevention of coagulation to improve tissue ischemia. This accelerates repair and enhances nutrition in hepatic cells.[2]

More than 70% of chronic hepatitis patients responded to danshen therapy in relief of symptoms such as nausea, malaise, liver pain, and abdominal distention.[2] Another report confirms danshen's therapeutic effects in chronic active hepatitis as well.[10]

Other effects of danshen include: Cytotoxic activities (of tanshinone analogs) against certain carcinoma cell lines, many of which were effective at concentrations < 1 mcg/ml;[11] marked protective action against gastric ulceration;[12] and CNS effects[13] including neurasthenia and insomnia treatments.[1]

TOXICOLOGY: Coadministration of danshen and warfarin result in exaggerated warfarin adverse effects. Both pharmacodynamic and pharmacokinetic parameters were affected when studied in rats. Observed interactions such as increased warfarin bioavailability, decreased warfarin clearance, and prolonged prothrombin times are all indicative of clinically important interactions if danshen and warfarin are taken together.[14,15] Severe clotting abnormalities have been reported in a case where danshen induces overcoagulation in a patient with rheumatic heart disease.[16] Another case report is available describing an interaction between danshen and methylsalicylate medicated oil.[17]

[1] *A Barefoot Doctor's Manual (The American Translation of the Official Chinese Paramedical Manual)*. Philadelphia, PA: Running Press, 1997;657.

[2] Zhang Z, et al. *Chung Kuo Chung Yao Tsa Chih* 1990;15(3):177–81.

[3] Feng S, et al. *Chung Hsi I Chieh Ho Tsa Chih* 1989;9(11):650–52.

[4] Han Q, et al. *J Tongji Med Univ* 1995;15(2):120–24.

[5] Anon. *Chin Med J* 1977;3(4):224–26.

[6] Zhou W, et al. *Am J Chin Med* 1990;18(1–2):19–24.

[7] Yu W, et al. *Yao Hsueh Hsueh Pao* 1994;29(6):412–16.

[8] Chang H, et al, ed. *Advances in Chinese Medical Materials Research Symposium*, 1984;217, 559–80.

[9] Zou Z, et al. *Yao Hsueh Hsueh Pao* 1993;28(4):241–45.

[10] Bai Y. *Chung Hsi I Chieh Ho Tsa Chih* 1984;4(2):86–87.

[11] Wu W, et al. *Am J Chin Med* 1991;19(3–4):207–16.

[12] Gu J. *Chung Hua I Hsueh Tsa Chih* (Taipei) 1991;71(6):630–32.

[13] Liao J, et al. *Proc Natl Sci Counc Repub China B* 1995;19(3):151–58.

[14] Lo A, et al. *Eur J Drug Metab Pharmacokinet* 1992;17(4):257–62.

[15] Chan K, et al. *J Pharm Pharmacol* 1995;47(5):402–6.

[16] Yu C, et al. *J Intern Med* 1997;241(4):337–39.

[17] Tam L, et al. *Aust N Z J Med* 1995;25(3):258.

SCIENTIFIC NAME(S): *Harpagophytum procumbens* D.C. Family: Pediliaceae

COMMON NAME(S): Devils' claw, grapple plant

ᏱᏱᏱ PATIENT INFORMATION ᏱᏱᏱ

Uses: Devil's claw is a folk remedy for an extensive range of diseases, including arthritis and rheumatism. Research suggests it may be useful as a hypotensive, antiarrhythmic, anti-inflammatory, and analgesic.

Side Effects: Significant toxicity has not been observed in limited use.

BOTANY: Devil's claw grows naturally in the Kalahari desert and Namibian steppes of southwest Africa. The secondary roots are used in decoctions and teas.

HISTORY: Devil's claw has been used in South Africa as a folk remedy for liver and kidney disorders, allergies, headaches, and rheumatisms, and in Canada and Europe for arthritis.[1,2]

PHARMACOLOGY: Studies of the crude methanolic extract of the secondary roots of *Harpagophytum procumbens* indicate that its effect on smooth muscles is caused by a complex interaction of the different active principles of the drug at the cholinergic receptors.[3] The dried crude methanolic component, harpagoside, interferes with the mechanisms that regulate the influx of calcium in cells of smooth muscles.[3] The methanolic extract also causes a mild decrease in the heart rate with a concomitant and positive inotropic effect at higher doses. The coronary flow decreases at higher doses only.

The negative chronotropic and positive inotropic effects of harpagoside are comparatively higher with respect to that of the extract, whereas harpagide has only a slight negative chronotropic effect and a considerable negative inotropic one.[4]

Aqueous extract of devil's claw reduces carrageenan-induced edema at 400 and 800 mg/kg 4 hours after carrageenan injection. Orally administered extracts are inefficient, which could be attributed to the time in transition in the stomach, where the pH is acidic, causing a decrease in activity of the extract.[4]

The results of a German clinical study indicate that devil's claw has anti-inflammatory activity comparable to that of phenylbutazone. Analgesia was observed, along with a reduction in abnormally high uric acid and cholesterol levels.[5]

TOXICOLOGY: Harpagoside has been found to be of low toxicity with an LD-50 of greater than 13.5 g/kg in mice. Although no chronic toxicity studies have been reported, rats given oral doses of 7.5 g/kg/day harpagoside showed no clinical, hematologic, or gross pathologic changes.[6] Adverse effects in human trials have been rare, generally consisting of headache, tinnitus, or anorexia.

---

[1] Ragusa S, et al. *J Ethnopharmacol* 1984;11(3):245.

[2] Moussard C, et al. *Prostaglandins Leuko Essent Fatty Acids* 2993;46(4):283.

[3] Occhiuto F, et al. *J Ethnopharmacol* 1985;13(2):201.

[4] Soulimani R, et al. *Can J Physiol Pharmacol* 1994;72:1532.

[5] Kampf R. *Schweitz Apothek Zeitung* 1976;114:337.

[6] Whitehouse LW, et al. *Can Med Assoc J* 1983;129(3):249.

SCIENTIFIC NAME(S): *Angelica polymorpha* Maxim. var. *sinensis*; *A. dahurica; A. atropurpurea.* Family: Umbelliferae

COMMON NAME(S): Dong quai, tang-kuei, Dang-gui, Chinese Angelica

---

ᏒᏒᏒ PATIENT INFORMATION ᏒᏒᏒ

Uses: Derivatives of dong quai have been found to stimulate the CNS and uterus, suppress the immune system, and provide analgesic activity.

Side Effects: Components of dong quai can cause cancer or skin problems ranging from photosensitization to skin cancer.

BOTANY: Dong quai is an aromatic herb widely distributed throughout the Orient. The root of this plant is used medicinally.

HISTORY: The plant has been used for centuries in traditional Asian medicine where a decoction is used to treat gynecologic problems (eg, menstrual cramps, irregular menses). Historically, it has been used as an antispasmodic, a blood purifier, and to manage hypertension, rheumatisms, ulcers, anemia, and constipation.[1] Dong quai has been used for the prevention and treatment of allergic attacks.

PHARMACOLOGY: Many coumarins of dong quai have been shown to exert vasodilatory and antispasmodic effects. One of the coumarins, osthol, is a CNS stimulant. The recognized pharmacologic activities of this class of compounds suggest that appropriate doses of dong quai could exert demonstrable pharmacologic effects.

Coumarins, found in dried roots of *Angelica dahurica,* were found to initiate induced lipolysis of epinephrine and corticotropin as well as inhibit insulin-induced lipogensis.[2]

An aqueous extract of dong quai has been found to inhibit experimentally induced IgE titers, suggesting that components of the plant may have immunosuppressive activity.[1]

The anti-inflammatory, analgesic and antipyretic actions, and acute toxicity of the Chinese medicinal plant *Angelica dahurica* are further discussed.[3]

TOXICOLOGY: The furocoumarins, psoralen, and bergapten, compounds of dong quai, can induce photosensitization, resulting in potentially severe photodermatitis. These episodes have generally been confined to people collecting plants of the family Umbelliferae. Psoralens, in the presence of light, induce melanization in human skin and have been used medicinally in the treatment of skin depigmentation and psoriasis. However, these agents are photocarcinogenic and are mutagenic even in the absence of light.[10] There is no firm evidence that ingestion of plants containing psoralens is dangerous, but the potential toxicity should be considered by the user. It should also be recognized that safrole, found in the essential oil, is carcinogenic and is not recommended for ingestion.

---

[1] Sung CP, et al. *J Nat Prod* 1982;45:398.
[2] Kimura Y, et al. *Planta Medica* 1982(Jul);45:183–87.

[3] Li HY, et al. *China J Chin Materia Medica* 1991;16(9):560–62.
[4] Ivie GW et al. *Science* 1981;213:909.

SCIENTIFIC NAME(S): *Echinacea angustifolia* DC. The related species *E. purpurea* (L.) Moench and *E. pallida* (Nutt.) Britton have also been used in traditional medicine. Family: Compositae

COMMON NAME(S): American cone flower, black susans, comb flower, Echinacea, hedgehog, Indian head, Kansas snakeroot, narrow-leaved purple coneflower, purple cone flower, scurvy root, snakeroot

---

❧❧❧ PATIENT INFORMATION ❧❧❧

Uses: Echinacea is used today for topical wound healing and internal stimulation of the immune system.

Side Effects: There are no known side effects associated with echinacea. Its extracts and components have been injected at high doses without toxic effects.

BOTANY: Echinacea is native to Kansas, Nebraska, and Missouri. There has been significant confusion regarding the naming and identification of the *Echinacea* species. Because of this confusion, it should be recognized that much of the early research conducted on this plant (and in particular with European *E. angustifolia)* was probably conducted on *E. pallida.*[1] At least a half dozen synonyms have been documented for these plants.

E. angustifolia is a perennial herb with narrow leaves and a stout stem that grows to 90 cm in height. The plant terminates in a single colorful flower head. The plant imparts a pungent, acrid taste when chewed and causes tingling of the lips and tongue.

Echinacea products have been found to be adulterated with another member of the family Compositae, *Parthenium integrifolium* L. This plant has no pharmacologic activity.

HISTORY: Echinacea is a popular herbal remedy in the central US, where it is indigenous. The plant was used in traditional medicine by the American Indians and quickly adopted by the settlers. During the 1800s, claims for the curative properties of the plant ranged from a blood purifier to a treatment for dizziness and rattlesnake bites.[2] During the early part of the 20th

century, extracts of the plant were used as anti-infectives; however, the use of these products fell out of favor after the discovery of modern antibiotics.

The plant and its extracts continue to be used topically for wound-healing action and internally to stimulate the immune system. Most of the research during the past 10 years has focused on the immunostimulant properties of this plant.

PHARMACOLOGY: A small but growing body of evidence is evolving to support the traditional uses of echinacea as a wound-healing agent and immunostimulant.

Most studies have indicated that the lipophilic fraction of the root and leaves contains the most potent immunostimulating components. Although a number of pharmacologically active components have been isolated, no single compound appears to be responsible for the plant's activity.

Several caffeoyl conjugates have been isolated from *E. angustifolia* that demonstrate antihyaluronidase activity; these include chicoric acid, cynarine, chlorogenic acid, and caftaric acid.[3] The inhibition of this enzyme is believed to limit the progression of certain degenerative inflammatory diseases.

Perhaps the most intriguing activity of this plant rests in the ability of its extracts to enhance the immune response. A number of in vitro and animal studies have documented the activation of immunologic activity. These extracts appear to exert their effects by stimulating phagocytosis, increasing cellular respiratory activity, and increasing the mobility of leukocytes.

Extracts of *E. purpurea* have been found to increase the phagocytosis of *Candida albicans* by granulocytes and monocytes in vitro,[4] although the extract had no effect on the intracellular killing of bacteria.

The root oil inhibits leukemia cells in vitro and in vivo. The compound (Z)-1,8-pentadecadiene appears to be the active principle and can account for up to 44% of the root oil of some species. Its trans isomer is less active.[5]

The purified polysaccharide arabinogalactan, isolated from *E. purpurea*, was effective in activating macrophages to cytotoxicity against tumor cells and microorganisms following intraperitoneal injection in mice.[6] This polysaccharide induces macrophages to produce tumor necrosis factor, interleukin-1, and interferon beta–2. Polysaccharides derived from *E. purpurea* enhance the cytotoxic activity of treated macrophages aginst tumor cells and the intracellular parasite *Leishmania enrietti*.[7] The research suggested that this activity may be of clinical value in the defense against tumors and infectious diseases particularly in immunocompromised patients.

One study found the administration of *Echinacea* extracts to man stimulated cell-mediated immunity following a single dose, but that repeated daily doses suppressed the immune response.[8] In a more recent German study conducted in a small number of patients (15) with advanced metastasized colorectal cancer, echinacin (a component of the plant) was added to treatment consisting of cyclophosphamide and thymostimulin; the mean survival time was 4 months, and 2 patients survived for > 8 months, suggesting that this form of immunotherapy may have some value in treating these ill patients.[9]

Although the results are encouraging, they are too preliminary to draw conclusions about the appropriate therapeutic uses of *Echinacea* extracts. Similarly, there are no well-controlled studies that have evaluated the effects of *otc Echinacea* supplements. Consequently, dosages are not well defined.

TOXICOLOGY: Little is known about the toxicity of this plant despite *Echinacea's* widespread use in many countries. It has been documented in American traditional medicine for more than a century and has not generally been associated with acute or chronic toxicity. Purified *Echinacea* polysaccharide is relatively non-toxic. Acute toxicity studies found that doses of arabinogalactan as high as 4 g/kg injected intraperitoneally or intravenously were essentially devoid of toxic effects.[6]

[1] Bauer R, et al. *Planta Medica* 1988;54:426.

[2] Tyler VE. *The New Honest Herbal.* Philadelphia: G.F. Stickley Co., 1987.

[3] Facino RM, et al. *Farmaco* 1993;48(10):1447.

[4] Wildfeuer A, et al. *Arzneimittelforschung* 1994;44(3):361.

[5] Voaden DJ, et al. *J Medicinal Chem* 1972;15(6):619.

[6] Luettig B, et al. *J Nat Cancer Instit* 1989;81(9):669.

[7] Steinmuller C, et al. *Int J Immunopharmacol* 1993;15(5):605.

[8] Coeugniet EG, et al. *Onkologie* 1987;10(Suppl 3):27.

[9] Lersch C, et al. *Cancer Invest* 1992;10(5):343.

SCIENTIFIC NAME(S): *Sambucus canadensis* L. (American elder) and *Sambucus nigra* L. (European elder). Family: Caprifoliaceae

COMMON NAME(S): Sweet elder, common elder, elderberry, sambucus[1]

·ﻬ· PATIENT INFORMATION ·ﻬ·

Uses: Elder flowers and berries have been used in flavorings and are considered to have diuretic and laxative properties.

Side Effects: There have been reports of toxicity, particularly involving the stems and leaves.

BOTANY: The American elder is a tall shrub that grows to 3.6 m. It is native to North America. The European elder grows to ≈ 9 m and while native to Europe, it has been naturalized to the US.

HISTORY: Elder flowers and berries have been used in traditional medicine and as flavorings for centuries. In folk medicine, the flowers have been used for their diuretic and laxative properties and as an astringent. Various parts of the elder have been used to treat cancer and a host of other unrelated disorders.[2] Distilled elder flower water has been used as a scented vehicle for topical preparations and extracts are used to flavor foods, including alcoholic beverages. The fruits have been used to prepare elderberry wine.

PHARMACOLOGY: Elder flowers are considered to have diuretic and laxative properties; however, the specific compounds responsible for these activities have not been well established. The compound sambuculin A and a mixture of alpha- and beta-amyrin palmitate have been found to exhibit strong antihepatotoxic activity against liver damage induced experimentally by carbon tetrachloride.[3]

TOXICOLOGY: Because of the cyanogenic potential of the leaves, extracts of the plant may be used in foods, provided HCN levels do not exceed 25 ppm in the flavor. Toxicity in children who used pea shooters made from elderberry stems has been reported.[2]

One report of severe illness following the ingestion of juice prepared from elderberries has been recorded by the Centers for Disease Control.[4] People attending a picnic, who ingested several glasses of juice made from berries picked the day before, reported nausea, vomiting, weakness, dizziness, numbness, and stupor. One person who consumed 5 glasses of juice was hospitalized for stupor. All recovered. Although cyanide levels were not reported, there remains the possibility of cyanide-induced toxicity in these patients. While elderberries are safe to consume, particularly when cooked (uncooked berries may produce nausea), leaves and stems should not be crushed when making elderberry juice.

[1] Leung AY. *Encyclopedia of Common Natural Ingredients Used in Food, Drugs, and Cosmetics.* New York, NY: John Wiley and Sons, 1980.

[2] Duke JA. *Handbook of Medicinal Herbs.* Boca Raton, FL: CRC Press, 1985.

[3] Lin C-N, Tome W-P. *Planta Medica* 1988;54(3):223.

[4] Anonymous. *Mor Mortal Wkly Rep* 1984;33(13):173.

SCIENTIFIC NAME(S): *Acanthopanax senticosus* (Rupr. et Maxim. ex Maxim.) Harms. This plant is commonly referred to as *Eleutherococcus senticosus* Maxim., but has been referred to as *Hedera senticosa* in some texts. Family: Araliaceae

COMMON NAME(S): Devil's shrub, eleuthera, eleutherococ, shigoka, Siberian ginseng, touch-me-not, wild pepper

---

PATIENT INFORMATION

Uses: Eleutherococcus bears similarities to ginseng in its properties and alleged effects. It has been used as a hypotensive, immunostimulant, and energy enhancer.

Side Effects: Although side effects seem rare, it should not be used by patients in febrile states, hypertonic crisis, or MI. In some individuals it may produce drowsiness or nervousness.

BOTANY: *Eleutherococcus* belongs to the same family as the ginseng genus *Panax*. *Eleutherococcus* is found in forests of broadleaf trees and broadleafs with spruce and cedar. It grows at elevations of ≈ 800 meters above sea level. The plant is a shrub, commonly attaining a height of 2 to 3 m or, less commonly, 5 to 7 m. It has gray or grayish brown bark and numerous thin thorns. The leaves are long–stalked and palmate. *Eleutherococcus* has male and female forms, with flowers arranged in a globular umbrella. Male plants produce violet flowers; female plants have yellowish flowers. The berries are oval and black. The root is used in herbal medicine. Because eleutherococcus grows abundantly in areas such as Russia, it has become a popular substitute for ginseng.

HISTORY: Eleutherococcus has been studied intensively in Russia. It is used as a health food in China. As with ginseng, extracts of the plant have been promoted as "adaptogens" that aid the body in responding to environmental stress. The plant and extracts have been used to normalize high or low blood pressure, stimulate the immune system, and increase work capacity. Reputed

effects include increasing body energy levels, protection against toxins, reduction of tumors, and control of atherosclerosis.[1]

PHARMACOLOGY: In vitro experiments have some activity of eleutherococcus against L1210 murine leukemia cells. When root extract was added to cytarabine or N-6-(delta-2–isopentenyl)-adenosine, the extract had an additive effect with conventional antimetabolite drugs, with an ED-50 of ≈ 75 mcg/ml. This suggests that addition of the extract to anticancer regimens might possibly reduce doses of toxic drugs.[2]

P. ginseng has been shown to protect cell cultures from the effects of gamma irradiation. The mechanism seems to involve alteration of cellular metabolism, rather than DNA repair. Eleutherococcus extract has a similar action, but to only a slight degree.[3]

Eleutherococcus extracts, like those of *P. ginseng*, bind to progestin, mineralocorticoid, and glucocorticoid receptors. In addition, eleutherococcus extracts bind estrogen receptors. This may explain the observed glucocorticoid-like activity of the extracts.[4]

There is evidence of therapeutic benefits of eleutherococcus. In one study of

36 healthy volunteers, an injection of an ethanolic extract given 3 times daily for 4 weeks produced drastic increases in the absolute numbers of immuno-competent cells, particularly T-cells. The increase was most marked for helper/inducer cells, although cytotoxic and natural killer cells also increased in numbers. A general enhancement of the activation state of T-cells was evident.[5]

In hypotensive children between 7 and 10 years of age, an eleutherococcus extract improved subjective signs, raised systolic and diastolic blood pressures, and increased total peripheral resistance.[6]

Other recent studies have verified the wide range of *Eleutherococcus* properties including the effect on the human physical working capacity,[7] the immune systems of cancer patients,[8] the heart structure in MI,[9] malignant arrhythmias,[10] myocarditis and other coronary heart diseases,[11] radiation recovery,[12] diabetes,[13] hyperlipemia,[14] for its antimicrobial actions,[15] and for prenatal prevention of congenital developmental anomalies in rats.[16]

TOXICOLOGY: Use of eleutherococcus extract has been associated with little or no toxicity. However, use is not recommended for patients in febrile states, hypertonic crisis, or MI. Rare reported side effects have included slight languor or drowsiness immediately after administration; this may be the result of a hypoglycemic effect of the extract.[1]

It is sometimes suggested by lay literature that eleutherococcus represents an "improved ginseng" preparation, in that it imparts the adaptogenic effect of ginseng without the potential for annoying side effects. There are no good comparative studies to support such claims.[17]

[1] Brekhman II, et al. *Farmatsiia* 1991;40(1):39.
[2] Hacker B, et al. *J Pharm Sci* 1984;73(2):270.
[3] Ben-Hur E, et al. *Am J Chin Med* 1981;9(1):48.
[4] Pearce PT, et al. *Endocrinol Jpn* 1982;29(5):567.
[5] Bohn B, et al. *Arzneimittelforschung* 1987;37(10):1193.
[6] Kaloeva ZD. *Farmakol Toksikol* 1986;49(5):73.
[7] Asano K, et al. *Planta Med* 1986;48(3):175.
[8] Kupin VI, et al. *Vopr Onkol* 1986;32(7):21.
[9] Afanas'eva TN, et al. *Bull Eksper Bio Med* 1987;103(2):212.
[10] Tian BJ, et al. *Chung Kuo Chun Yao Tsa Chih* 1989;14(8):493.
[11] Shang YS, et al. *Chung Hsi i Chih Ho Tsa Chih* 1991;11(5):280.
[12] Minkova M, et al. *Acta Physiol Pharmacol Bulg* 1987;13(4):66.
[13] Molokovskii DS, et al. *Probl Endokrinol* 1989;35(6):82.
[14] Shi Z, et al. *Chung Hsi i Chieh Ho Tsa Chih* 1990;10(3):155.
[15] Tarle D, et al. *Farma Glasnik* 1993;49:161.
[16] Godeichuk TN, et al. *Ontogenez* 1993;24(1):48.
[17] Connert J. *Dtsch Apoth Ztg* 1980;120;735.

The Ephedras

SCIENTIFIC NAME(S): Many members of the genus *Ephedra* have been used medicinally. The most common of these include *E. altissima*, *E. sinica* Stapf., *E. intermedia* Schrenk and Meyer, and *E. nevadensis* Watson. Family: Ephedraceae (Gnetaceae)

COMMON NAME(S): Sea grape, ma-huang, yellow horse, yellow astringent, joint fir, squaw tea, Mormon tea, popotillo, teamster's tea.

⋙ PATIENT INFORMATION ⋙

Uses: Ephedra preparations are traditionally used to relieve colds, improve respiratory function, and treat a range of ills from headaches to venereal disease. Evidence shows that plant parts of various species exert hypoglycemic, hypo- and hypertensive, diuretic, and anti-inflammatory effects.

Side Effects: Large doses may cause a variety of ill effects from skin reactions to toxic psychosis and mutagenic effects. Those with high blood pressure and diabetes should exercise caution before using ephedra.

BOTANY: *Ephedra* species have a worldwide distribution. They are generally erect evergreen plants, often resembling small shrubs. The plants resemble a bunch of jointed branches covered with minute leaves. These plants generally have a strong pine odor and astringent taste. They have been suggested as an economic cash crop for the southwestern US.[1]

HISTORY: The Ephedras have a long history of use as stimulants and for the management of bronchial disorders. It is believed that these plants were used more than 5000 years ago by the Chinese to treat asthma.[2] Ephedra has been used in Asian medicine to treat colds, flu, fevers, chills, headaches, edema, lack of perspiration, nasal congestion, aching joints and bones, coughing, and wheezing.[3] Today, Ephedra continues to find a place in herbal preparations designed to relieve cold symptoms and to improve respiratory function. However, the use of standardized ephedrine/ pseudoephedrine preparations has supplanted the use of the crude drug in most developed countries.

North American species which are alkaloid-free (eg, *E. nevadensis*) have been made into refreshing, non-stimulating beverages used to treat venereal diseases. The fruits of some species are eaten, while ashes of *E. intermedia* are mixed with chewing tobacco in Pakistan.[4]

PHARMACOLOGY: Ephedrine and its related alkaloids are CNS stimulants. Ephedrine is active when given orally, parenterally, or ophthalmically. It stimulates the heart, causing increased blood pressure and heart rate and is an effective bronchodilator. It can stimulate contraction of the uterus and has diuretic properties. Because it constricts peripheral blood vessels, it can relieve congestion in mucous tissues. Pseudoephedrine has a weaker cardiac effect but a greater diuretic activity.[4] Administration of the fluid extract and decoction of Mormon tea has resulted in diuresis, most likely caused by compounds other than ephedrine. Teas of these plants can cause constipation as a result of their tannin content.

Crude aerial parts of Ephedra (known in Chinese as mao) cause hyperglycemia, most likely induced by the ephedrine alkaloids. However, investigations into the crude drug found a fraction that exhibited repeated hypoglycemic effects.[5]

Although crude Ephedra aerial parts (mao) can induce hypertension, crude ephedra root (mao-kon) causes hypotension. This effect is caused by several related macrocyclic spermine alkaloids designated ephedradines.[6]

Others studies of the hypotensive effect of the root preparation have isolated L-tyrosine betaine (maokonine), a compound that induces hypertension, suggesting that, depending on the species, a variable effect on blood pressure may be observed.[7]

TOXICOLOGY: In large doses, ephedrine causes nervousness, headache, insomnia, dizziness, palpitations, skin flushing, tingling, vomiting, anxiety, and restlessness. Toxic psychosis could be induced by ephedrine. Skin reactions have been observed in sensitive patients.[4,8] Patients with high blood pressure and diabetes should exercise caution when using these plants.

E. altissima yields several mutagenic n-nitrosamines under simulated gastric conditions. For example, N-nitrosephedrine causes metastasizing liver-cell carcinomas, as well as cancer of the lung and forestomach in animals. However, the investigators noted that the potential for endogenous formation of these compounds following ingestion of the tea is extremely small.[9]

The FDA warns consumers not to purchase or consume ephedrine-containing dietary supplements with labels that often portray the products as apparent alternatives to illegal street drugs such as "ecstacy," because these products pose health risks to consumers.

[1] McLaughlin SP. *Economic Botany* 1985;39(4):473.

[2] Weiss RF. *Herbal Medicine*. Gothenburg, Sweden: AB Arcanum, 1988.

[3] Blumenthal M, et al. *HerbalGram* 1995;34:22.

[4] Morton JF. *Major Medicinal Plants: Botany, Culture and Uses*. Springfield, IL: Charles C. Thomas, 1977.

[5] Shabana MM, et al. *Arch Exp Veterinarmed* 1990;44(3):389.

[6] Hikino H, et al. *Planta Med* 1983;48(4):290.

[7] Tamada M, et al. *Planta Medica* 1978;34(3):291.

[8] Kalix P. *J Ethnopharmacol* 1991;32(1–3):201.

[9] Tricker AR, et al. *Toxicol Lett* 1987;38(1–2):45.

SCIENTIFIC NAME(S): *Oenothera biennis* L. Family: Onagraceae

COMMON NAME(S): Evening primrose, EPO, OEP

◌◌◌◌ PATIENT INFORMATION ◌◌◌◌

Uses: EPO has been used to treat cardiovascular disease, breast disorders, premenstrual syndrome, mastalgia, rheumatoid arthritis, multiple sclerosis, atopic eczema, dermatological disorders, and other illnesses.

Side effects: No adverse effects have been attributed to evening primrose oil.

BOTANY: The evening primrose is a large, delicate wildflower native to North America and is not a true primrose. The blooms usually last one evening. Primrose is an annual or biennial and can grow in height from 1 to 3 m. The flowers are yellow, and the fruit is a dry pod ≈ 5 cm long, which contains many small seeds.[3] The small seeds contain an oil characterized by its high content of gamma-linolenic acid (GLA).[1] Wild varieties of *O. biennis* contain variable amounts of linoleic acid and GLA; however, extensive cross-breeding has produced a commercial variety that consistently yields an oil with 72% cis-linoleic acid and 9% GLA. This is perhaps the richest plant source of GLA, though a commercially grown fungus has been reported to produce an oil containing 20% GLA, and newer strains may produce even greater yields.[2]

PHARMACOLOGY: Essential fatty acids (EFAs) are important cellular structural elements and precursors of prostaglandins, which regulate metabolic functions.[3] EFAs are the biologically active parts of polyunsaturated fats. EFA ingestion is believed to help reduce the incidences of cardiovascular disease and obesity. EFAs cannot be manufactured by the body and must be provided by the diet in relatively large amounts. It has been recommended that 1% to 3% of total daily caloric intake be EFAs.[4] The World Health Organization recommends an increased level of 5% for children and pregnant or lactating women.[5]

Animal studies have shown that dietary EFA-deprivation can lead to eczema-like lesions, hair loss, a generalized defect in connective tissue synthesis with poor wound healing, failure to respond immunologically to infection, infertility (especially in males), fatty degeneration of the liver, renal lesions with a lack of normal water balance, and atrophy of lacrimal and salivary exocrine glands. This suggests that human illnesses with similar symptoms may result, in part, from poor EFA metabolism or insufficient dietary EFA. Because EPO represents a rich source of EFAs, particularly GLA, its use has been suggested in the treatment of these deficiency syndromes. It has been postulated that GLA, DGLA (the prostaglandin precursor dl-homo-GLA), and arachidonic acid are present in human milk for an important and specific purpose.[6,7] It is believed that the conversion of linoleic acid to GLA in humans is a rate-limiting metabolic step,[8] with only a relatively small amount of dietary linoleic acid (LA) being converted to GLA and to other metabolites.[9] The delta-6-desaturase enzyme is required for this conversion.

Factors interfering with this GLA production include aging, diabetes, high alcohol intake, high-fat diets, certain vitamin deficiencies, hormones, high cholesterol levels, and viral infections.[5] The essential fatty acids beyond this rate-limiting step are crucial for proper development of many body tissues, especially the brain. The brain contains $\approx$ 20% of 6-desaturated EFAs by weight. Infants cannot form an adequate amount of EFAs if linoleic acid is the only dietary source of n-6-EFA; this may be why preformed GLA, DGLA, and arachidonic acid are present in human milk. Studies have compared fatty acids in the phospholipids of red blood cells from infants fed human milk with those from infants fed commercial milk formulas. Infants fed commercial formulas showed phospholipids containing higher levels of linoleic acid and significantly lower levels of DGLA and arachidonic acid. Dietary supplementation to pregnant women with EPO results in an increase of total fat and EFA content in breast milk.[10] The presence of linoleic acid metabolites in human milk can affect the composition of red blood cell membranes.[11]

Taking large amounts (30 to 40 g/day) of linoleic acid has little effect on DGLA or arachidonic acid blood levels.[12-14] However, taking < 500 mg GLA/day can produce a significant increase in DGLA concentration and a smaller increase in arachidonic acid in plasma phospholipids.[9] These elevated levels do not exceed normal amounts found in the US diet.[15] Therefore, GLA, not linoleic acid, is capable of elevating the levels of linoleic acid metabolites in human blood. Below-normal plasma or adipose-tissue concentrations of GLA, DGLA, or arachidonic acid may occur in healthy middle-aged men who will later develop heart disease,[16-19] healthy middle-aged people who will later suffer stroke,[20] diabetic patients,[21,22] patients with atopic dermatitis,[22-24] heavy drinkers,[25,26] females with premenstrual syndrome,[27] and older people.[28,29]

Cardiovascular disease: Linoleic acid can reduce elevated serum cholesterol levels, but GLA has cholesterol-lowering activity $\approx$ 170 times greater than the parent compound.[30] In 79 patients who took 4 g *Efamol*/day in a placebo-controlled study, a significant (p < 0.001) decrease of $\approx$ 32% in serum cholesterol was noted after 3 months of treatment. A nonsignificant (NS) decrease was observed in the placebo group.[31] In some studies, GLA has lowered plasma cholesterol and triglycerides and inhibited in vivo platelet aggregation.[32] Elevated plasma lipids and in vivo platelet aggregation are risk factors for heart disease and stroke, and GLA lowers both of these.[33] In a report of 20 hyperlipidemic patients, 2.4 to 7.4 ml/day of *Pre-Glandin* I (containing 9% GLA) was administered. There were no changes in serum cholesterol, HDL cholesterol, or triglyceride levels.[34]

Breast cancer and related disorders: Improvement in serum fatty acid levels by EPO supplementation in women with benign breast disorders has not been associated with a clinical response.[35] In women with proven recurrent breast cysts, EPO treatment for 1 year resulted in a slightly lower (NS) recurrence rate compared with placebo.[36]

Premenstrual syndrome (PMS) and mastalgia: Clinical studies investigating EPO use in these conditions have had positive results. It has been suggested that an abnormal sensitivity to prolactin or a deficiency of PGE1 (thought to attenuate the biologic activity of prolactin) may contribute to PMS. Levels of GLA and subsequent metabolites were lower in women with PMS than in controls, indicating a possible defect in the conversion of linoleic acid to GLA. This may result in an exceptional sensitivity to normal changes in prolactin levels.[37] In 19 PMS patients receiving evening primrose oil each morning and evening during the last 14 days before menstruation for 5 consecutive cycles, PMS symptoms were decreased. The greatest effect was seen during the fifth cycle.[38] PMS and breast pain are common with high fat intake. Women with breast pain may be unable to convert LA to GLA.[5] In some studies, PMS and premenstrual breast pain (cyclic mastalgia) have been relieved by GLA to a significantly greater degree than with placebo.[39] However, a placebo-controlled evaluation of EPO found the oil to have no effect and that the effects observed in women with moderate PMS were solely due to a placebo effect.[40] A number of clinical studies have evaluated the effect of EPO in women with nodular or polycystic breast disease. Treatments with agents such as bromocriptine, danazol, or EPO have been associated with improvement in breast pain in up to 77% of patients with cyclical mastalgia and 44% of those with noncyclical mastalgia.[41]

Rheumatoid arthritis: A double-blind, placebo-controlled study investigated the effects of altering dietary EFAs on requirements for nonsteroidal anti-inflammatory drugs (NSAIDs) in patients with rheumatoid arthritis. The major aim was to determine whether EPO or EPO/fish oil could replace NSAIDs. An initial 1-year treatment period was followed by 3 months of placebo. At 1 year, EPO and EPO/fish oil produced significant subjective improvement compared with placebo. Furthermore, by 1 year, the patients taking EPO or EPO/fish oil had significantly reduced their use of NSAIDs. Following 3 months of placebo, those receiving initial NSAID treatment had relapsed. Despite decreased NSAID use, measures

of disease activity did not worsen. However, there was no evidence that EPO and EPO/fish oil acted as disease-modifying agents.[42] EPO therapy for rheumatoid arthritis requires longer than 3 months for any beneficial effects.[5] A study of EPO vs olive oil found that EPO use resulted in a significant reduction in morning stiffness after 3 months.[43]

Multiple Sclerosis: In MS there is abnormality in EFA metabolism and lymphocytic function. Several studies have shown slight but variable improvement in patients fed diets high in linoleic acid. In an open trial of EPO, 3 of 8 patients with MS showed improvement in the manual dexterity test, but no improvement was noted in grip strength. When the oil was given with colchicine, 4 of 6 patients improved in their general physical tone.[44] Others have noted similar improvement with GLA therapy.[45-47]

Atopic dermatitis and dermatologic disorders: In atopic dermatitis, GLA was more effective than placebo in improving skin condition, providing relief from pruritus, and allowing reduced reliance on corticosteroid medication.[48,49] Other reports exist (most double-blind, crossover, randomized, or placebo-controlled) that evaluate EPO in atopic dermatitis treatment. All reports suggest improvement in atopic eczema, regarding factors such as itch, scaling, disease severity, grade of inflammation, percent of body surface area involvement, dryness, erythema, and surface damage.[48-53] Women with "premenstrual flare" of eczema reported improvement in their condition.[53] A meta-analysis involving 311 patients (1 to 60 years of age) in 9 randomized, double-blind, placebo-controlled studies determined EPO to be more effective than placebo.[54] A defect in the function of delta-6-desaturase, the enzyme responsible for the conversion of linoleic acid to GLA, has been found in patients with atopic dermatitis.[55] Forty-eight children (2 to 8 years of age) administered 0.5 g/kg/day of *Epogam* showed significant improvement in disease severity independent of whether the patients had IgE-mediated allergy manifestations. EPO also increased content of n-6 fatty acids in red blood cell membranes, without affecting membrane microviscosity.[56] EPO doses of 6 g/day in a double-blind, placebo-controlled study of 102 patients improved the lipid profile of the epidermis in patients with atopic dermatitis[57] but it was not effective in treatment of the disease itself.[58]

Other diseases: In diabetic patients, GLA reversed neurological damage.[59] GLA supplementation to children with type 1 diabetes mellitus (insulin-dependent) indicated that favorable and statistically significant increases in serum essential fatty acid levels and decreases in PGE2 levels occurred, which may provide a therapeutic benefit.[60] One study demonstrated that GLA accelerated recovery of liver function in alcoholics and reduced the severity of withdrawal symptoms.[26] EPO has been tested for use in diagnosis and symptom relief of myalgic encephalomyelitis (Tapanui flu).[61] EPO may prevent or slow the development of hypertension in pregnancy by its pressor response to angiotensin II.[62] In combination therapy, 3 patients with Crohn's disease remained in relapse-free remission after EPO administration.[63]

The value of a drug that is effective in a wide variety of EFA-deficiency disorders cannot be overstated. The treatment of several unique medical conditions with EPO has been undertaken, often with excellent results. Many of the published studies have been open trials that require confirmation through

double-blind testing; however, these studies generally have been well designed and their results adequately analyzed. The disorders treated include autoimmune diseases, childhood hyperactivity, chronic inflammation, ethanol-induced toxicity and acute alcohol withdrawal syndrome, icthyosis vulgaris, scleroderma, Sjogren's syndrome, Sicca syndrome, brittle nails, mastalgia, psychiatric syndromes, tardive dyskinesia, ulcerative colitis, and migraine headaches. GLA has shown in vitro antitumor activity against primary liver cancer cells, but this effect was not demonstrated in a clinical trial.[64] Reviews of evening primrose oil are listed in the bibliography.[65-75]

TOXICOLOGY: As a nutritional supplement, the maximum label-recommended daily dose of EPO is ≈ 4 g. This dose contains 300 to 360 mg GLA, which contributes: (1) 6 to 7 mg GLA/kg/day likely to be produced from linoleic acid in the healthy adult female, (2) 23 to 65 mg GLA/kg/day consumed by a breastfed baby, or (3) 70 to 400 mg/kg/day of all the metabolites of linoleic acid consumed by a breastfed infant. According to these estimates, the amounts of GLA in the recommended doses of EPO are in the same range as the amounts of GLA and other related EFAs present in widely consumed foods. Thus, there is little concern about the safety of EPO as a dietary supplement in the recommended dosage range. There are considerable data on the safety of EPO from Efamol, Ltd., a commercial supplier of oil derived from hybridized forms of *Oenothera* species. In toxicological studies carried out for 1 year, EPO at doses up to 2.5 ml/kg/day in rats and 5 ml/kg/day in dogs was found to possess no toxic properties. Similar results were obtained in 2-year carcinogenicity and teratological investigations. With ≈ 1000 tons of EPO sold in several countries as a nutritional supplement since the 1970s, there have been no complaints concerning the safety of the product.[76]

[1] DerMarderosian A, et al. *Natural Product Medicine*. Philadelphia, PA: G. F. Stickley Co., 1988.

[2] *Market Letter* 1986 Aug 4:21.

[3] Leung A. *Encyclopedia of Common Natural Ingredients*, 2nd ed. New York, NY: John Wiley and Sons, Inc., 1996.

[4] Horrobin DF. *Holistic Med* 1981;3:118.

[5] Winther M. *Nat Pharm* 1996 Oct/Nov:8-9,27.

[6] Clandinin M, et al. *Lipid Res* 1982;20:901.

[7] Crawford MA. *Progr Food Nutr Sci* 1980;4:755.

[8] Brenner RR. *Progr Lipid Res* 1982;20:41.

[9] Manku MS, et al. *Eur J Clin Nutr* 1988;42:55.

[10] Cant A, et al. *J Nutr Sci Vitaminol* 1991;37:573.

[11] Putnam JC, et al. *Am J Clin Nutr* 1982;36:106.

[12] Dayton S, et al. *J Lipid Res* 1966;7:103.

[13] Lasserre M, et al. *Lipids* 1983;20:227.

[14] Singer P, et al. *Prostaglandins Leukotr Med* 1984;15(2):159.

[15] Holman RT. *Am J Clin Nutr* 1979;32:2390.

[16] Horrobin DF, et al. *Intl J Cardiol* 1987;17:241.

[17] Miettinen TA, et al. *BMJ* 1982;285:993.

[18] Salonen JT, et al. *Am J Cardiol* 1985;58:226.

[19] Wood DA, et al. *Lancet* 1984;2:117.

[20] Miettinen TA. *Monogr Atheroscler* 1986;4:19.

[21] Jones DB, et al. *BMJ* 1983;286:178.

[22] Mercuri O, et al. *Biochem Biophys Acta* 1988;116:407.

[23] Manku MS, et al. *Br J Dermatol* 1984;110:643.

[24] Strannegard IL, et al. *Intl Arch Allergy Appl Immunol* 1987;82:423.

[25] Glen L, et al. *Clin Exp Res* 1987;11:37.

[26] Nervi AM, et al. *Lipids* 1980;15:263.

[27] Bruch MG, et al. *Am J Obstet Gynecol* 1984;150:363.

[28] Darcet P, et al. *Ann Nutr Alim* 1980;34:277.

[29] Horrobin DF. *Rev Pure Appl Pharmacol Sci* 1983;4:339.

[30] Horrobin DF, et al. *Lipids* 1983;18:558.

[31] Horrobin DF, et al. Intern conference on oils, fats and waxes 1983, Auckland, New Zealand.

[32] van Doormal JJ, et al. *Diabetologia* 1986;29:A603.

[33] Puolaka J, et al. *J Reprod Med* 1985;30:149.

[34] Viikari J, et al. *Int J Clin Pharmacol Ther Toxicol* 1986 Dec;24:668-70.

[35] Gateley CA, et al. *Br J Surg* 1992;79:407.

[36] Mansel RE, et al. *Ann NY Acad Sci* 1990;586:288.

[37] Horrobin DF. Abstract, Int. Symposium on Premenstrual Tension and Dysmenorrhea (1983), Charleston, SC.

[38] Larsson B, et al. *Curr Ther Res* 1989 Jul;46:58-63.

[39] Pye J, et al. *Lancet* 1985 Aug 17;2:373-77.

[40] Khoo S, et al. *Med J Aust* 1990 Aug 20;153:189-92.

[41] Gateley CA, et al. *Br Med Bull* 1991;47:284.

[42] Belch JJF, et al. *Ann Rheum Dis* 1988;47:96.

[43] Brzeski M, et al. *Br J Rheumatol* 1991;30:370.

[44] Horrobin DF. *Med Hypoth* 1979;5:365.

[45] Field EF. *Lancet* 1978;1:780

[46] Millar JHD, et al. *BMJ* 1973;1:765.

[47] Field EF, et al. *Eur Neurol* 1983;22:78.

[48] Schalin-Karrila M. *Br J Dermatol* 1987;117:11.

[49] Wright S, et al. *Lancet* 1982;2:1120.

[50] Lovell C, et al. *Lancet* 1981 Jan 31;1:278.

[51] Bordoni A, et al. *Drugs Exp Clin Res* 1988;14(4):291-97.

[52] Biagli P, et al. *Drugs Exp Clin Res* 1988;14(4):285-90.

[53] Humphreys F, et al. *Eur J Dermatol* 1994;4(8):598-603.

[54] Morse P, et al. *Br J Dermatol* 1989 Jul;121:75-90.

[55] Kerscher MJ, et al. *Clin Investig* 1992;70:167.

[56] Biagli P, et al. *Drugs Exp Clin Res* 1994;20(2):77-84.

[57] Schafer L, Kragballe K. *Lipids* 1991;26:557.

[58] Berth-Jones J. *Lancet* 1993 Jun 19;341:1557-60.

[59] Jamal GA. *Lancet* 1986;1:1098.

[60] Arisaka M, et al. *Prostaglandins Leukot Essent Fatty Acids* 1991;43:197.

[61] Simpson L. *N Z Pharm* 1985 Jan;5:14.

[62] O'Brien P, et al. *Br J Clin Pharmacol* 1985 Mar;19:335-42.

[63] Novak E. *Can Med Assoc J* 1988 Jul 1;139:14.

[64] van der Merwe CF, et al. *Prostaglandins Leukot Essent Fatty Acids* 1990;40:199.

[65] Ballentine C, et al. *FDA Consumer* 1987 Nov;21:34–35.

[66] Sinclair B. *N Z Pharm* 1988 Jan;8:28-29, 31.

[67] Barber A. *Pharm J* 1988 Jun 4;240:723-25.

[68] Anonymous. *S Afr Pharm J* 1989 Feb;56:55-75.

[69] Barber A. *Ir Pharm Union Rev* 1989 Apr;14:121-22, 124.

[70] Kleijnen J. *Pharm Weekbl* 1989 Jun 9;124:418-23.

[71] Po A. *Pharm J* 1991 Jun 1;246:676-78.

[72] Pittit J. *Ir Pharm Union Rev* 1991 Oct;16:248,250-51, 253-56, 258-59.

[73] Anonymous. *Ir Pharm Union Rev* 1992 Sep;17:199, 201.

[74] Docherty M. *Aust J Pharm* 1994 Jan;75:48-53.

[75] Kleijnen J. *Br Med J* 1994 Oct;309:824-25.

[76] Carter JP. *Food Technol* 1988;(6):72.

SCIENTIFIC NAME(S): *Euphrasia officinalis* L. Other species include *E. rostkoviana* Hayne and *E. stricta* J.P. Wolff ex J.F. Lehm. Family: Scrophulariaceae

COMMON NAME(S): Eyebright

ᴁᴁ PATIENT INFORMATION ᴁᴁ

Uses: Eyebright preparations have been used to treat a variety of complaints, especially inflammatory eye disease.

Side Effects: Adverse effects outweigh the benefits.

BOTANY: This small European annual plant grows to ≈ 30 cm. It has oval leaves but can have a variable appearance. Its flowers are arranged in a spike; the white petals often have a red tinge, but may be purple-veined or have a yellow spot on the lower petal. It blooms from July to September. The flowers have the appearance of bloodshot eyes.

HISTORY: Eyebright was prescribed by Theophrastus and Dioscorides for the treatment of eye infections. This was perhaps a result of the similarity of the "bloodshot" petals to irritated eyes. The plant has been used in homeopathy to treat conjunctivitis and other ocular inflammations. The plant continues to find use in black herbal medicine.[1]

Further historic data on the use of Euphrasia includes a 14th century cure for "all evils of the eye." An eyebright ale was described in Queen Elizabeth's era. It was in British Herbal Tobacco and smoked for chronic bronchial conditions and colds. Other early uses include treatments for allergies, cancers, coughs, conjunctivitis, earaches, epilepsy, headaches, hoarseness, inflammation, jaundice, ophthalmia, rhinitis, skin ailments, and sore throats.

PHARMACOLOGY: There are no controlled studies in man to evaluate its effectiveness in the treatment of ocular irritations.

Eyebright is commonly used in European folk medicine for blepharitis and conjunctivitis, as well as a poultice for styes and the general management of eye fatigue. It is also used internally for coughs and hoarseness, as well as a homeopathic remedy for conjunctivitis.[2] The phenol-carboxylic acids are thought to play a role in the antibacterial effects of eyebright.

TOXICOLOGY: While there are no known risks associated with eyebright, its purported activities have not been clinically substantiated and the folkloric use is hygienically unacceptable.

German studies suggest that eyebright tincture can induce confusion, cephalalgia, eye pressure with tearing, itching, redness, and swelling of the margins of the lids, photophobia, dim vision, weakness, sneezing, coryza, nausea, toothache, constipation, hoarseness, cough, expectoration, dyspnea, yawning, insomnia, polyuria, and diaphoresis.[3] Hence, ophthalmic use is strongly discouraged.

---

[1] Boyd EL, et al. *Home Remedies and the Black Elderly.* Ann Arbor, MI: University of Michigan, 1984.

[2] Bisset NG, ed. *Herbal Drugs and Phytopharmaceuticals.* Stuttgart: Medpharm Scientific Publishers, 1994.

[3] Duke JA. *Handbook of Medicinal Herbs.* Boca Raton, FL: CRC Press, 1985.

SCIENTIFIC NAME(S): *Foeniculum vulgare* Mill. syn. F. *officinale* All. and *Anethum foeniculum.* Family: Apiaceae (Umbelliferae). A number of subspecies have been identified and their names add to the potential confusion surrounding the terminology of these plants.

COMMON NAME(S): Common, sweet or bitter fennel, carosella, Florence fennel, finocchio, garden fennel, large fennel, wild fennel[1,2]

ಜಜಜ PATIENT INFORMATION ಜಜಜ

Uses: Fennel has been used as a flavoring, scent, insect repellent, herbal remedy for poisoning and GI conditions, and as a stimulant to promote lactation and menstruation.

Side Effects: Fennel may cause photodermatitis, contact dermatitis, and cross reactions. The oil may induce hallucinations and seizures. Poison hemlock is sometimes mistaken for fennel.

BOTANY: Fennel is an herb native to southern Europe and Asia Minor. It is cultivated in the US, Great Britain, and temperate areas of Eurasia. All parts of the plant are aromatic. When cultivated, fennel stalks grow to a height of ≈ 90 cm. Plants have finely divided leaves composed of many linear or awl-shaped segments. Grayish, compound umbels bear small, yellowish flowers. The fruits or seeds are oblong ovals ≈ 6 mm long and greenish or yellowish brown; they have 5 prominent dorsal ridges. The seeds have a taste resembling that of anise. Besides *F. vulgare*, *F. dulce* ("carosella") is grown for its stalks, while *F. vulgare* var *azoricum* Thell. ("finocchio") is grown for its bulbous stalk bases.

HISTORY: According to Greek legend, man received knowledge from Mount Olympus as a fiery coal enclosed in a stalk of fennel. The herb was known to the ancient Chinese, Indian, Egyptian, and Greek civilizations, and Pliny recommended it for improving the eyesight. The name foeniculum is from the Latin word for "fragrant hay." Fennel was in great demand during the Middle Ages. The rich added the seed to fish and vegetable dishes, while the poor reserved it as an appetite suppressant to be eaten on feast days. The plant was introduced to North America by Spanish priests and the English brought it to their early settlements in Virginia.[3] All parts of the plant have been used for flavorings, and the stalks eaten as a vegetable. The seeds serve as a traditional carminative. Fennel has been used to flavor candies, liqueurs, medicines, and food, especially pastries, sweet pickles, and fish. The oil can be used to protect stored fruits and vegetables against infection by pathogenic fungi.[4] Beekeepers have grown it as a honey plant.[3] Health claims have included its use as a purported antidote to poisonous herbs, mushrooms, and snakebites,[5] and for the treatment of gastroenteritis, indigestion, to stimulate lactation, and as an expectorant and emmenagogue.[1] Tea made from crushed fennel seeds has been used as an eyewash.[3] Powdered fennel is said to drive fleas away from kennels and stables.[4]

PHARMACOLOGY: As an herbal medicine, fennel is reputed to increase milk secretion, promote menstruation, facilitate birth, ease the male climacteric, and increase the libido. These supposed properties led to research on fennel for the development of synthetic estrogens during the 1930s. The principal estrogenic component of fennel was

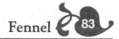

originally thought to be anethole, but it is now believed to be a polymer of anethole, such as dianethole or photoanethole.[6] The volatile oil of fennel increases the phasic contraction of ileal and tracheal smooth muscle in the guinea pig. The effect was generally greater with ileal muscle.[7]

TOXICOLOGY: Administration of the volatile oil to rats has exacerbated experimentally-induced liver damage.[8] Ingestion of the volatile oil may induce nausea, vomiting, seizures, and pulmonary edema.[9] Its therapeutic use in Morocco has occasionally induced epileptiform madness and hallucinations.[4] The principal hazards with fennel itself are photodermatitis and contact dermatitis. Some individuals exhibit cross-reactivity to several species of Apiaceae, characteristic of the so-called

celery-carrot-mugwort-condiment syndrome.[10] Rare allergic reactions have been reported following the ingestion of fennel.

Fennel oil was found to be genotoxic in the *Bacillus subtilis* DNA-repair test.[11] Estragole, present in the volatile oil, has been shown to cause tumors in animals.

A survey of fennel samples in Italy found viable aerobic bacteria, including coliforms, fecal streptococci, and *Salmonella* species, suggesting the plant may serve as a vector of infectious GI diseases.[12]

A serious hazard associated with fennel is that poison hemlock can easily be mistaken for the herb. Hemlock contains highly narcotic coniine, and a small amount of hemlock juice can cause vomiting, paralysis, and death.[5]

[1] Locock RA. *CPJ/RPC* 93/94;12/1:503.

[2] Meyer JE. *The Herbalist.* Hammond, IN: Hammond Book Co., 1934.

[3] Dobelis IN, ed. *Magic and Medicine of Plants.* Pleasantville, NY: Reader's Digest Assoc., 1986.

[4] Duke JA. *Handbook of Medicinal Herbs.* Boca Raton, FL: CRC Press, 1985.

[5] Loewenfeld C, et al. *The Complete Book of Herbs and Spices.* London: David E. Charles, 1974.

[6] Albert-Puleo M. *J Ethnopharmacol* 1980;2:337.

[7] Reiter M, et al. *Arzneimittelforsch* 1985;35(1A):408.

[8] Gershbein LL. *Food Cosmet Toxicol* 1977;15:173.

[9] Marcus C, et al. *J Agric Food Chem* 1979;27:1217.

[10] Wuthrich B, et al. *Dtsch Med Wochenschr* 1984;109:981.

[11] Sekizawa J, et al. *Mutat Res* 1982;101:127.

[12] Ercolani GL. *Appl Environ Microbiol* 1976;31:847.

Fenugreek

SCIENTIFIC NAME(S): *Trigonella foenum-graecum* L. Family: Leguminosae

COMMON NAME(S): Fenugreek

⠶⠶⠶ PATIENT INFORMATION ⠶⠶⠶

Uses: Fenugreek has been used as a flavoring, animal forage, insect repellent, and folk medicine for boils, diabetes, and tuberculosis. In lab animals, it has been shown to lower blood cholesterol and glucose, and to exert anti-inflammatory and diuretic effects.

Side Effects: Ingestion of large quantities may result in hypoglycemia.

BOTANY: Fenugreek spice is commonly sold as the dried ripe seed. The plant is an annual that is native to Asia and southeastern Europe.

HISTORY: The European herb has been used for centuries as a cooking spice and in folk medicine for treating boils, diabetes, cellulitis, and tuberculosis. Extracts of the seeds are used to flavor maple syrup substitutes. The seeds are rich in protein and the plant is grown as an animal forage. Following commercial extraction of diosgenin (which is used as a natural precursor in commercial steroid synthesis), the nitrogen and potassium-rich seed residue is used as an agricultural fertilizer.

PHARMACOLOGY: Fenugreek seeds reduce serum cholesterol levels in lab animals. In one study, fractions of fenugreek seeds were added to the diets of diabetic hypercholesterolemic and healthy dogs for 8 days. The defatted fraction, which is rich in fibers ($\approx$ 54%) and contains about 5% steroidal saponins, lowered plasma cholesterol, blood glucose, and plasma glucagon levels from pretreatment values in both diabetic hypercholesterolemic and healthy dogs.[1] The hypocholesterolemic effect has also been reproduced in rats. When fenugreek seeds replaced 50% of their diet for 2 weeks, healthy rats showed a 42% decreased and hypercholesterolemic rats showed a 58% decrease from baseline in cholesterol levels.[2]

The hypoglycemic effect of the seeds was evaluated further in dogs. Fractions of the seeds were administered orally to healthy and diabetic dogs for 8 days. The lipid extract had no pharmacologic effects. The defatted fraction lowered blood glucose levels, plasma glucagon, and somatostatin levels, and reduced carbohydrate-induced hyperglycemia. When this fraction was added to the insulin treatment of diabetic dogs, a decrease in hyperglycemia and insulin dose was noted. It is not clear if these changes are caused by the common effect of dietary fiber on blood glucose or by a pharmacologically active compound.[3]

Water and alcoholic extracts have been shown to stimulate the isolated guinea pig uterus, indicating that these extracts may have oxytocic activity.

A French patent (2,073,285 Oct 1972) has been granted to a product purported to have antitumor activity, especially against "fibromas." The product contains extracts of tansy, juniper berries, fenugreek seeds, cinnamon, sedum, St. John's wort flowers, bitter orange rind, and hydrated ferric oxide. No clinical studies have been reported using this or any other fenugreek extract in the treatment of cancers.

Fenugreek extracts have been shown to exhibit some anti-inflammatory and diuretic activity in animal models.[4]

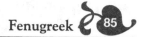

Fenugreek leaf extracts have been shown to repel numerous common insects.[5]

A recent study demonstrated that the steroid saponins of fenugreek enhance food consumption and motivation to eat, and reduce plasma cholesterol levels in rats.[6] Studies continue on the ability of fenugreek to lower blood glucose both in healthy as well as in diabetic rats, dogs, and humans.[7-11] Similarly, the hypocholesterolemic properties of fenugreek continue to be studied.[12-13] Another property of the plant is under investigation, namely its ability to decrease the quantity of calcium oxalate deposited in the kidneys.[14]

TOXICOLOGY: When ingested in usual culinary quantities, fenugreek is essentially devoid of adverse reactions. An interesting syndrome was noted in a 9-day-old boy who was admitted to the hospital for the treatment of gastroenteritis. Nurses noted that the boy's urine and entire body smelled distinctly of maple syrup. Laboratory tests ruled out the presence of "maple syrup urine" disease (an inborn error of metabolism that results in the abnormal accumulation of leucine, isoleucine, and valine and their ketoacid metabolites in the blood and urine). The mother told the physicians that she had been giving the child a tea prepared by boiling fenugreek seeds in water, a common Ethiopian folk remedy for diarrhea and vomiting. The smell of the tea was found to be indistinguishable from that of the child's urine.[15]

The acute toxicity from a large dose of fenugreek has not been characterized, but may result in potentially severe hypoglycemia. Fenugreek may also cause a new type of occupational asthma.[16] Finally, myositis and peritonitis have occurred in chickens given fenugreek crude saponins intramuscularly or intraperitoneally.[17]

[1] Valette G, et al. *Atherosclerosis* 1984;50(1):105.
[2] Singhal PC, et al. *Curr Sci* 1982;51:136.
[3] Ribes G, et al. *Ann Nutr Metab* 1984;28(1):37.
[4] Totte J, et al. *Farm Tijdschr Belg* 1983;60:203.
[5] Jilani G, et al. *J Econ Entomol* 1983;76:154.
[6] Petit PR, et al. *Steroids* 1995;60(10):674.
[7] Khosla P, et al. *Indian J Physiol Pharmacol* 1995;39(2):173.
[8] Sharma RD, et al. *Eur J Clin Nutr* 1990;44(4):301.
[9] Madar Z, et al. *Eur J Clin Nutr* 1988;42(1):51.
[10] Ajabnoor MA, et al. *J Ethnopharmacol* 1988;22(1):45.
[11] Ribes G, et al. *Proc Soc Exp Biol Med* 1986;182(2):159.
[12] Stark A, et al. *Br J Nutr* 1993;69(1):277.
[13] Sauvaire Y, et al. *Lipids* 1991;26(3):191.
[14] Ahsan SK, et al. *J Ethnopharmacol* 1989;26(3):249.
[15] Bartley GB, et al. *N Engl J Med* 1981;305(8):467.
[16] Dugue P, et al. *Presse Med* 1993;22(19):922.
[17] Nakhla HB, et al. *Vet Hum Toxicol* 1991;33(6):561.

SCIENTIFIC NAME(S): *Tanacetum parthenium* Schulz-Bip. synonymous with *Chrysanthemum parthenium* L. Bernh., *Leucanthemum parthenium* (L.) Gren and Godron, and *Pyrethrum parthenium* (L.) Sm.[1] Alternately described as a member of the genus *Matricaria*. Family: Asteraceae/Compositae

COMMON NAME(S): Feverfew, featherfew, altamisa, bachelor's button, featherfoil, febrifuge plant, midsummer daisy, nosebleed, Santa Maria, wild chamomile, wild quinine[2-5]

⚘⚘ PATIENT INFORMATION ⚘⚘

Uses: Traditionally an antipyretic, feverfew has been used in recent times to avert migraines and relieve menstrual pain, asthma, dermatitis, and arthritis.

Drug Interactions: Possible interaction with anticoagulants.

Side Effects: Patients withdrawn from feverfew experienced a syndrome of ill effects. Most adverse effects of treatment with feverfew are mild, although some patients experience increased heart rate. Feverfew should not be used by pregnant or lactating women or children under 2 years of age.

BOTANY: A short bushy perennial that grows from 15 to 60 cm tall along fields and roadsides, the feverfew's yellow-green leaves and yellow flowers resemble those of chamomile *(Matricaria chamomilla)*,. The flowers bloom from July to October.

HISTORY: The herb feverfew has had a long history of use in traditional and folk medicine, especially among Greek and early European herbalists. However, during the last few hundred years feverfew had fallen into general disuse, until recently.[6] It has now become popular as a prophylactic treatment for migraine headaches and its extracts have been claimed to relieve menstrual pain, asthma, dermatitis, and arthritis. Traditionally, the herb has been used as an antipyretic, from which its common name is derived. The leaves are ingested, fresh or dried, with a typical daily dose of 2 to 3 leaves. These are bitter and are often sweetened before ingestion. It has also been planted around houses to purify the air because of its strong, lasting odor. A tincture of its blossoms doubles as an insect repellant and balm for insect bites.[3] It was once used as an antidote for overindulgence in opium.[2]

PHARMACOLOGY: Feverfew extracts affect a wide variety of physiologic pathways.

In vitro: Feverfew may inhibit prostaglandin synthesis. Extracts of the above-ground portions of the plant suppress prostaglandin production; leaf extracts inhibit prostaglandin production; however, this effect is not moderated by cyclooxygenase.[7]

Aqueous extracts prevent the release of arachidonic acid and inhibit in vitro aggregation of platelets stimulated by adenosine diphosphate (ADP) or thrombin.[8] It is controversial whether these extracts block the synthesis of thromboxane, a prostaglandin involved in platelet aggregation.[9-10] Data suggest that feverfew's mechanism of prostaglandin synthesis inhibition differs from that of the salicylates. Extracts may inhibit platelet behavior via effects on platelet sulfhydryl groups.[11-12]

Feverfew extracts are potent inhibitors of serotonin release from platelets and polymorphonuclear leucocyte granules, providing a plausible connection between the claimed benefit of feverfew in migraines and arthritis. Feverfew may produce an antimigraine effect similar to methysergide maleate (*San-*

sert), a known serotonin antagonist.[13-14] Extracts of the plant also inhibit the release of enzymes from white cells found in inflamed joints (a similar anti-inflammatory effect may occur in the skin) providing a rationale for the use of feverfew in psoriasis.

In addition, feverfew extracts inhibit phagocytosis, the deposition of platelets on collagen surfaces, and mast cell release of histamine,[15] exhibit antithrombotic potential and cytotoxic activity,[16] and have in vitro antibacterial activity. Monoterpenes in the plant may exert insecticidal activity, and alphapinene derivatives may possess sedative and mild tranquilizing effects.

Clinical Uses: Much interest has been focused on the activity of feverfew in the treatment and prevention of migraine headaches.[17] The first account of its use as a preventative for migraine appeared in 1978 about a woman who had suffered from severe migraine since 16 years of age. At the age of 68, she began using 3 leaves of feverfew daily, and after 10 months her headaches ceased altogether. This case prompted studies by Dr. E. Stewart Johnson.[6]

A study in 8 feverfew-treated patients and 9 placebo-controlled patients found that fewer headaches were reported by patients taking feverfew for up to 6 months of treatment. Patients in both groups had self-medicated with feverfew for several years before enrolling in the study. The incidence of headaches remained constant in those patients taking feverfew but increased almost 3-fold in those switched to placebo during the trial (p < 0.02).[18] Abrupt discontinuation of feverfew in patients switched to placebo caused incapacitating headaches in some patients. Nausea and vomiting were reduced in patients taking feverfew. The statistical analysis has been questioned but the results provide a unique insight into the activity of feverfew.[19] These results were confirmed in a more recent placebo-controlled study[20] It was predicted that feverfew will be useful not only for the classical migraine and cluster headache, but for premenstrual, menstrual, and other headaches as well.[21]

However, some studies found that the experimental observations may not be clinically relevant to migraine patients taking feverfew.[22] Ten patients who had taken extracts of the plant for up to 8 years to control migraine headaches were evaluated for physiologic changes. The platelets of all treated patients aggregated characteristically to ADP and thrombin and similarly to those of control patients. However, aggregation in response to serotonin was greatly attenuated in the feverfew users.

Canada's Health Protection Branch has granted a Drug Identification Number (DIN) for a British feverfew (*Tanacetum parthenium*) product. This allows the manufacturer, Herbal Laboratories, Ltd., to claim, as a nonprescription drug, the product's effectiveness in the prevention of migraine headache. Canada's Health Protection Branch recommends a daily dosage of 125 mg of a dried feverfew leaf preparation, from authenticated *Tanacetum parthenium* containing at least 0.2% parthenolide for the prevention of migraine.[23]

TOXICOLOGY: In one study, patients received 50 mg/day, roughly equivalent to 2 leaves.[18] Adverse effects during 6 months of continued feverfew treatment were mild and did not result in discontinuation. Four of the 8 patients taking the plant had no adverse effects. Heart rate increased by up to 26 beats/min in 2 treated patients. There were no differences between treatment groups in laboratory test results.

Patients who were switched to placebo after taking feverfew for several years experienced a cluster of nervous system reactions (rebound of migraine symptoms, anxiety, poor sleep patterns) along with muscle and joint stiffness, which was referred to as "postfeverfew syndrome."

In a larger series of feverfew users, 18% reported adverse effects, the most troublesome being mouth ulceration (11%). Feverfew can induce more widespread inflammation of the oral mucosa and tongue, often with lip swelling and loss of taste.[18] Dermatitis has been associated with this plant.[15,24]

The leaves of the plant have been shown to possess potential emmenagogue activity and is not recommended for pregnant or lactating mothers or children < 2 years of age.[23] Although an interaction with anticoagulants is undocumented, this may be clinically important in sensitive patients.

Analysis of the frequency of chromosomal aberrations and sister chromatid exchanges in circulating lymphocytes from patients who ingested feverfew for 11 months did not find any aberrations, which suggested that the plant does not induce chromosomal abnormalities.[25]

[1] Awang DVC. *Can Pharm J* 1989;122:266.

[2] Duke JA. *Handbook of Medicinal Herbs*. Boca Raton, FL: CRC Press, 1985.

[3] Dobelis IN, ed. *Magic and Medicine of Plants*. Pleasantville, NY: Reader's Digest Assoc., 1986.

[4] Meyer JE. *The Herbalist*. Hammond, IN: Hammond Book Co., 1934.

[5] Castleman M. *The Healing Herbs*. Emmaus, PA: Rodale Press, 1991.

[6] Hobbs C. *National Headache Foundation Newsletter* Winter 1990:11.

[7] Collier HOJ, et al. *Lancet* 1980;2:922.

[8] Loecshe EW, et al. *Folia Haematol* 1988;115:181.

[9] Makheja AN, et al. *Lancet* 1981;2:1054.

[10] Heptinstall S, et al. *Lancet* 1985;1:1071.

[11] Heptinstall S, et al. *J Pharm Pharmacol* 1987;39:459.

[12] Voyno-Yesenetskaya TA, et al. *J Pharm Pharmacol* 1988;40:501.

[13] Tyler VE. *The New Honest Herbal*. Philadelphia, PA: GF Stickley Co., 1987.

[14] Olin BR, Hebel SK, eds. *Drug Facts and Comparisons*. St. Louis: Facts and Comparisons, 1991(Oct):257.

[15] Hayes NA, et al. *J Pharm Pharmacol* 1987;39:466.

[16] Hobbs C. *HerbalGram* 1989;20:26.

[17] *Lancet* 1985;1:1084.

[18] Johnson ES, et al. *BMJ* 1985;291:569.

[19] Waller PC, et al. *BMJ* 1985;291:1128.

[20] Murphy JJ, et al. *Lancet* 1988;2:189.

[21] Hobbs C. *National Headache Foundation Newsletter* Winter 1990:10.

[22] Biggs, et al. *Lancet* 1982;2:776.

[23] Awang DVC. *HerbalGram* 1993;29:34.

[24] Vickers HR. *BMJ* 1985;291:827.

[25] Anderson D, et al. *Human Toxicol* 1988;7:145.

SCIENTIFIC NAME(S): *Linum usitatissimum* L. Family: Linaceae

COMMON NAME(S): Flax, flaxseed, linseed, lint bells,[1] linum

---

❧❧❧ PATIENT INFORMATION ❧❧❧

Uses: Linseed oil, derived from flaxseed, has been used as a topical demulcent and emollient, laxative, and as treatment for coughs, colds, and urinary tract infections. Flaxseed cakes have been used as cattle feed. Research suggests dietary flaxseed may improve blood lipid profile.

Side Effects: Ingestion of large amounts may be harmful. Many workers exposed to flax show immunologically positive antigens.

BOTANY: The flax plant grows as a slender annual and reaches 30 to 90 cm in height. It branches at the top and has small, pale green alternate leaves that grow on the stems and branches. Flax was introduced to the North American continent from Europe and grows in Canada and the northwestern US. Each branch is tipped with 1 or 2 delicate blue flowers that bloom from February through September.[2]

HISTORY: Flax has been used for more than 10,000 years as a source of fiber for weaving.[2] It was one of the earliest plants recognized for purposes other than as food. Flax is prepared from the fibers in the stem of the plant.[3] Linseed oil, derived from the flaxseed, has been used as a topical demulcent and emollient and as a laxative, particularly for animals. Linseed oil is used in paints and varnishes as a waterproofing agent. Flaxseed cakes have been used as cattle feed.

Traditional medicinal uses of the plant have varied. One text notes that the seeds have been used to remove foreign material from the eye. A moistened seed would be placed under the closed eyelid for a few moments allowing the material to adhere to the seed, thereby facilitating removal.[4] Other uses include the treatment of coughs and colds, constipation, and urinary tract infections.[2] The related *L. catharticum* yields a purgative decoction.[4]

PHARMACOLOGY: Significant interest has centered on the ability of diets rich in flax to improve the blood lipid profile. Preliminary work indicated that egg yolk was enriched with alpha-linolenic acid by feeding hens diets containing flax. Furthermore, the cholesterol content of the liver tissue of the chicks born to the flax-fed hens was lower ($p > 0.05$) than in chicks hatched from control hens.[5]

More recent evidence indicates that flax-supplemented diets reduce atherogenic risk factors. When hyperlipemic subjects ate 3 slices of bread containing flaxseed plus 15 g of ground flaxseed daily for 3 months, serum total and low-density lipoprotein cholesterol levels were reduced. However, high-density lipoprotein cholesterol levels did not change. In addition, thrombin-stimulated platelet aggregation decreased with the flax supplement. These changes suggest beneficial improvement in plasma lipid and related cardiovascular risk factors.[6]

When healthy female volunteers supplemented their diet with 50 g/day of ground flaxseed for 4 weeks, the diet raised alpha-linolenic acid levels in both plasma and erythrocytes; serum total cholesterol decreased by 9% and low-density lipoprotein cholesterol dropped by 18%. Similar results were obtained when either flaxseed oil or flour was used, suggesting high bioavailability of the alpha-linolenic acid from ground flaxseed. No cyanogenic glucosides were detected in baked flax muffins.[7]

Flax contains lignans (phytochemicals shown to have weakly estrogenic and antiestrogenic properties). When healthy women ingested flaxseed powder for 3 menstrual cycles, the ovulatory cycles had a longer luteal phase. There were no differences between control and flax in estradiol or estrone levels, although the luteal phase progesterone/estradiol ratios were higher with flax. These findings suggest a specific role for flax lignans in the relationship between diet and sex steroid action, and possibly between diet and the risk of breast and other hormone-dependent cancers.[8]

TOXICOLOGY: The cyanogenic properties of some of the constituents of flax suggest that ingestion of large amounts of the plant may be harmful. However, this is primarily a veterinary problem encountered in grazing animals.

In one survey, $\approx$ 50% of the workers exposed to flax at their jobs demonstrated immunologically positive antigen tests.[9] No other significant toxicity has been associated with dietary levels of flax.

[1] Meyer JE. *The Herbalist*. Hammond, IN: Hammond Book Co., 1934.

[2] Dobelis IN. *Magic and Medicine of Plants*. Pleasantville, NY: Reader's Digest Association, 1986.

[3] Lewis WH, Elvin-Lewis MPF. *Medical Botany: Plants Affecting Man's Health*. New York: John Wiley & Sons, 1977.

[4] Evans WC. *Trease and Evans' Pharmacognosy*. 13th ed. London: Balliere Tindall, 1989.

[5] Cherian G, Sim JS. *Lipids* 1992;27:706.

[6] Bierenbaum ML, et al. *J Am Coll Nutr* 1993;12:501.

[7] Cunnane SC, et al. *Br J Nutr* 1993;69:443.

[8] Phipps WR, et al. *J Clin Endocrinol Metab* 1993;77:1215.

[9] Zuskin E, et al. *Environ Res* 1992;59:350.

Fo-ti

SCIENTIFIC NAME(S): *Polygonum multiflorum* Thunb. (Polygonaceae)

COMMON NAME(S): He shou wu, flowery knotweed, climbing knotweed, Chinese cornbind. This plant should not be confused with the commercial product *Fo-ti Tieng*, which does not contain fo-ti.

✽✽✽ PATIENT INFORMATION ✽✽✽

Uses: Fo-ti has been used in China for its rejuvenating and toning properties, to increase liver and kidney function, and to cleanse the blood. It is also used for insomnia, weak bones, constipation, and atherosclerosis. It can increase fertility and blood sugar levels, relieve muscle aches, and exhibit antimicrobial properties against tuberculosis bacillus and malaria.

Side Effects: Little information exists on fo-ti's side effects. Discourage use in pregnant women.

BOTANY: Fo-ti is native to central and southern China and distributed in Japan and Taiwan. It is a perennial climbing herb, which can grow to 9 m in height. The plant has red stems, heart-shaped leaves, and white or pink flowers. The roots of 3- to 4-year-old plants are dried in autumn. The stems and leaves are also used.[1,2]

HISTORY: Fo-ti is a popular Chinese tonic herb, dating back to 713 A.D.[1] It is considered one of the country's great four herbal tonics (along with angelica, lycium, and panax).[3] Regarded as a rejuvenating plant, fo-ti has been thought to prevent aging and promote longevity.[1]

PHARMACOLOGY: In China, fo-ti is used for its rejuvenating and toning properties. It is used to increase liver and kidney function and cleanse the blood. The plant is also prescribed for symptoms of premature aging such as gray hair.[1] It is also indicated for insomnia, weak bones, constipation, and atherosclerosis.[2]

Fo-ti has been shown to reduce blood cholesterol levels in animals.[1] The root portion of the plant has exhibited an inhibitory effect on triglyceride accumulation and reduced enlargement of mice livers.[4] In a human clinical trial, fo-ti had similar cholesterol-lowering effects.[1]

Fo-ti exhibits antimicrobial properties against tuberculosis bacillus and malaria.[1] Other uses of the plant include: To increase fertility,[1] increase blood sugar levels,[1] treat anemia, and relieve muscle aches.[3]

TOXICOLOGY: There is little information in the area of toxicology from fo-ti. However, all plants that contain anthraquinone cathartic compounds should be used cautiously to prevent developing dependence on their laxative effects. One case report describes herb-induced hepatitis in a 31-year-old pregnant Chinese woman from medicine prepared from the plant.[5] The use of these compounds in pregnant women should be discouraged.

[1] Chevallier A. *Encyclopedia of Medicinal Plants.* New York, NY: DK Publishing, 1996;121.
[2] Reid D. *Chinese Herbal Medicine.* Boston, MA: Shambhala Publishing, Inc., 1994;150.
[3] Duke J. *CRC Handbook of Medicinal Herbs.* Boca Raton, FL: CRC Press, Inc., 1989;163-64.
[4] Liu C, et al. *Chung Kuo Chung Yao Tsa Chih* 1992;17(10):595-96.
[5] Hong, et al. *Am J Chin Med* 1994;22(1):63-70.

Garlic

SCIENTIFIC NAME(S): *Allium sativum* L. Family: Liliacea

COMMON NAME(S): Garlic, allium, stinking rose, rustic treacle, nectar of the gods, camphor of the poor, poor man's treacle[1,2]

❦❦❦ PATIENT INFORMATION ❦❦❦

Uses: Evidence suggests garlic lowers blood sugar, cholesterol, and lipids. Among its traditional uses, it has been used for its antiseptic and antibacterial properties.

Side Effects: Garlic may affect those requiring stringent blood glucose control or being treated with anticoagulants.

BOTANY: A perennial, odiferous bulb with a tall, erect flowering stem growing from 60 to 90 cm, garlic produces pink to purple flowers that bloom from July to September.

HISTORY: The name *Allium* comes from the Celtic word "all" meaning "burning or smarting." Garlic was valued as an exchange medium in ancient Egypt and described in Cheops pyramid inscriptions. The folk uses of garlic have ranged from the treatment of leprosy in humans to managing clotting disorders in horses. During the Middle Ages, physicians prescribed the herb to cure deafness, while the American Indians used garlic as a remedy for earaches, flatulence, and scurvy.

PHARMACOLOGY: Researchers at Shandong Academy of Medical Science reported that allicin, a compound in garlic, increased the levels of 2 important antioxidant enzymes in the blood, catalase and glutathione peroxidase. This discovery confirmed the antioxidant and free-radical scavenging potential of allicin. Researchers in Japan found 5 sulfur compounds in aged garlic extract that inhibited lipid peroxidation in the liver, preventing a reaction that is considered to be one of the main features of aging in liver cells. The sulfur compounds appeared to be $\approx$ 1000 times more potent in antioxidant activity than the crude, aged garlic extract.[3]

Garlic has received attention for its ability to slow the process of atherosclerosis and control hypertension.[4]

In one study, 10 healthy subjects received a fatty meal containing 100 g of butter either alone or with the juice of 50 g of garlic. After 3 hours, the garlic-treated group showed mean serum cholesterol levels 7% lower than baseline compared to the untreated group, which was 7% above baseline (the changes were significant, $p < 0.001$ for both groups). Furthermore, the garlic-treated group had a 15% increase in fibrinolytic activity compared to controls (49% decrease) ($p < 0.001$ for both groups).[5]

In one study, 20 healthy subjects were fed garlic for 6 months. The oil significantly lowered mean serum cholesterol and triglyceride levels while raising high-density lipoprotein (HDL) levels. Sixty-two patients with coronary artery disease and elevated cholesterol levels were also studied. Garlic decreased the serum cholesterol, triglyceride, and low-density lipoprotein (LDL) levels ($p < 0.05$) while increasing the HDL fraction ($p < 0.001$).[6]

The organic disulfides found in the oil can reduce activity of the thiol group found in many enzymes and oxidize nicotinamide adenine dinucleotide phosphate (NADPH). As such, these compounds can inactivate thiol enzymes such as coenzyme A and HMG-CoA reductase, and can oxidize

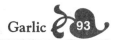

NADPH, all of which are factors normally required for lipid synthesis.

Garlic oil inhibits platelet function, probably by interfering with thromboxane synthesis.[7] Ariga et al[8] isolated a component of garlic oil that inhibits platelet aggregation and identified it as methylallyltrisulphide (MATS). MATS is present in natural oil in a concentration of 4% to 10%. The purified compound inhibits ADP-induced platelet aggregation at a concentration of < 10 mcmol/L in plasma.

Further studies indicate that the most potent antithrombotic compound in garlic is ajoene, which is formed by an acid-catalyzed reaction of 2 allicin molecules followed by rearrangement. Unlike other antithrombotics, ajoene appears to inhibit platelet aggregation regardless of the mechanism of induction.[9]

Scientists have demonstrated the effect of ajoene in preventing clot formation caused by vascular damage. The experiment mimicked the conditions of blood flow in small- and medium-sized arteries by varying the velocity of the blood; the compound proved to be effective in both conditions. The authors suggested that ajoene may be useful in situations where emergency treatment is needed to prevent clot formation produced by vascular damage.[3]

The inhibition of platelet aggregation is also observed in people who ingest fresh garlic. In one study, the platelets from subjects who had eaten garlic cloves (100 to 150 mg/kg) showed complete inhibition to aggregation induced by 5-hydroxytryptamine. The effect was no longer detectable 2.5 hours after ingestion.[10]

Although an earlier study concluded that dried garlic, administered in the form of sugar-coated tablets, had no effect on blood lipids, apolipoproteins, and blood coagulation parameters in patients with primary hyperlipoproteinemia,[11] more recent studies have found that garlic tablets produce a significantly greater reduction in total cholesterol and LDL-C than with placebo.

Another study stated that total cholesterol levels in those taking garlic tablets dropped by 6% and LDL cholesterol was reduced by 11%. Researchers have discovered that garlic tablets reduced the susceptibility of LDL oxidation by 34% vs the placebo group.[12-13]

Some investigators believe that garlic's ability to reduce cholesterol, triglycerides, and LDL, increase HDL, reduce platelet adhesiveness, and increase fibrinolytic activity can combine to decrease the risk of atherosclerotic disease.[12] Some demographic data suggest that the lower-than-normal incidence of atherosclerotic disease in parts of Spain and Italy may be caused by the routine consumption of garlic.

A recent study concluded that a garlic preparation of 1.3% allicin appeared to lower diastolic blood pressure in a large dose.[14]

Garlic has reduced blood-sugar levels.[15] Researchers noted an increase in serum insulin and improvement in liver glycogen storage after garlic administration.[16]

As recently as World War II, garlic extracts were used to disinfect wounds. During the 1800s, physicians routinely prescribed garlic inhalation for the treatment of tuberculosis. Garlic extracts inhibit the growth of numerous strains of *Mycobacterium*, but at concentrations that may be difficult to achieve in human tissues.[16]

Preparations containing garlic extracts are used in Russia and Japan. Gram-positive and gram-negative organisms are inhibited in vitro by garlic extracts.

The potency of garlic is such that 1 mg is equivalent to 15 Oxford units of penicillin, making garlic about 1% as active as penicillin.[16]

Garlic extracts have shown antifungal activity when tested in vitro and has been suggested in the treatment of oral and vaginal candidiasis.[16] In an attempt to quantitate the in vivo activity of garlic extracts, volunteers were administered 25 ml of fresh garlic extract orally.[17] Serum and urine samples were tested for antifungal activity against 15 species of fungal pathogens. While serum exhibited anticandidal and anticryptococcal activity within 30 minutes after ingestion, no biological activity was found in urine. The findings suggest that while garlic extracts may exhibit some antifungal activity in vivo, they are probably of limited use in the treatment of systemic infections.

The antineoplastic activity of garlic has been studied in mice injected with cancer cells that had been pretreated with a garlic extract. No deaths occurred in this treatment group for up to 6 months, while mice injected with untreated cancer cells died within 16 days.[16] It is believed that the reaction of allicin with sulfhydryl groups may contribute to this inhibitory effect.

Garlic contains the trace elements germanium and selenium, which have been thought to play a role in improving host immunity and "normalizing" the oxygen utilization of neoplastic cells. Researchers studied the effects of garlic oil in preventing skin tumors. The study found that 2 oil-soluble compounds from garlic, diallyl sulfide and diallyl disulfide, when applied topically, protected mice against carcinogen-induced skin tumors and increased survival rate.[3]

TOXICOLOGY: Although garlic is used extensively for culinary purposes with essentially no ill effects, the long-term safety of concentrated extracts is unclear.

A single 25 ml dose of fresh garlic extract has caused burning of the mouth, esophagus, and stomach, nausea, sweating, and lightheadedness, and the safety of repeated doses of this amount has not been defined. Repeated exposure to garlic dust can induce asthmatic reactions.[16]

There are no studies that evaluate the effect of garlic and its extracts in people who require stringent blood glucose control or in those being treated with anticoagulants (coumarins, salicylates, "antiplatelet" drugs), but the potential for serious interactions should be kept in mind.

[1] Dobelis IN. *Magic and Medicine of Plants.* Pleasantville, NY: The Reader's Digest Association, 1986.

[2] Osol A, Farrar GE Jr, ed. *The Dispensatory of the United States of America,* 25th ed. Philadelphia: JB Lippincott, 1955:1538.

[3] McCaleb R. *Herbal Gram* 1993;29:18.

[4] Kamanna VS, et al. *Ind J Med Res* 1984;79:580.

[5] Bordia A, et al. *Lancet* 1973;ii:1491.

[6] Bordia A. *Am J Clin Nutr* 1981;34:2100.

[7] Makheja AN, et al. *Lancet* 1979;i:781.

[8] Ariga T, et al. *Lancet* 1980;i:150.

[9] *Chem Eng News* 1985;63(1):34.

[10] Boullin DJ. *Lancet* 1981;i:776.

[11] Luley C, et al. *Arzneimittelforschung* 1986;36:766.

[12] Jain AK, et al. *Am J Med* 1993;94:632.

[13] Glorious Garlic. *NARD Journal* 1993;9:13.

[14] McMahon FG, et al. *Pharmacotherapy* 1993;13(4):406.

[15] Castleman, M. *The Healing Herbs.* Emmaus, PA: Rodale Press, 1991.

[16] Pareddy SR, et al. *Hospital Pharmacist Report* 1993;8:27.

[17] Caporaso, et al. *Antimicrob Agents Chemother* 1983;23:700.

SCIENTIFIC NAME(S): *Gentiana lutea* L. Stemless gentian is derived from *G. acaulis* L. Family: Gentianaceae

COMMON NAME(S): Gentian, stemless gentian, yellow gentian, bitter root, pale gentian, gall weed

---

❧❧❧ PATIENT INFORMATION ❧❧❧

Uses: Gentian is used to stimulate the appetite, improve digestion, and treat GI complaints. It has also been used to treat wounds, sore throat, arthritic inflammations, and jaundice.

Side Effects: The extract may cause gastric irritation and not be tolerated by pregnant women or those with hypertension.

BOTANY: Native to Europe and western Asia, *G. lutea*, a perennial herb with erect stems and oval leaves, grows to 1.8 m in height. The plant produces a cluster of fragrant orange-yellow flowers. *G. acaulis* is a small herb with a basal rosette of lance-shaped leaves and grows to 10 cm in height. It is native to the European Alps at 900 to 1500 m above sea level. The roots and rhizomes are nearly cylindrical, sometimes branched, varying in thickness from 5 to 40 mm. The root and rhizome portions are longitudinally wrinkled. The color of the rhizomes, ranging from dark brown to light tan, appears to be related to its bitter principal content.[1] The roots and rhizome of *G. lutea* are used medicinally, whereas the entire plant of *G. acaulis* is used.

HISTORY: Gentians have been used to stimulate the appetite, improve digestion, and treat GI problems.[2,3] Gentian and stemless gentian are approved for food use. Stemless gentian is used as a tea or alcoholic extract such as *Angostura bitters*. Extracts are used in foods, cosmetics, and antismoking products. The plant has been used externally to treat wounds and internally to treat sore throat, arthritic inflammations, and jaundice.

PHARMACOLOGY: Ingestion of bitter substances may improve the appetite and aid in digestion. However, since gentian is most often consumed as an ingredient in an alcoholic beverage, it is difficult to distinguish the effects of gentian from those of alcohol.[4]

TOXICOLOGY: Usually, the extract is taken in small doses that do not cause adverse effects. One author suggested that gentian may not be well tolerated in hypertension or pregnancy.[5] The extract may cause gastric irritation, resulting in nausea and vomiting.

The highly toxic white hellebore (*Veratrum album* L.) often grows in close proximity to gentian. At least 5 cases of acute veratrum alkaloid poisoning has been reported in people preparing homemade gentian wine accidentally contaminated by veratrum.[6]

---

[1] Meyer JE. *The Herbalist.* Hammond, IN: Hammond Book Co., 1934.

[2] Leung AY. *Encyclopedia of Common Natural Ingredients Used in Food, Drugs, and Cosmetics.* New York, NY: John Wiley and Sons, 1980.

[3] DerMarderosian A, et al. *Natural Product Medicine.* Philadelphia, PA: G.F. Stickley Co., 1988.

[4] Tyler VE. *The New Honest Herbal.* Philadelphia, PA: G.F. Stickley Co., 1987.

[5] Tyler VE. *The Honest Herbal.* Philadelphia, PA: G.F. Stickley Co., 1982.

[6] Garnier R, et al. *Ann Med Interne* 1985;136:125.

SCIENTIFIC NAME(S): *Zingiber officinale* Roscoe; occasionally *Z. capitatum* and *Z. zerumbet* Smith are used. Family: Zingiberaceae

COMMON NAME(S): Ginger

❧❧❧ PATIENT INFORMATION ❧❧❧

Uses: Ginger roots and rhizomes are used as seasoning. In traditional medicine, it has been used as a carminative, stimulant, diuretic, and antiemetic. It also has been used as an insecticide and fungicide.

Side Effects: Excessive amounts may cause CNS depression and cardiac arrhythmias.

BOTANY: This perennial grows in warm climates such as India, Jamaica, and China, and is native to southeast Asia. The plant carries a green-purple flower in terminal spikes; the flowers are similar to orchids. The rhizome is aromatic and the source of the dried powdered spice.[1]

HISTORY: The roots and rhizomes of ginger have been used as a seasoning and have played an important role in Chinese, Indian, and Japanese medicine. Ginger is thought to possess carminative, stimulant, diuretic, and antiemetic properties.[2] Fluid extracts of ginger have been used since the 1500s for the treatment of GI distress. In China, ginger root and stem are used as pesticides against aphids and fungal spores.[3]

PHARMACOLOGY: The gingerols and the related compound shogaol have been found to possess cardiotonic activity. Crude methanol extracts of ginger are known to have a powerful positive inotropic effect on animal hearts. The gingerols have been found to exert a dose-dependent positive inotropic action at doses as low as 10^{-4}g/ml when applied to isolated atrial tissue.[2]

Administration of [6]-gingerol and [6]-shogaol (1.75 to 3.5 mg/kg IV and 70 to 140 mg/kg orally) inhibited spontaneous motor activity, produced antipyretic and analgesic effects and pro-longed hexobarbital-induced sleeping time in laboratory animals. [6]-shogaol was generally more potent than [6]-gingerol and showed an intense antitussive effect when compared to dihydrocodeine phosphate. Interestingly, [6]-shogaol inhibited intestinal motility when given IV, but facilitated GI motility after oral administration. Both compounds were cardiodepressant at low doses and cardiotonic at higher doses.[4] [6]-gingerol, the dehydrogingerdiones, and the gingerdiones are potent inhibitors of prostaglandin biosynthesis through the inhibition of prostaglandin synthetase.[5]

The volatile oil of ginger root was capable of inhibiting the growth of bacteria in a closed chamber,[6] and commercial applications of this activity are being investigated.

The cytotoxic compound zerumbone and its epoxide have been isolated from the rhizomes of *Z. zerumbet*. This plant, also a member of the family Zingiberaceae, has been used traditionally in China as an antineoplastic. The isolates inhibited the growth of a hepatoma tissue culture.[7] In addition, juice prepared from ginger root has been found to inactivate the mutagenicity of tryptophan pyrolysis products in vitro.[8]

The root stock of the related *Z. capitatum* contains a heat-stable interferon

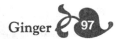

that possesses some immune-stimulating activity. It has no direct virucidal or antitumor activity.[9]

Little is known about the human pharmacology of ginger. One widely publicized double-blind study was conducted to compare the effect of 940 mg of powdered ginger root, 100 mg dimenhydrinate (eg, *Dramamine*, an antihistamine), and placebo (chickweed herb) in the prevention of motion sickness. Thirty-six subjects were given the preparations and placed blindfolded in a rotating chair. Subjects who received ginger root remained in the chair an average of 5.5 minutes, compared to 3.5 minutes for the dimenhydrinate group and 1.5 minutes for the placebo group. Half of the ginger-treated subjects remained in the chair for the full 6 minutes of the test; none of the subjects in the other groups completed the test. In general, it took longer for the ginger group to begin feeling sick, but once the vomiting center was activated, sensations of nausea and vomiting progressed at the same rate in all groups. The authors postulated that, unlike an-

tihistamines which act on the CNS, the aromatic, carminative, and possibly absorbent properties of ginger ameliorate the effects of motion sickness in the GI tract itself. It may increase gastric motility, blocking GI reactions and subsequent nausea feedback.[10]

More recently, pregnant women suffering from hyperemesis gravidarum received ginger (250 mg 4 times daily) or placebo for 4 days. A significant (p = 0.003) percentage of women (70.4%) subjectively preferred ginger treatment, with greater symptomatic relief being observed compared to placebo.[11]

TOXICOLOGY: There are no reports of severe toxicity in humans from the ingestion of ginger root. In culinary quantities, the root is generally devoid of activity. Large overdoses carry the potential for causing CNS depression and cardiac arrhythmias. Reports that ginger extracts may be mutagenic or antimutagenic in experimental test models require confirmation.[11] There is no good evidence regarding the safety of ingesting large amounts of this material by pregnant women.

[1] Schauenberg P, et al. *Guide to Medicinal Plants*. New Canaan, CT: Keats Publishing, Inc., 1977.

[2] Shoji N, et al. *J Pharm Sci* 1982;71 (10):1174.

[3] Yang RZ, et al. *Econ Bot* 1988;42(3):376.

[4] Suekawa M, et al. *J Pharmacobiodyn* 1984;7(11):836.

[5] Kiuchi F, et al. *Chem Pharm Bull* 1982;30(2):754.

[6] Inouye S, et al. *Microbial Biochem* 1984;100:232.

[7] Matthes HWD, et al. *Phytochemistry* 1980;19:2643.

[8] Morita K, et al. *Agric Biol Chem* 1978;42(6):1235.

[9] Babbar OP. *Indian J Exp Biol* 1982;20:572.

[10] Mowrey DB, et al. *Lancet* 1982(March 20);i:655.

[11] Fischer-Rasmussen W, et al. *Eur J Obstet Gynecol Reprod Biol* 1991;38(1):19.

Ginkgo

SCIENTIFIC NAME(S): *Ginkgo biloba* L. Family: Ginkgoaceae

COMMON NAME(S): Ginkgo, maidenhair tree, kew tree, ginkyo, yinhsing (Silver Apricot-Japanese)

⚘⚘⚘ PATIENT INFORMATION ⚘⚘⚘

Uses: Ginkgo has been used to treat Raynaud's disease, cerebral insufficiency, anxiety/stress, tinnitus, dementias, circulatory disorders/asthma. It has positive effects on memory and diseases associated with free radical generation.

Side Effects: Severe side effects are rare; possible effects include headache, dizziness, heart palpitations, and GI and dermatologic reactions. Ginkgo pollen can be strongly allergenic. Contact with the fleshy fruit pulp causes allergic dermatitis, similar to poison ivy.

BOTANY: The ginkgo is the world's oldest living tree species and can be traced back more than 200 million years to fossils of the Permian period. It is the sole survivor of the family Ginkgoaceae. Individual trees may live as long as 1000 years. They grow to a height of ≈ 3750 cm and have fan-shaped leaves. The species is dioecious; male trees > 20 years old blossom in the spring. Adult female trees produce a plum-like gray-tan fruit that falls in late autumn. Its fleshy pulp has a foul, offensive odor and causes contact dermatitis. The edible inner seed resembles an almond and is sold in Asian markets.[1]

HISTORY: In China, where the species survived the ice age, ginkgo was cultivated as a sacred tree, and is still found decorating Buddhist temples throughout Asia. It has not been found in the wild. Preparations have been used for medicinal purposes for > 1000 years. Traditional Chinese physicians used ginkgo leaves to treat asthma and chillblains, which is the swelling of the hands and feet from exposure to damp cold. The ancient Chinese and Japanese ate roasted ginkgo seeds, and considered them a digestive aid and preventive against drunkenness.[2] The flavonoids act as free radical scavengers and the terpenes (ginkgolides) inhibit platelet activating factor.[3] Currently,

oral and IV forms are available in Europe, where it is one of the most widely prescribed medications. Neither form has been approved for medical use in the US, where ginkgo is sold as a nutritional supplement.

PHARMACOLOGY: Numerous studies on the pharmacological actions of ginkgo have been reported, including treatment of cerebral insufficiency, dementia, circulatory disorders, and asthma. The plant is also known for its antioxidant and neuroprotective effects.

Cerebral insufficiency: Cerebral insufficiency may cause anxiety and stress, memory, concentration, and mood impairment, and hearing disorders, all of which may benefit from ginkgo therapy. IV injection of ginkgo biloba extract (GBE) increased cerebral blood flow in ≈ 70% of the patients evaluated. This increase was age-related: Patients between the ages of 30 and 50 years had a 20% increase from baseline, compared with 70% in those 50 to 70 years old. Further, the time to reach peak blood flow was shorter in the elderly.[4] Cerebral insufficiency in 112 patients (average age 70.5 years) treated with ginkgo leaf extract (120 mg) for 1 year, resulted in reduced symptoms such as headache, dizziness, short-term memory, vigilance, and disturbance.[5] Electroencephalographic effects of different preparations of GBE

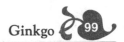

have been measured.[6] A review of 40 clinical trials, most evaluating 120 mg GBE per day for 4 to 6 weeks, reported positive results in treating cerebral insufficiency. Only 8 studies did not have major methodological flaws; the results from these studies were, nevertheless, difficult to interpret. They suggested that long-term treatment (> 6 weeks) is required and that any effect is similar to that observed following treatment with ergoloids.[7] A meta-analysis of 11 placebo-controlled, randomized, double-blinded studies, concluded GBE (150 mg/day) was superior to placebo in patients with cerebrovascular insufficiency.[8]

Antianxiety/stress: MAO inhibition in rats produced by extracts of ginkgo (dried and fresh leaves) was detected, suggesting a mechanism by which the plant exerts its antistress actions.[9] Glucocorticoid synthesis, regulated by ACTH (adrenocorticotropic hormone), which accelerates cholesterol transport, can lead to neurotoxicity. Ginkgolides A and B decrease cholesterol transport, resulting in decreased corticosteroid synthesis. The antistress and neuroprotective effects of GBE may also be caused by this mechanism of action.[10] The anxiolytic effects of GBE in combination with *Zingiber officinale*, was compared in animals. Results showed effects to be comparable to diazepam, but in high doses, the combination may have anxiolytic properties.[11] Social behavior in animals has been evaluated using GBE, diazepam, and ethyl beta-carboline-3-carboxylate.[12]

Memory improvement: In elderly men with slight age-related memory loss, ginkgo supplementation reduced the time required to process visual information.[13] Effects of GBE on event-related potentials in 48 patients with age-associated memory impairment has been measured.[14] Significant improvement in memory (as measured by a series of

psychological testing), in 8 patients (average age, 32 years) was found one hour after administration of 600 mg GBE vs placebo, again confirming the plant's usefulness in this area.[5]

Tinnitus hearing disorder therapy: Because of the diverse etiology of tinnitus and lack of objective method to measure its symptoms, results using GBE for treatment of this disease are contradictory. GBE may have positive effects in some individuals.[15]

In patients with hearing disorders secondary to vascular insufficiency of the ear, $\approx$ 40% of those treated orally with a leaf extract for 2 to 6 months showed improvement in auditory measurements. The extract was also effective in relieving vertigo associated with vestibular dysfunction.[16]

Dementias: Therapeutic effectiveness of ginkgo biloba in dementia syndromes has been demonstrated.[17-18] One report recommends early GBE therapy in dementias, especially because there are no side effects associated with other dementia drugs.[19] Effects of 240 mg/day GBE in $\approx$ 200 patients with dementia of Alzheimer type and multi-infarct dementia, have been investigated in a randomized, double-blinded, placebo-controlled, multi-center study. Parameters such as psychopathological assessment, attention, memory, and behavior were monitored, resulting in clinical efficacy of the extract in dementias of both types.[20] In another set of patients with moderate dementias (of Alzheimer, vascular, or mixed type), short-term IV infusion therapy with GBE also had positive results, improving psychopathology and cognitive performance.[21] In a 52-week, randomized, double-blinded, placebo-controlled, multi-center study, mild-to-severe Alzheimer or multi-infarct dementia patients received 120 mg/day GBE vs placebo. Results of this report again confirm improved cognitive performance and social functioning in a number of cases.[22]

Circulatory disorders/asthma: Ginkgolides competitively inhibit the binding of platelet-activating factor (PAF) to its membrane receptor.[5,23] Effects of this mechanism are useful in the treatment of allergic reaction and inflammation (asthma and bronchospasm) and also in circulatory diseases.

In one double-blinded, randomized, crossover study in asthma patients, ginkgolides were effective in early and late phases of airway hyperactivity.[5]

A meta-analysis evaluating GBE in peripheral arterial disease, concludes a highly significant therapeutic effect of the plant in this area.[24] Numerous studies are available concerning GBE and circulatory disorders including its ability to protect against cardiac ischemia reperfusion injury,[25] to adjust fibrinolytic activity,[26] and, in combination with aspirin, to treat thrombosis.[27] It also appears useful in management of peripheral vascular disorders such as Raynaud's disease, acrocyanosis, and post-phlebitis syndrome.[16] IV injection of 50 to 200 mg of ginkgo extract caused a dose-dependent increase in microcirculation and blood viscoelasticity in patients with pathologic blood flow disorders.[28]

A 6-month, double-blind trial suggested some efficacy in treating obliterative arterial disease of the lower limbs. Patients who received extract showed a clinically and statistically significant improvement in pain-free walking distance, maximum walking distance, and plethysmorgraphic recordings of peripheral blood flow.[29] GBE improves walking performance in 60 patients with intermittent claudication, with good tolerance to the drug.[30] However, another report concludes that GBE 120 mg/day has no effect on walking distance or leg pain in intermittent claudication patients (but finds other cognitive functions to be improved).[31] A review of 10 controlled trials evaluating treatment of the plant for this condition, found poor methodological quality, but did note all the studies to show clinical effectiveness of GBE in treating intermittent claudication.[32]

Antioxidant/neuroprotective effects: GBEis known to improve diseases associated with free radical generation. The ginkgolides may contribute to neuroprotective effects. The flavonoid fraction contains free radical scavengers, both of which are important in areas such as hypoxia, seizure activity, and peripheral nerve damage.[33]

GBE exerts a restorative effect in aged rats caused by its protective action on neuronal membrane.[34] It was also shown to protect rat cerebellar neurons suffering from oxidative stress induced by hydrogen peroxide.[35] GBE may be a potent inhibitor of nitric oxide production under tissue-damaging inflammatory conditions in murine macrophage cell lines.[36] GBE was found to be more effective than water-soluble antioxidants and as effective as lipid-soluble antioxidants, in an in vitro model using human erythrocyte suspensions.[37]

Numerous other reports exist concerning this topic, including GBE's effect against lipid peroxidation and cell necrosis in rat hepatocytes,[38] its effect as an oxygen radical scavenger and antioxidant,[39] and its powerful effects on copper-mediated LDL oxidative modification.[40] In Chernobyl accident recovery workers, GBE's antioxidant effects were also studied. Clastogenic factors (risk factors for development of late effects of irradiation) were successfully reduced by the plant.[41]

A number of potentially beneficial effects have been observed for ginkgo, including its ability to prevent the deterioration of lipid profiles when sub-

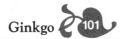

jects were challenged with high-cholesterol meals over an extended holiday season,[42] improvement in the symptoms of PMS, particularly breast-related symptoms,[43] GBE's use in eye problem,s[23] and its scavenging abilities to reduce functional and morphological retina impairments.[44] In addition, GBE has in vitro and in vivo activity against *Pneumocystis carinii,*[45] and has been studied in animals with diabetes[46-47] and human diabetic patients. When GBE extract was given, peripheral blood flow increased by 40% to 45%, compared with an increase of 35% after administration of nicotinic acid.[48] Other reports suggest GBE to be effective in arresting fibrosis development (in 86 chronic hepatitis patients),[49] promoting hair regrowth in mice,[50] and relaxing penile tissue, suggesting a possible use as a drug for impotence.[51] Seed extracts of the plant possess antibacterial and antifungal activity.[23]

TOXICOLOGY: Ingestion of the extract has not been associated with severe side effects. Adverse events from clinical trials of up to 160 mg/day for 4 to 6 weeks did not differ from the placebo group. German literature lists ginkgo's possible side effects as headache, dizziness, heart palpitations, and GI and dermatologic reactions. Injectable forms of ginkgo may cause circulatory disturbances, skin allergy, or phlebitis. Willmar Schwabe Co. has withdrawn its parenteral ginkgo product *Tebonin* from the market because of the possible severity of side effects from this form.[23]

A toxic syndrome, ("Gin-nan" food poisoning) has been recognized in Asia in children who have ingested ginkgo seeds. Approximately 50 seeds produce tonic/clonic seizures and loss of consciousness.[52] Seventy reports (between 1930 and 1960) found 27% lethality, with infants being most vulnerable. Ginkgotoxin (4-O-methylpyridoxine), found only in the seeds, was responsible for this toxicity.[5,23]

Contact with the fleshy fruit pulp has been known since ancient times to be a skin irritant. Constituents alkylbenzoic acid, alkylphenol, and their derivatives cause reactions of this type. Allergic dermatitis such as erythema, edema, blisters, and itching have all been reported.[23] A cross-allergenicity exists between ginkgo fruit pulp and poison ivy. Ginkgolic acid and bilobin are structurally similar to the allergens of poison ivy, mango rind, and cashew nut shell oil. Contact with the fruit pulp causes erythema and edema, with the rapid formation of vesicles accompanied by severe itching. Symptoms last 7 to 10 days. Ingestion of two pieces of pulp has been reported to cause perioral erythema, rectal burning, and painful spasms of the anal sphincter.[1]

Allergans ginkgols and ginkgolic acids can cause contact reactions of mucous membranes, resulting in cheilitis and GI irritation. However, oral ginkgo preparations do not have this ability.[5,23] Ginkgo pollen can be strongly allergenic.[53]

In one report, spontaneous bilateral subdural hematomas have been associated with ingestion of the plant.[54]

Since no human data are available about pregnancy and lactation, ginkgo should be avoided by this population.[5,23]

[1] Becker LE, et al. *JAMA* 1975;231:1162.

[2] Castleman M. *The Herb Quarterly* 1990 Spring:26.

[3] Z'Brun A. *Schweiz Rundsch Med Prax* 1995;84(1):1–6.

[4] Pistolese GR. *Minerva Med* 1973;79:4166.

[5] Newall C, et al. *Herbal Medicines.* London, England: Pharmaceutical Press, 1996;138–40.

[6] Kunkel H. *Neuropsychobiology* 1993;27(1):40–45.

[7] Kleijnen J, et al. *Br J Clin Pharmacol* 1992;34(4):352–58.

[8] Hopfenmuller W. *Arzneimittelforschung* 1994;44(9):1005–13.

[9] White H, et al. *Life Sci* 1996;58(16):1315–21.

[10] Amri H, et al. *Endocrinology* 1996;137(12):5707–18.

[11] Hasenohrl R, et al. *Pharmacol Biochem Behav* 1996;53(2):271–75.

[12] Chermat R, et al. *Pharmacol Biochem Behav* 1997;56(2):333–39.

[13] Allain H, et al. *Clin Ther* 1993;15:549-58.

[14] Semlitsch H, et al. *Pharmacopsychiatry* 1995;28(4):134–42.

[15] Holgers K, et al *Audiology* 1994;33(2):85–92.

[16] Nazzaro P, et al. *Minerva Med* 1973;79:4198.

[17] Herrschaft H. *Pharm Unserer Zeit* 1992;21(6):266–75.

[18] Itil T, et al. *Psychopharmacol Bull* 1995;31(1):147–58.

[19] Reisecker F. *Wien Med Wochenschr* 1996;146(21–22):546–48.

[20] Kanowski S, et al. *Pharmacopsychiatry* 1996;29(2):47–56.

[21] Haase J, et al. *Z Gerontol Geriatr* 1996;29(4):302–9.

[22] LeBars P, et al. *JAMA* 1997;278(16):1327–32.

[23] DeSmet P, et al. Ginkgo Biloba. Berlin: Springer-Verlag 1997;51–66.

[24] Schneider B. *Arzneimittelforschung* 1992;42(4):428–36.

[25] Haramaki N, et al. *Free Radic Biol Med* 1994;16(6):789–94.

[26] Shen J, et al. *Biochem Mol Biol Int* 1995;35(1):125–34.

[27] Belougne E, et al. *Thromb Res* 1996;82(5):453–58.

[28] Koltringer P, et al. *Fortschr Med* 1993;111:170.

[29] Bauer U. *Arzneimittelforschung* 1984;34:716.

[30] Blume J, et al. *VASA* 1996;25(3):265–74.

[31] Drabaek H, et al. *Ugeskr Laeger* 1996;158(27):3928–31.

[32] Ernst E. *Fortschr Med* 1996;114(8):85–87.

[33] Smith P, et al. *J Ethnopharmacol* 1996;50(3):131–39.

[34] Huguet F, et al. *J Pharm Pharmacol* 1994;46(4):316–18.

[35] Oyama Y, et al. *Brain Res* 1996;712(2):349–52.

[36] Kobuchi H, et al. *Biochem Pharmacol* 1997;53(6):897–903.

[37] Kose K, et al. *J Int Med Res* 1995;23(1):9–18.

[38] Joyeux M, et al. *Planta Med* 1995;61(2):126–29.

[39] Maitra I, et al. *Biochem Pharmacol* 1995;49(11):1649–55.

[40] Yan L, et al. *Biochem Biophys Res Commun* 1995;212(2):360–66.

[41] Emerit I, et al. *Radiat Res* 1995;144(2):198–205.

[42] Kenzelmann R, et al. *Arzneimittelforschung* 1993;43:978.

[43] Tamborini A, et al. *Ref Fr Gynecol Obstet* 1993;88:447-57.

[44] Droy-Lefaix M, et al. *Int J Tissue React* 1995;17(3):93–100.

[45] Atzori C, et al. *Antimicrob Agents Chemother* 1993;37:1492.

[46] Agar A, et al. *Int J Neurosci* 1994;76(3–4):259–66.

[47] Punkt K, et al. *ACTA Histochem* 1997;99(3):291–99.

[48] Bartolo M. *Minerva Med* 1973;79:4192.

[49] Li W, et al. *Chung Kuo Chung Hsi I Chieh Ho Tsa Chih* 1995;15(10):593–95.

[50] Kobayashi N, et al. *Yakugaku Zasshi* 1993;113(10):718–24.

[51] Paick J, et al. *J Urol* 1996;156(5):1876–80.

[52] Yagi M, et al. *Yakugaku Zasshi* 1993;113:596.

[53] Long R, et al. *Hua Hsi I Ko Ta Hsueh Hsueh Pao* 1992;23:429.

[54] Rowin J, et al. *Neurology* 1996;46(6):1775–76.

BOTANY: Ginseng commonly refers to *Panax quinquefolium* L. or *Panax ginseng* C. A. Meyer, 2 members of the family Araliaceae. The ginsengs were classified as members of the genus *Aralia* in older texts. A number of species of ginseng grow around the world and are used in local traditional medicine. The roots or rhizomes of these plants are used medicinally.

Scientific Name	Common Name	Distribution
P. quinquefolium L.	American ginseng	US
P. ginseng C. A. Meyer	Korean ginseng	N.E. China, Korea, East Siberia
P. pseudoginseng Wall. var. *notoginseng*	Sanchi ginseng	S.W. China
P. pseudoginseng var. major	Zhuzishen	China
P. pseudoginseng (Will.) subsp. *japonicus*	Chikusetsu ginseng	Japan
P. pseudoginseng subsp. *himalaicus*	Himalayan ginseng	Japan
P. trifolius L.	Dwarf ginseng	US

In the US, ginseng is found in rich, cool woods; a significant crop is also grown commercially. The short plant grows from 3 to 7 compound leaves that drop in the fall. It bears a cluster of red or yellowish fruits from June to July. The roots mature slowly and are usually harvested only after the first 3 years of growth. The shape of the root can vary between species and has been used to distinguish types of ginseng.

Approximately 45,000 kg of dried cultivated *P. quinquefolium* root and an equal amount of wild root are shipped abroad from the US annually. About 5% of the root crop is retained for domestic use.[1]

HISTORY: For more than 2000 years, various forms of ginseng have been used in medicine. The name Panax derives from the Greek word "all healing." Ginseng root's man-shaped figure (shen-seng means "man-root") led proponents of the "Doctrine of Signatures" to believe that the root could strengthen any part of the body. Through the ages, the root has been used in the treatment of asthenia, atherosclerosis, blood and bleeding disorders, colitis, and for the relief of symptoms of aging, cancer, and senility.

Evidence that the root possesses a general strengthening effect, raises mental and physical capacity, exerts a protectant effect against experimental diabetes, neurosis, radiation sickness, and some cancers has been reported. Today, its popularity is due to the "adaptogenic" (stress-protective) effect of the saponin content.

PHARMACOLOGY: It has been claimed that ginseng exerts a strengthening effect while also raising physical and mental capacity for work. These properties have been defined as an "adaptogenic effect" or a non-specific increase in resistance to the noxious effects of physical, chemical, or biological stress.[2] The panaxosides, a ginseng component, may alter the activity of hormones produced by the pituitary,[3] adrenal,[4] or gonadal tissue.[5]

Despite the shortcomings of many animal studies, a significant body of experience describes some of the pharmacologic effects of the panaxosides. For example, ginsenoside Rb-1 has CNS activity (depressant, anticonvulsant, analgesic, antipsychotic), protects against the development of stress ulcers, and accelerates glycolysis and nuclear RNA synthesis. Ginseng appears to potentiate the normal function of the adrenal gland, for some "anti-stress" activity.

Five glycans with strong hypoglycemic activity have been isolated from the root.[6,7] Ginsenoside Rg-1 given to postoperative gynecologic patients caused a greater increase in hemoglobin and hematocrit levels among treated women than in placebo-treated controls. Serum protein and body weight also increased to a greater degree in the treated patients. The adaptogenic effect has not been well documented in humans, although there is a strong body of evidence from traditional medicine.

TOXICOLOGY: Through its extensive history of use in popular herbal products, ginseng has established a remarkable record of safety. It is estimated that > 6 million people ingest ginseng regularly in the US alone. Nevertheless, there have been a few reports of severe reactions. One controversial report described a "ginseng-abuse syndrome" among 133 patients who took relatively large doses of the root (> 3 g/day) for up to 2 years.[8] Patients reported a feeling of stimulation, well-being, and increased motor and cognitive efficiency, but also often noted diarrhea, skin eruptions, nervousness, sleeplessness, and hypertension. This was an open study and the simultaneous intake of other drugs (eg, caffeine) confounded interpretation of the data.

Other reports have implicated ginseng as having an estrogen-like effect in women.[9] One case of diffuse mammary nodularity has been reported,[10] as well as a case of vaginal bleeding in a 72-year-old woman.[11]

The most common ginseng side effects are nervousness and excitation, which usually diminish after the first few days of use or with dosage reduction. Inability to concentrate has also been reported following long-term use.[12]

The hypoglycemic effect of the whole root and individual panaxosides has been reported. Although no cases of serious reactions in diabetic patients have been reported, those who must control their blood glucose levels should take ginseng with caution.

A patient receiving warfarin experienced a decrease in the international normalized ratio 2 weeks after starting ginseng, which reversed within 2 weeks of stopping the gingseng.[13]

[1] Lewis WH. *JAMA* 1980;243:31.
[2] Brekham II, et al. *Lloydia* 1969;32:46.
[3] Fulder SJ. *Am J Chin Med* 1981;9:112.
[4] Hiai S, et al. *Endocrinol Jap* 1979;26:737.
[5] Fahim MS, et al. *Arch Androl* 1982;8:261.
[6] Konno C, et al. *Planta Medica* 1984;50:434.
[7] Masashi T, et al. *Planta Medica* 1984;50:436.
[8] Siegal RK. *JAMA* 1979;241:1614.
[9] Punnonen R, Lukola A. *BMJ* 1980;281:1110.
[10] Palmer BV, et al. *Br Med J* 19781:1284.
[11] Greenspan EM. *JAMA* 1983;249:2018.
[12] Hammond TG, et al. *Med J Aust* 1981;1:492.
[13] Janetzky K, et al. *Am J Health Syst Pharm* 1997;54:692-93.

Glucomannan

105

SCIENTIFIC NAME(S): *Amorphophallus konjac* Koch. Family: Araceae

COMMON NAME(S): Konjac, Konjac mannan, glucomannan

❧❧ PATIENT INFORMATION ❧❧

Uses: Glucomannan reportedly alleviates constipation, reduces intestinal flora, lowers blood sugar and cholesterol, and may possibly promote weight loss and inhibit cancer.

Side Effects: Severe esophageal and GI obstruction have been reported with tablets. The hypoglycemic effects are potentially dangerous to diabetic patients.

SOURCE: Konjac mannan is a polysaccharide derived from the tubers of konjac. It is purified from konjac flour by repeated treatment with cupric hydroxide and subsequent washings with ethanol[1] or by dialysis against water.[2]

PHARMACOLOGY: Polysaccharides such as guar gum (composed of galactose and mannose, galactomannan), tragacanth, cellulose, methylcellulose, pectin, and wheat bran have found use as foodstuffs and dietary and therapeutic agents. Their ability to swell by the absorption of water has made them useful as laxatives. Konjac mannan has been reported to alleviate moderate constipation in 1 to 2 days.

By increasing the viscosity of the intestinal contents, slowing gastric emptying time, and acting as a barrier to diffusion, agents such as guar gum have been shown to delay the absorption of glucose from the intestines.[3] Several small studies have shown that diabetics fed a diet consisting largely of raw vegetables, uncooked seeds, fruits, and goat's milk were able to reduce or discontinue their insulin requirements.[4] Similarly, konjac mannan has been reported to reduce the need for hypoglycemic agents. When 13 diabetic patients received 3.6 or 7.2 g of konjac mannan daily for 90 days, their mean fasting glucose levels fell by 29% and insulin or hypoglycemic agent doses were reduced in most patients.[5] Five healthy men enrolled in the same study

underwent a glucose tolerance test with or without a single dose of 2.6 g konjac mannan. The polysaccharide reduced mean blood glucose levels by 7.3% at 30 minutes with a concomitant decrease in serum insulin concentration. Another study of 72 type 2 diabetic patients showed a significant reduction in fasting blood glucose and postprandial blood glucose after consuming konjac with food for 30 and 65 days.[6]

Konjac mannan is gaining popularity as a weight-reducing agent and is often included in "grapefruit diet" tablets. Some research has indicated that patients treated with oral glucomannan have decreased body weight compared with control groups. In one study involving an 8-week cardiac rehabilitation program, patients were given 1.5 grams of glucomannan twice daily.[7] Body weight among treated patients decreased by 1.5 kg at the end of 4 weeks and 2.2 kg at the end of 8 weeks. These losses were significant when compared with the placebo group.

Hydrophilic gums have found some use as diet aids based on the theory that the feeling of fullness provided by their swelling leads to a decrease in appetite. Such agents are generally considered to be only marginally effective.

Konjac mannan has been shown to reduce plasma cholesterol levels in rats.[8] Interestingly, only water-soluble konjac mannan has this effect.

In a study of 10 overweight patients, the daily administration of 100 ml of 1% konjac mannan solution for 11 weeks resulted in decreases in serum cholesterol levels of 0% to 39% (mean, 18%).[9] In a separate double-blind crossover trial involving 63 men, total cholesterol was reduced by 10% among subjects given a daily dose of 3.9 g konjac glucomannan for a 4-week period.[10] The diabetic patients treated in another study showed a reduction in mean serum cholesterol levels of 11% after 20 days of konjac mannan treatment.[5] Several other studies confirm the effects of konjac mannan on lipid metabolism.[11-13]

The activity of this polysaccharide cannot be explained by a simple interaction with bile acids since konjac mannan shows no in vitro or in vivo bile-binding activity. Rather, it appears to inhibit the active transport of cholesterol in the jejunum and the absorption of bile acids in the ileum.[14] A study on bile output in rats fed a diet of 5% konjac mannan showed an increase in the volume of bile juice secreted and the release of bile acids, protease, and amylase compared to animals fed a control diet without fiber.[15] This effect was only observed for prolonged feeding of the experimental diet with konjac mannan and could not be produced with a single dose.

TOXICOLOGY: Four cases of severe esophageal obstruction caused by glucomannan diet tablets have been reported.[16-17] Glucomannan-containing tablets have been banned in Australia since May 1985 because they also carry the potential for inducing lower GI obstruction. Encapsulated and powder forms remain available.

Glucomannan use is associated with a reduction in the need for hypoglycemic agents, and the product may result in a loss of glycemic control in diabetic patients. It should be used with great care by diabetic patients.

[1] Kiriyama S, et al. *J Nutr* 1972;102(12):1689.
[2] US patents 3,973,008 [Aug 3, 1976] and 3,856,945 [Dec 24, 1974].
[3] Jenkins DJ, et al. *BMJ* 1978;1(6124):1392.
[4] Anonymous. *Med Letter Drugs Ther* 1979;21(12):51.
[5] Doi K, et al. *Lancet* 1979(May 5);1:987.
[6] Huang CY, et al. *Biomed Environ Sci* 1990;3(2):123.
[7] Reffo GC, et al. *Curr Ther Res* 1990(May);47:753.
[8] Kiriyama S, et al. *J Nutr* 1969;97(3):382.
[9] Arvill A, Bodin L. *Am J Clin Nutr* 1995;61(3):585.
[10] US patents 3,973,008 [Aug 3, 1976] and 3,856,945 [Dec 24, 1974].
[11] Zhang MY, et al. *Biomed Environ Sci* 1990;3(1):99.
[12] Hou YH, et al. *Biomed Environ Sci* 1990;3(3):306.
[13] Shimizu H, et al. *J Pharmacobiodyn* 1991;14(7):371.
[14] Kiriyama S, et al. *J Nutr* 1974;104(1):69.
[15] Ikegami S, et al. *J Nutr Sci Vitaminol* 1984;30(6):515.
[16] Gaudry P. *Med J Austr* 1985;142(3):204.
[17] Henry DA, et al. *BMJ* 1986;292(6520):591.

SCIENTIFIC NAME(S): 2–Amino-2–deoxyglucose

COMMON NAME(S): Chitosamine

PATIENT INFORMATION

Uses: Glucosamine is being investigated extensively as an antiarthritic in osteoarthritis.

Side Effects: Well-tolerated. No side effects have been directly associated with glucosamine.

BIOLOGY: Glucosamine is found in mucopolysaccharides, mucoproteins, and chitin. Chitin is found in yeasts, fungi, arthropods, and various marine invertebrates as a major component of the exoskeleton. It also occurs in other lower animals and members of the plant kingdom.[1]

PHARMACOLOGY: Chitin has been described as a vulnerary or wound-healing polymer,[2] while glucosamine has been referred to as a pharmaceutical aid and antiarthritic.[1] There is a progressive degeneration of cartilage glycosaminoglycans (GAG) in osteoarthritis. The idea of using glucosamine orally is to provide a "building block" for its regeneration. Glucosamine is the rate-limiting step in GAG biosynthesis. It is biochemically formed from the glycolytic intermediate fructose-6-phosphate by way of amination of glutamine as the donor, ultimately yielding glucosamine-6-phosphate. This is subsequently converted or acetylated to galactosamine before being incorporated into growing GAG. Hopefully, this will stimulate the production of cartilage components and bring about joint repair.[3] Several double-blind studies indicate that glucosamine sulfate may be better than some nonsteroidal anti-inflammatory drugs (NSAIDs) and placebos in relieving both pain and inflammation caused by osteoarthritis.[3–5] The efficacy and safety of IM glucosamine sulfate in osteoarthritis of the knee was studied in a randomized, placebo-controlled double-blind study and revealed that the treatment was well tolerated and effective.[4] Other double-blind clinical studies of intra-articular glucosamine were conducted and resulted in reduced pain, increased angle of joint flexion, and restored articular function compared with placebo.[5] The relative efficacy of ibuprofen and glucosamine sulfate was compared in the management of osteoarthritis of the knee.[6] At 8 weeks, glucosamine was more effective in reducing pain (1.5 g daily dose orally). Oral glucosamine sulfate therapy vs placebo in osteoarthritis was studied, and researchers found (80 patients, 1.5 g daily dose orally) decreased symptoms and improved autonomous motility with glucosamine.[7] These investigators also employed electron microscopy studies on cartilage and found that patients who had placebo showed a typical picture of established osteoarthrosis, while those on glucosamine showed a picture similar to healthy cartilage. They concluded that glucosamine tends to rebuild damaged cartilage, thus restoring articular function in most chronic arthrosic patients.

Other studies showed that glucosamine can be safe and effective in the treatment of various forms of osteoarthritis. Standard drug therapy is only of palliative benefit and may worsen loss of cartilage. Glucosamine is an intermediate in mucopolysaccharide synthesis, and its availability in cartilage tissue culture can be rate-limiting for proteoglycan production. Reviews of related literature also demonstrate glucosamine's effectiveness in decreasing pain and improving mobility in osteoarthritis without side effects. Further, by mechanisms still unknown, the natural methyl donor 5-adenosylmethionine also promotes production of cartilage proteoglycans and is likewise therapeutically beneficial in osteoarthritis in well-tolerated oral doses. One researcher promotes the use of glucosamine and other safe nutritional measures supporting proteoglycan synthesis because these may offer a practical method of preventing or postponing the onset of osteoarthritis in athletes and older people.[8]

Other studies on glucosamine show its pharmacokinetics (radiolabeled glucosamine was quickly and completely absorbed either orally or by IV);[9] attempt to synthesize derivatives of glucosamine that have immunomodulating activity;[10] demonstrate the ability of glucosamine to inhibit the development of viral cytopathic effects and the production of infective viral particles;[11] and show the inhibitory effects of D-glucosamine on a carcinoma and protein, RNA, and DNA synthesis.[12]

TOXICOLOGY: No direct toxic effects of glucosamine could be found in the scientific literature; however, one report shows potential bronchopulmonary complications of antirheumatic drugs including glucosamine.[13]

[1] Budavari S, ed. *The Merck Index*, 11th ed. Merck & Co., Inc., Rahway, NJ. 1989;4353.

[2] Budavari S, ed. *The Merck Index*, 11th ed. Merck & Co., Inc., Rahway, NJ. 1989;2049.

[3] Anonymous. *Am J Natl Med* 1994;1(1):10-14.

[4] Reichelt A, et al. *Arzneimittelforschung* 1994;44(1):75-80.

[5] Vajaradul Y. *Clin Ther* 1981;3(5):336-43.

[6] Vaz A. *Curr Med Res Opin* 1982;8(3):145-9.

[7] Drovanti A, et al. *Clin Ther* 1980;3(4):260-72.

[8] McCarty M. *Med Hyp* 1994;42(5):323-37.

[9] Setnikar I, et al. *Arzneimittelforschung* 1986(Apr);36:729-35.

[10] Valcavi U, et al. *Arzneimittelforschung* 1989;39(10):190-95.

[11] Delgadillo R, et al. *J Pharm Pharmacol* 1988(Jul);40:488-93.

[12] Bekesi J, et al. *Can Res* 1970(Dec);30:2905-912.

[13] Larget-Piet B, et al. *Ther* 1986;41(4):269-77.

SCIENTIFIC NAME(S): *Hydrastis canadensis* L. Family: Ranunculaceae

COMMON NAME(S): Eye balm, eye root, goldenseal, ground raspberry, Indian dye, jaundice root, orange root, tumeric root, yellow Indian paint, yellow puccoon, yellow root[1]

❧❧❧ PATIENT INFORMATION ❧❧❧

Uses: Goldenseal has been used as an eyewash, antispasmodic, for the treatment for dysmenorrhea, minor sciatica, and rheumatic and muscular pain.

Side Effects: Large doses may be toxic, causing a variety of problems including GI distress, hypertension, convulsions, and respiratory failure. Goldenseal should not be used during pregnancy.

BOTANY: Goldenseal is a stout perennial found in deep, rich woods from Vermont to Arkansas. The 5- to 9-lobed palmate leaves can grow to ≈ 25 cm. It produces dark red berries in April and May from green-white flowers. The rhizomes are golden-yellow and knotted in appearance.

HISTORY: The use of goldenseal dates to the settlers who learned of its use from the American Indians who used it as a dye and for its medicinal properties. It had been used as a bitter stomachic for the relief of catarrhal conditions and as an eye wash. After the Civil War, goldenseal was an ingredient in many patent medicines. It was collected to the point of near extinction.[2] Today, it is farmed but still costly,[2] and in many places it has been almost exterminated by commercial wild harvesting.[1] Preparations containing goldenseal have been marketed for the treatment of menstrual disorders, pain of minor sciatica, rheumatic or muscular pain, and as an antispasmodic.[1] Today goldenseal finds some use as an ingredient in commercial sterile eye washes.

Goldenseal had gained the reputation of being able to prevent the detection of morphine in urine samples.[3] This notion arose from a plot in John Uri Lloyd's novel *Stringtown on the Pike* (Dodd Mead, 1900), and was given further credence by the fact the Lloyd was an internationally known plant pharmacist.[4] However, studies have found no basis for this belief.[5]

PHARMACOLOGY: The activity of goldenseal is largely because of the presence of alkaloid hydrastine and to a lesser extent from berberine.[6] Goldenseal has been used as a uterine hemostatic but was found to be unreliable in its action; its activity was inferior to that of the ergot alkaloids in the treatment of postpartum hemorrhage. Berberine stimulates bile secretion. It has weak antibiotic activity and some antineoplastic activity.[7] Several reports show berberine to be effective against many bacteria that cause diarrhea, including cholera bacteria.

Hydrastine constricts peripheral blood vessels and has been investigated for the treatment of gastric inflammation. Hydrastine administered internally can result in a rise in blood pressure, whereas berberine can induce hypotension.[6] The plant has been associated with a hypoglycemic effect.[8] Empirical evidence and clinical experiences suggest goldenseal may be useful in helping to "cleanse" the liver or blood and restore digestive function in alcoholics.[4]

TOXICOLOGY: In higher doses, hydrastine can cause exaggerated reflexes, hypertension, convulsions, and death from respiratory failure. Large doses of the plant irritate the mouth and throat and cause nausea, vomiting, diarrhea, and paresthesias. CNS stimulation and respiratory failure induced by the plant can be fatal. Moderate doses of the alkaloid hydrastine cause peripheral vasoconstriction and increase cardiac output. A 10% solution of hydrastine causes pupillary dilation.[9]

[1] Dobelis IN, ed. *Magic and Medicine of Plants.* Pleasantville, NY: Readers Digest, 1986.

[2] Castleman M. *The Healing Herbs.* Emmaus, PA: Rodale Press, 1991.

[3] Hamon, NW. *CPJ-RPC* 1990;11:508.

[4] Foster S. *Herbal Gram* 1989;21:7.

[5] Ostrenga JA, Perry D. *Pharm Chem Newsletter* 1975;4(1):1

[6] Genest K, et al. *Can J Pharm Sci* 1969;4:41.

[7] Hartwell, JL. *Lloydia* 1971;34:103.

[8] Farnsworth NR, et al. *Tile and Till* 1971;57:52.

[9] Henry TA. *The Plant Alkaloids.* Philadelphia, PA: Blakiston CO, 1949.

SCIENTIFIC NAME(S): *Centella asiatica* (L.) Urb. Also: *Hydrocotyle asiatica* Family: Umbelliferae (Apiaceae).

COMMON NAME(S): Gotu kola, hydrocotyle, Indian pennywort, talepetrako

---

❧❧❧ PATIENT INFORMATION ❧❧❧

Uses: Traditionally used as treatment for a variety of ills and as an aphrodisiac, gotu kola has demonstrated some efficacy in treating wounds and varicose veins. Evidence suggests it has antifertility, hypotensive, and sedative effects.

Side Effects: Gotu kola causes contact dermatitis in some individuals.

BOTANY: *Centella asiatica* is a slender, creeping plant that grows in swampy areas of India, Sri Lanka, Madagascar, South Africa, and the tropics.

HISTORY: Gotu kola has been widely used to treat a variety of illnesses, particularly in traditional Eastern medicine. Sri Lankans noticed that elephants, renowned for their longevity, munched on the leaves of the plant. Thus the leaves became known as a promoter of long life, with a suggested "dosage" of a few leaves each day. Among the ailments purported to be cured or controlled by gotu kola are mental problems, high blood pressure, abscesses, rheumatism, fever, ulcers, leprosy, skin eruptions, nervous disorders, and jaundice. Gotu kola has been touted as an aphrodisiac. Gotu kola should not be confused with the dried seed of *Cola nitida* (Vent.), the plant used in cola beverages. *Cola nitida* contains caffeine and is a stimulant, while gotu kola has no caffeine and has sedative properties.[1]

PHARMACOLOGY:

Wound healing: Gotu kola extracts have promoted wound healing.[2] Cell culture experiments have shown that the total triterpenoid fraction of the extracts, at a concentration of 25 mcg/ml, does not affect cell proliferation, total cell protein synthesis, or the biosynthesis of proteoglycans in human skin fibroblasts. However, the fraction increases the collagen content of cell layer fibronectin, which may explain the wound healing action.[3] The glycoside madecassoside has anti-inflammatory properties, while asiaticoside appears to stimulate wound healing.

Titrated extract of gotu kola (TECA, 100 mg/kg) has been used as a scarring agent to stimulate wound healing in patients with chronic lesions (eg, cutaneous ulcers, surgical wounds, fistulas, gynecologic lesions). A clinical study evaluated TECA for treating bladder lesions in 102 patients with bilharzial infections. Injections of TECA 2%, usually administered IM for 1 to 3 months, produced cure or improvement in 75% of the cases, as determined from symptoms and urinary and cystoscopic findings. Healing occurred with little scar formation, thus avoiding much of the loss of bladder capacity resulting from bilharzial infections.[4]

Gotu kola has also shown promise in treatment of psoriasis. When creams containing oil and water extracts of the leaves were administered each morning to 7 psoriatic patients, 5 showed complete clearance of lesions within 3 to 7 weeks. One patient showed clearance of most lesions, and one showed improvement without clearance. One patient experienced a mild recurrence 4 months after treatment. Although this study was not controlled, a placebo effect was considered unlikely. The creams were nontoxic and cosmetically acceptable, making them suitable for long-term use.[1]

Antihypertensive Effects: The efficacy of Centellase from gotu kola in the treatment of venous hypertension has been evaluated, using a combined microcirculatory model.[5] The researchers conducted a single-blind, placebo-controlled randomized study of the effects of the total triterpenoid fraction in 89 patients with venous hypertension microangiopathy. The effects of Centellase were found to be significantly different from placebo in hypotensive activity on all the microcirculatory parameters investigated. No side effects were noted.

Varicose Veins: The effects of gotu kola extract on mucopolysaccharide metabolism were noted in subjects with varicose veins.[6] The total triterpenic fraction of the plant (60 mg/day for 3 months) elevated the basal levels of uronic acids and of lysosomal enzymes, indicating an increased mucopolysaccharide turnover in varicose vein patients. These results confirm the regulatory properties of *C. asiatica* extract on the metabolism in the connective tissue of the vascular wall.

Miscellaneous Effects: A preliminary study showed TECA to produce histologic improvement in 5 of 12 patients with chronic hepatic disorders.[7] One study of 94 patients with venous insufficiency of the lower limbs indicated that TECA produced clinical improvement in this condition. Improvement occurred in the subjective measures of the sensation of heaviness and pain in the legs, edema, and overall patient assessment of efficacy, and in the objective measure of vein distensibility. The researchers concluded that TECA stimulated collagen synthesis in the vein wall, thus increasing vein tonicity and reducing the capacity of the vein to distend. In contrast, patients receiving placebo exhibited an increase in vein distensibility.[8]

The pharmacokinetics of the total triterpenic fraction of gotu kola have been studied, after single and multiple administrations to healthy volunteers.[9] Using an HPLC procedure for detection of asiatic acid, researchers found that after two chronic treatment doses, the peak plasma concentration, area under the curve, and half-life were higher than those observed after the corresponding single-dose administration.

Relatively large doses of extract have been found to be sedative in small animals; this property is attributed to the presence of two saponin glycosides, brahmoside, and brahminoside.

TOXICOLOGY: Preparations of gotu kola have a reputation for having a relative lack of toxicity. However, contact dermatitis has been reported in some patients using preparations of fresh or dried parts of the plant.[10] This is not surprising in light of the topical irritant qualities of certain components of the plant. In the cited study of bilharzial patients, some who received SC injections rather than IM injections experienced pain at the injection site with blackish discoloration of the SC tissues. These side effects may have been diminished with IM injections.[3]

[1] Natarajan S, et al. *Ind J Dermatol* 1973;18(4):82.
[2] Poizot A, et al. *C R Acad Sci* 1978;286(10):789.
[3] Tenni R, et al. *Ital J Biochem* 1988;37(2):69.
[4] Fam A. *Intern Surg* 1973;58:451.
[5] Becaro G, et al. *Curr Ther Res* 1989;46:1015.
[6] Arpaia MR, et al. *Int J Clin Pharma Res* 1990;10(4):229.
[7] Darnis F, et al. *Sem Hop* 1979;55(37–38):1749.
[8] Pointel JP, et al. *Angiology* 1987;38(1 Pt 1):46.
[9] Grimaldi R, et al. *J Ethnopharmacol* 1990;28(2):235.
[10] Eun HC, et al. *Contact Dermatitis* 1985;13(5):310.

SCIENTIFIC NAME(S): *Citrus paradisi* Macfad., Rutaceae

COMMON NAME(S): Grapefruit

꘎꘎꘎ PATIENT INFORMATION ꘎꘎꘎

Uses: Grapefruit juice is used as a nutritional supplement for potassium loss. Grapefruit pectin can help reduce cholesterol and promote regression of atherosclerosis. Other effects include induction of red cell aggregation by constituent naringin, reduction of hemocrits, and possible anti-cancer effects.

Drug Interactions: Grapefruit juice ingestion may increase plasma concentrations and pharmacologic and toxic effects of astemizole, midazolam, triazolam, the dihydropyridine calcium channel blockers (eg, amlodipine, felodipine, nifedipine, nimodipine, nisoldipine), cyclosporine, and ethinyl estradiol. The onset of quinidine action may be delayed.

Side Effects: Grapefruit juice can reduce metabolism of drugs by the CYP3A4 enzyme system (eg, some nonsedating antihistamines, benzodiazepines, selected calcium channel blockers, estrogens, quinidine, cyclosporine), thereby markedly increasing drug levels.

BOTANY: The grapefruit is a large, dimpled citrus fruit, measuring ≈ 7 to 15 cm in diameter. It most likely descends from a cross between a pomelo (pummelo) or shaddock (*C. grandis*), a large Malaysian citrus, and a sweet orange. The fruit grows in clusters similar to grapes, and this may be how the grapefruit received its name. Grapefruits can be considered a "New World" product, a species only a few hundred years old.[1-3] The juice of the fruit, including concentrate, accounts for ≈ 42% of all US processed grapefruit products. In the US, the grapefruit is popular as a breakfast fruit. Approximately 50% of the world's grapefruit crop is made into juice.[2]

HISTORY: In 1310 B.C., Greek historian Theophrastus wrote how Citron was thought to be an antidote to poison and how it could also "sweeten the breath." Pliny, a Roman naturalist, labeled the fruit as a medicine.[4] In 1750, the grapefruit, then called small shaddock, was first mentioned by Griffith Hughes as the forbidden fruit of Barbados.[1,2] The name grapefruit was said to have been first used in Jamaica in 1814. In 1823, the grapefruit was introduced in Florida by a French count, Odette Phillippe, but did not begin to gain popularity until the end of the 19th century.[1] Worldwide production of grapefruit today averages 4.3 million metric tons.[2]

In the 1930s, Hollywood's "Grapefruit Diet" came into vogue with calorie intake of ≈ 800 per day, including grapefruit consumption at each meal. Weight was lost from this diet, but any diet based primarily on one food is not healthy and lacks nutrients.[5]

PHARMACOLOGY: Nutrition studies have discovered grapefruit to be of value as a dietary supplement.[6] Grapefruit has also been used as a nutritional supplement for patients experiencing potassium loss.[7]

Grapefruit pectin has been found to reduce cholesterol and promote regression of atherosclerosis.[4,8] Because the pectin resides in the cell walls of the fruit and not in the juice, the juice itself does not decrease blood cholesterol.[4] Other grapefruit effects include the induction of red cell aggregation by constituent naringin (per in vitro observation) and reduction of hematocrits in 36 human subjects who ingested 1 grapefruit per day.[9]

The Swedes have studied grapefruit for its anti-cancer effects. In a 1986 analysis, subjects who consumed citrus fruit daily had lower incidences of pancreatic cancer.[2]

A pharmacokinetic study suggests citrus flavanones undergo glucuronidation before urinary excretion.[10]

Grapefruit juice has increased the bioavailability of certain drugs by inhibition of the cytochrome P450 3A4 (CYP3A4) isozyme found in the liver and gut wall.[11-15] The effects of grapefruit juice are primarily on the isozyme found in the gut wall. As a result of this inhibition, more of the drug is absorbed and the plasma concentration increases. The elevated drug concentration may lead to an increase in the drug's activity and side effects. In some cases, the drug concentration increase may be beneficial (see Toxicology).

TOXICOLOGY: Grapefruit juice has interacted with certain nonsedating antihistamines, benzodiazepines, the dihydropyridine class of calcium channel blockers, cyclosporine, estrogens, and quinidine. The mechanism of the interaction probably involves inhibition of gut wall enzymes, specifically the CYP3A4 isozyme.

Antihistamines: Grapefruit ingestion may increase the bioavailability of terfenadine and astemizole.[16-19] Altered cardiac repolarization (in poor metabolizers of terfenadine)[17] and increases in the QT interval[16] have been reported when terfenadine was taken with grapefruit juice compared with water. More than one metabolic pathway appears to be inhibited.[19] There is considerable patient variability in the pharmacokinetic effect of the interaction.[19]

Benzodiazepines: In healthy subjects taking midazolam or triazolam with grapefruit juice, it has increased plasma concentrations and the area under the plasma concentration-time curve (AUC) of these benzodiazepines.[20-21] However, the clinical effects of taking midazolam or triazolam with grapefruit juice are likely to be minor.[20-22]

Calcium channel blockers: The bioavailability of the dihydropyridine calcium channel blockers, including amlodipine, felodipine, nifedipine, nimodipine, and nisoldipine, may be increased by concurrent ingestion of grapefruit juice.[23-32] While the increases in peak plasma concentrations for amlodipine were slight (15%),[29] peak plasma concentrations of felodipine increased > 300%,[23-24,27,33] nifedipine increased by nearly 35% and the hypotensive effects were enhanced,[21] nimodipine levels increased by 24%,[23] and nisoldipine plasma levels increased by 400%.[14] The bioavailability of diltiazem, a different class of calcium channel blocker (eg, a benzothiazepine), was not affected by grapefruit juice ingestion.[34]

Cyclosporine: Studies have demonstrated that grapefruit juice alters the pharmacokinetics of cyclosporine.[35-39] Taking cyclosporine with grapefruit juice may result in an increase in plasma concentrations[38-39] and AUC of cyclosporine.[35,39] In addition, concentrations of a cyclosporine metabolite may be increased.[39] An increase in neurologic side effects, including tremors, was reported when cyclosporine was taken with grapefruit juice.[39] Some patients are instructed by their physicians to take cyclosporine with grapefruit juice to administer a lower dose of cyclosporine and reduce cost to the patient.[35] Thus, grapefruit juice may provide an inexpensive, nontoxic method to reduce the cyclosporine dose.[35] In this situation, patients should avoid fluctuations in their grapefruit juice ingestion.

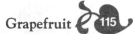

Estrogens: In 13 healthy female volunteers, grapefruit juice increased plasma concentration of ethinyl estradiol by 37% and the AUC by 28% compared with ingestion of the estrogen with herbal tea.[40]

Quinidine: In one study, administration of quinidine with grapefruit juice delayed the absorption of quinidine and inhibited the metabolism of quinidine to its major metabolite, 3-hydroxyquinidine.[41] The effects of quinidine on the QT_c interval were delayed and reduced by ingestion with grapefruit juice.

Miscellaneous: Other reports are available regarding the effect of grapefruit juice on caffeine metabolism,[42] inhibition of 11-beta-hydroxysteroid dehydrogenase,[43] and shifting the metabolic ratios of clomipramine.[44] Grapefruit juice has been associated with hypotension in one patient.[45]

[1] Davidson A, et al. *Grapefruit, Pomelo, Ugli. Fruit-A Connoiseur's Guide and Cookbook.* New York, NY: Simon and Schuster Inc. 1991:66.

[2] Ensminger A, et al. *Grapefruit Foods and Nutrition Encyclopedia*, 2nd ed. Boca Raton, FL:CRC Press Inc. 1994;1097-99.

[3] Simpson B, et al. *Fruits and Nuts of Warm Regions. Economic Botany-Plants in our World.* New York, NY: McGraw-Hill Inc. 1995:124.

[4] Carper J. Grapefruit. *The Food Pharmacy.* New York, NY: Bantam Books. 1988:213-15.

[5] http://countryliving.com/gh/health/07nutrb3.htm

[6] Staroscik J, et al. *J Am Diet Assoc* 1980;77(5):567-69.

[7] Boner G, et al. *Harefuah* 1980;98(6):251-52.

[8] Cerda J. *Trans Am Clin Climatol Assoc* 1987;99:203-13.

[9] Robbins R, et al. *Int J Vitam Nutr Res* 1988;58(4):414-17.

[10] Ameer B, et al. *Clin Pharmacol Ther* 1996;60(1):34-40.

[11] Bailey D, et al. *Clin Pharmacokinet* 1994;26(2):91-98.

[12] Anon. *Med Lett Drugs Ther* 1995;37(955):73-74.

[13] Fuhr U, et al. *Clin Pharmacol Ther* 1995;58(4):365-73.

[14] Spence J. *Clin Pharmacol Ther* 1997;61(4):395-400.

[15] Ameer B, et al. *Clin Pharmacokinet* 1997;33(2):103-21.

[16] Benton R, et al. *Clin Pharmacol Ther* 1996;59(4):383-88.

[17] Honig P, et al. *J Clin Pharmacol* 1996;36(4):345-51.

[18] Clifford C, et al. *Eur J Clin Pharmacol* 1997;52(4):311-15.

[19] Rau S, et al. *Clin Pharmacol Ther* 1997;61(4):401-9.

[20] Hukkinen S, et al. *Clin Pharmacol Ther* 1995;58(2):127-31.

[21] Kupferschmidt MHT, et al. *Clin Pharmacol Ther* 1995;58(1):20-28.

[22] Vanakowski J, et al. *Eur J Clin Pharmacol* 1996;50(6):501-8.

[23] Bailey D, et al. *Lancet* 1991;337(8736):268-69.

[24] Edgar B, et al. *Eur J Clin Pharmacol* 1992;42(3):313-17.

[25] Miniscalco A, et al. *J Pharmacol Exp Ther* 1992;261(3):1195-99.

[26] Bailey D, et al. *Clin Pharmacol Ther* 1993;54(6):589-94.

[27] Bailey D, et al. *Br J Clin Pharmacol* 1995;40(2):135-40.

[28] Rashid T, et al. *Br J Clin Pharmacol* 1995;40(1):51-58.

[29] Josefsson M, et al. *Eur J Clin Pharmacol* 1996;51(2):189-93.

[30] Lundahl J, et al. *Eur J Clin Pharmacol* 1997;52(2):139-45.

[31] Fuhr U, et al. *Int J Clin Pharmacol Ther* 1998;36(3):126-32.

[32] Pisarik P. *Arch Fam Med* 1996;5(7):413-16.

[33] Bailey D, et al. *Clin Pharmacol Ther* 1996;60(1):25-33.

[34] Sigusch H, et al. *Pharmazie* 1994;49(9):675-79

[35] Yee G, et al. *Lancet* 1995;345(8955):955-56.

[36] Bennett W. *Pediatr Nephrol* 1995;9(1):10.

[37] Majeed A, et al. *Pediatr Nephrol* 1996;10(3):395-96.

[38] Hollander A, et al. *Clin Pharmacol Ther* 1995;57(3):318-24.

[39] Ioannides-Demos L, et al. *J Rheumatol* 1997;24(1):49-54.

[40] Weber A, et al. *Contraception* 1996;53(1):41-47.

[41] Min D, et al. *J Clin Pharmacol* 1996;36(5):469-76.

[42] Fuhr U, et al. *Int J Clin Pharmacol Ther* 1995;33(6):311-14.

[43] Lee Y, et al. *Clin Pharmacol Ther* 1996;59(1):62-71.

[44] Oesterheld J. *J Clin Psychopharmacol* 1997;17(1):62-63.

[45] Nilsson I. *Lakartidningen* 1997;94(3):112-13.

Grape Seed

SCIENTIFIC NAME(S): *Vitis vinifera* L. and *V. coignetiae* Family: Vitaceae

COMMON NAME(S): Grape seed, muskat

⊱⊰ PATIENT INFORMATION ⊱⊰

Uses: Grape seed oil has shown promise in lab research as a cleansing agent, anti-enzyme, nutritional supplement, and inhibitor of tooth decay.

Side Effects: Research has indicated hepatoxicity in mice.

SOURCE: Red grape seeds are generally obtained as a by-product of wine production. When ground, these seeds become the source of grape seed oil.

PHARMACOLOGY: Wine grape seeds are used as "health oils" because of their high content of essential fatty acids and tocopherols.[1] A methanol extract of the Asian medicinal plant *Vitis coignetiae* indicated protective effects for liver cells in an in vitro assay method using primary cultured rat hepatocytes. Activity-guided fractionation of this extract produced epsilon-viniferin as an active principle. Ampelopsin C and the mixture of vitisin A and cis-vitisin A were found to be strong hepatotoxins.[2]

The effects of dietary grape seed tannins on nutritional balance and on some enzymatic activities along the crypt-villus axis of rat small intestine have been studied.[3] This study did not reveal a significant tannin toxicity, except for a reduced dry matter and nitrogen digestibility. However, the tannins directly interfere with mucosal proteins, stimulating the cell renewal.[3]

Maffei et al[4] have studied the scavenging by procyanidins from *Vitis vinifera* seeds of reactive oxygen species involved in the onset and the maintenance of microvascular injury. They report that procyanidins have a remarkable dose-dependent antilipoperoxidant activity. They also inhibit xanthine oxidase activity. In addition, procyanidins non-competitively inhibit the proteolytic enzymes collagenase and elastase and the glycosidases hyaluronidase and beta-glucuronidase. These are involved in the turnover of the main structural components of the extravascular matrix collagen, elastin, and hyaluronic acid.[4]

Studies have shown that polyphenolic substances from the seeds and skin of the wine grapes ("Koshu") can strongly inhibit 5'nucleotidase activities from snake venom and rat liver membrane, have significant therapeutic activity in Ehrlich ascites carcinoma, have inhibitory action against the growth of *Streptococcus mutans*, a cariogenic bacteria, and inhibit glucan formation from sucrose.[5] The last 2 actions may indicate that these principles can aid in the prevention of dental caries.[5] Grape seed oil has been shown to be a safe and efficient hand-cleansing agent.[6]

TOXICOLOGY: No human toxicity has been reported in recent literature for the grape seed, the oil, or its isolated constituents.

[1] El-Mallah MH, et al. *Seifen-Oele-Fette-Wachse* 1993;119:45.

[2] Oshima Y, et al. *Experientia* 1995;51(1):63.

[3] Vallet J, et al. *Ann Nutr Metab* 1994;38(2):75.

[4] Maffei Facino R, et al. *Arzneimittelforschung* 1994;44(5):592.

[5] Toukairin T, et al. *Chem Pharm Bull* 1991;39(6):1480.

[6] Krogsrud NE, Larsen Al. *Contact Dermatitis* 1992;26(3):208.

SCIENTIFIC NAME(S): *Camellia sinensis* L. Kuntze. Family: Theaceae

COMMON NAME(S): Tea, green tea

⋙ PATIENT INFORMATION ⋙

Uses: Green tea retains many chemicals of the fresh leaf. It is thought to reduce cancer, lower lipid levels, help prevent dental caries, and possess antimicrobial, antimutagenic, and antioxidative effects.

Side Effects: The FDA advises those who are or may become pregnant to avoid caffeine. Tea may impair iron metabolism.

BOTANY: *C. sinensis* is a large shrub with evergreen leaves native to eastern Asia. The plant has leathery, dark green leaves and fragrant, white flowers with 6 to 9 petals.[1,2]

HISTORY: The dried, cured leaves of *C. sinensis* have been used to prepare beverages for > 4000 years.[3] The method of curing determines the nature of the tea to be used for infusion. Green tea is prepared from the steamed and dried leaves; by comparison, black tea leaves are withered, rolled, fermented, and then dried.[4] Oolong tea is semifermented and considered to be intermediate in composition between green and black teas.[2,5] The Chinese regarded the drink as a cure for cancer, although the tannin component is believed to be carcinogenic. The polyphenol presence in tea may play a role in lowering heart disease and cancer risk.[3]

PHARMACOLOGY:

Pharmacokinetics: Blood and urine levels have been investigated.[6] Drinking green tea daily may maintain plasma catechin levels that may exert antioxidant activity against lipoproteins in blood circulation.[7] High performance liquid chromatography (HPLC) determination of catechins and polyphenol components have been performed.[7-10]

Lipid effects: In vitro testing found that green tea markedly delays lipid peroxidation, with the polyphenol components having the strongest actions.[11] Green tea consumption has been associated with a decrease in total cholesterol levels but not in triglycerides or HDL cholesterol levels.[12] In this survey, ≥ 9 cups of tea had to be consumed per day for an significant effect.[13] One report did not support the tea's beneficial actions on serum lipid levels.[14]

Dental caries: Green tea exhibits antimicrobial actions against oral bacteria.[15] After 5 minutes of contact with a 0.1% green tea polyphenol solution, *Streptococcus mutans* was completely inhibited. Plaque and gingival index were decreased after a 0.2% solution was used to rinse and brush teeth.[16] Data suggest green tea's fluoride content may increase the cariostatic action, along with the other tea components.[17] After rinsing with green tea extract, the catechin components present in saliva have been determined by HPLC, and were present in the saliva for up to 1 hour.[18] Green tea consumption may also be effective in reducing the cariogenic potential of starch-containing foods by inhibiting salivary amylase, which hydrolyzes food starch to fermentable carbohydrates.[19]

Antimicrobial: Green tea inhibited the growth of diarrhea-causing bacteria *Staphylococcus aureus*, *S. epidermidis*, *Vibrio cholerae* O1, *V. cholerae* non-O1, *V. parahaemolyticus*, *V. mimicus*, *Campylobacter jejuni*, and *Plesiomonas shigelloides*.[20] In vitro antibiosis of green tea was demonstrated against 5 pathogenic fungi. When dilutions of 1:100 of culture filtrate green tea isolate were sprayed on infected plants, insect populations were also successfully controlled.[21] Green tea extract inhibits a wide range of pathogenic bacteria including methicillin-resistant *S. aureus*. This activity may be caused by the catechin and theaflavin components.[22] In addition, green tea extract had antibacterial actions against 24 bacterial strains in infected root canals.[23]

Antimutagenic: Antimutagenic activity against a variety of organisms has been evaluated from different tea components.[24,25] Flavonol constituents in both green and black teas contributed to antimutagenic potential against dietary carcinogens.[26] The catechin components have been shown to contribute to antimutagenicity as well.[27] The antimutagenic potential of green tea extracts may be caused by a direct interaction between reactive genotoxic species of various promutagens and nucleophilic tea components present in the aqueous extracts.[28]

Antioxidative: Antioxidative activity was studied in 25 tea types, actions due, in part, to catechins present.[29-31,32] Tea consumed with milk may affect in vivo antioxidation thought to be caused by the complexation of tea polyphenols by milk proteins.[33]

Anticancer: Some reports find that tea possesses anticarcinogenic effects, protecting against cancer risk.[29,34-38] One epidemiologic review explains favorable effects from tea only if high intake occurs in high-risk populations.[39] Another study finds data unsupportive in the hypothesis that black tea consumption protects against 4 major cancers.[40] One other epidemiological study suggests modest anticancer benefits with several investigations leading to the possibility of decreased risks of digestive tract cancer from tea.[41]

The polyphenol components of green tea may have chemopreventative properties.[42-49] The polyphenol content of green tea has been shown to inhibit the in vitro and in vivo formation of N-nitrosation by-products, which have been established as cancer-inducing compounds.[50] Various catechins exhibit inhibitory actions on tumor cell lines, including breast, colon, lung, and melanoma.[51] A report on the non-polyphenolic fraction of green tea finds pheophytins to be potent antigenotoxic substances as well.[52]

Tea and curcumin used in combination on certain cell types were noted to have a synergistic effect in chemoprevention.[53,54] There are many proposed mechanisms as to how green tea expresses its anticancer effects.[29,43,44,47,49]

Anticancer, GI reports: Green tea may offer protective effects against digestive tract cancers.[55] One study suggests a protective effect against esophageal cancer.[56] Findings of another report concluded that green tea may lower the risk of colon, rectum, and pancreas cancers, as well.[57] Affected stomach cells treated with green tea catechin extract led to growth inhibition and induction of apoptosis, suggesting possible stomach cancer protection.[58] Catechins have also contributed to inhibition of small intestine carcinogenesis.[59] In tube-fed patients positive effects were seen against colon carcinoma.[60] One conflicting study found a direct correlation between drinking ≥ 5 cups of green tea a day and the preference for salty foods as a risk factor for pancreatic cancer among Japanese men.[61]

Anticancer, skin: Green tea offers chemopreventative effects against skin cancers of varying stages and is useful against inflammatory responses in cancers caused by known skin tumor promoters such as chemicals or radia-

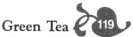
tion.[62] Green tea and its polyphenol fractions display a protective effect against UV radiation-induced skin cancer.[63]

Anticancer, various: Green tea's chemopreventative activities against hepatic and pulmonary carcinogenesis have been addressed,[64,65] as well as effects against lung tumorigenesis,[66] smoke-induced mutations,[67] pancreatic carcinogenesis,[68] and leukemia.[69] Green tea can inhibit the carcinogenic effects of female hormones, as well.[70] One report addresses the unconventional use of green tea to treat breast cancer.[71]

Miscellaneous effects: Two well-known components of green tea from a pharmacologic basis are caffeine and tannin. Caffeine is an effective CNS stimulant that can induce nervousness, insomnia, tachycardia, elevated blood sugar and cholesterol levels, high levels of stomach acid, and heartburn.[72] These components are also useful for headaches, enhancement of renal excretion of water, weight loss, and as a cardiotonic. Green tea is also used as an astringent, for wounds and skin disorders, and soothing insect bites, itching, and sunburn. Tea is also a sweat-inducer, a nerve tonic, and has been used for functional asthenia, eye problems, and as an analgesic.[1,2,4] Green tea has been employed in hepatitis treatment and for protection of the liver.[1,73] Green tea's role in stroke prevention,[74] as a thromboxane inhibitor,[75] and as a hypotensive has been described.[76]

TOXICOLOGY: The FDA has advised that women who are or may become pregnant should avoid caffeine-containing products.[72] Drinking moderate amounts of caffeine has shown inconsistent results, with more recent studies not demonstrating adverse effects on the fetus.[77,78] Caffeine-containing beverages may also alter female hormone levels, including estradiol.[79]

There is evidence that condensed catechin tannin of tea is linked to a high rate of esophageal cancer in regions of heavy tea consumption. This effect may be overcome by adding milk, which binds the tannin, possibly preventing its detrimental effects.[4] Catechins have also been linked to tea-induced asthma.[80] One study reports that catechins may have antiallergic effects, inhibiting type I allergic reactions.[81] Green tea workers experienced shortness of breath, stiffness, pain in neck and arms, and other occupation-related problems.[82]

The daily consumption of an average of 250 ml of tea by infants has been shown to impair iron metabolism, resulting in a high incidence of microcytic anemia.[83]

[1] Chevallier A. *Encyclopedia of Medicinal Plants.* New York, NY: DK Publishing, 1996;179.

[2] Bruneton J. *Pharmacognosy, Phytochemistry, Medicinal Plants.* Paris, France: Lavoisier, 1995; 885-87.

[3] Weisburger J. *Cancer Lett* 1997; 114(1-2):315-17.

[4] Duke JA. *Handbook of Medicinal Herbs.* Boca Raton, FL: CRC Press, 1985.

[5] Graham H. *Prev Med* 1992; 21(3):334–50.

[6] Yang CS, et al. *Cancer Epidemiol Biomarkers Prev* 1998;7(4):351-54.

[7] Nakagawa K, et al. *Biosci Biotechnol Biochem* 1997;61(12):1981-85.

[8] Unno T, et al. *Biosci Biotechnol Biochem* 1996;60(12):2066-68.

[9] Dalluge J, et al. *Rapid Commun Mass Spectrom* 1997;11(16):1753-56.

[10] Maiani G, et al. *J Chromatogr B Biomed Sci Appl* 1997;692(2):311-17.

[11] Yokozawa T, et al. *Exp Toxicol Pathol* 1997;49(5):329-35.

[12] Watanabe J, et al. *Biosci Biotechnol Biochem* 1998;62(3):532-34.

[13] Kono S, et al. *Prev Med* 1992;21(4):526.

[14] Tsubono Y, et al. *Ann Epidemiol* 1997;7(4):280-84.

[15] Saeki Y, et al. *Bull Tokyo Dent Coll* 1993;34(1):33-37.

[16] You S. *Chung Hua Kou Hsueh Tsa Chih* 1993;28(4):197-99.

[17] Yu H, et al. *Fukuoka Igaku Zasshi* 1992;83(4):174-80.

[18] Tsuchiya H, et al. *J Chromatogr B Biomed Sci Appl* 1997:703(1-2):253-58.

[19] Zhang J, et al. *Caries Res* 1998;32(3):233-38.

[20] Toda M, et al. *Nippon Saikingaku Zasshi* 1989;44(4):669-72.

[21] Bezbaruah B, et al. *Indian J Exp Biol* 1996;34(7):706-9.

[22] Yam T, et al. *FEMS Microbiol Lett* 1997;152(1):169-74.

[23] Horiba N, et al. *J Endod* 1991;17(3):122-24.

[24] Nagao M, et al. *Mutat Res* 1979;68(2):101-6.

[25] Yen G, et al. *Mutagenesis* 1996;11(1):37-41.

[26] Bu-Abbas A, et al. *Mutagenesis* 1996;11(6):597-603.

[27] Constable A, et al. *Mutagenesis* 1996:11(2):189-94.

[28] Bu-Abbas A, et al. *Mutagenesis* 1994;9(4):325-31.

[29] Katiyar S, et al. *J Cell Biochem Suppl* 1997;(27):59-67.

[30] Cheng T. *J Am Coll Cardiol* 1998;31(5):1214.

[31] Yamanaka N, et al. *FEBS Lett* 1997;401(2-3):230-34.

[32] Kumamoto M, et al. *Biosci Biotechnol Biochem* 1998;62(1):175-77.

[33] Serafini M, et al. *Eur J Clin Nutr* 1996;50(1):28-32.

[34] Mukhtar H, et al. *Prev Med* 1992;21(3):351-60.

[35] Yang C, et al. *J Natl Cancer Inst* 1993;85(13):1038-49.

[36] Mukhtar H, et al. *Adv Exp Med Biol* 1994;354:123-24.

[37] Mitscher L, et al. *Med Res Rev* 1997;17(4):327-65.

[38] Dreosti I, et al. *Crit Rev Food Sci Nutr* 1997;37(8):761-70.

[39] Kohlmeier L, et al. *Nutr Cancer* 1997;27(1):1-13.

[40] Goldbohm R, et al. *J Natl Cancer Inst* 1996;88(2):93-100.

[41] Blot W, et al. *Eur J Cancer Prev* 1996;5(6):425-38.

[42] Cheng S, et al. *Chin Med Sci J* 1991;6(4):233-38.

[43] Komori A, et al. *Jpn J Clin Oncol* 1993;23(3):186-90.

[44] Stoner G, et al. *J Cell Biochem Suppl* 1995;22:169-80.

[45] Han C. *Cancer Lett* 1997;114(1-2):153-58.

[46] Yang C, et al. *Environ Health Perspect* 1997;105 (Suppl. 4):971-76.

[47] Chan M, et al. *Biochem Pharmacol* 1997;54(12):1281-86.

[48] Ahmad N, et al. *J Natl Cancer Inst* 1997;89(24):1881-86.

[49] Tanaka K, et al. *Mutat Res* 1998;412(1):91-98.

[50] Wang H, et al. *IARC Sci Publ* 1991;105:546.

[51] Valcic S, et al. *Anticancer Drugs* 1996;7(4):461-68.

[52] Okai Y, et al. *Cancer Lett* 1997;120(1):117-23.

[53] Khafif A, et al. *Carcinogenesis* 1998;19(3):419-24.

[54] Conney A, et al. *Proc Soc Exp Biol Med* 1997;216(2):234-45.

[55] Inoue M, et al. *Cancer Causes Control* 1998;9(2):209-16.

[56] Gao Y, et al. *J Natl Cancer Inst* 1994;86(11):855-58.

[57] Ji B, et al. *Int J Cancer* 1997;70(3):255-58.

[58] Hibasami H, et al. *Oncol Rep* 1998;5(2):527-29.

[59] Ito N, et al. *Teratogenesis Carcinog Mutagen* 1992;12(2):79.

[60] Hara Y. *J Cell Biochem Suppl* 1997;27:52-58.

[61] Mizuno S, et al. *Jpn J Clin Oncol* 1992;22(4):286.

[62] Mukhtar H, et al. *J Invest Dermatol* 1994;102(1):3-7.

[63] Ley R, et al. *Environ Health Perspect* 1997;105(Suppl 4):981-84.

[64] Klaunig J, et al. *Prev Med* 1992;21(4):510-19.

[65] Cao J, et al. *Fundam Appl Toxicol* 1996;29(2):244-50.

[66] Katiyar S, et al. *Carcinogenesis* 1993;14(5):849-55.

[67] Lee I, et al. *J Cell Biochem Suppl* 1997;27:68-75.

[68] Majima T, et al. *Pancreas* 1998;16(1):13-18.

[69] Asano Y, et al. *Life Sci* 1997;60(2):135-42.

[70] Gao F, et al. *SCI CHINA B* 1994;37(4):418-29.

[71] Kaegie E. *CMAJ* 1998;158(8):1033-35.

[72] Tyler V. *The New Honest Herbal.* Philadelphia, PA: G.F. Stickley Co., 1987.

[73] Sugiyama K, et al. *Biosci Biotechnol Biochem* 1998;62(3):609-11.

[74] Sato Y, et al. *Tohoku J Exp Med* 1989;157(4):337-43.

[75] Ali M, et al. *Prostaglandins Leukot Essent Fatty Acids* 1990;40(4):281-83.

[76] Taniguchi S, et al. *Yakugaku Zasshi* 1988;108(1):77-81.

[77] Briggs G, et al. *Drugs in Pregnancy and Lactation,* 3rd ed. Baltimore, MD: Williams and Wilkins, 1990.

[78] Mills J, et al. *JAMA* 1993;269(5):593.

[79] Nagata C, et al. *Nutr Cancer* 1998;30(1):21-24.

[80] Shirai T, et al. *Ann Allergy Asthma Immunol* 1997;79(1):65-69.

[81] Shiozaki T, et al. *Yakugaku Zasshi* 1997;117(7):448-54.

[82] Mirbod S, et al. *Ind Health* 1995;33(3):101-17.

[83] Merhav H, et al. *Am J Clin Nutr* 1985;41:1210.

SCIENTIFIC NAME(S): *Paullinia cupana* Kunth var. *sorbilis* (Mart.) Ducke or *P. sorbilis* (L.) Mart. Family: Sapindaceae

COMMON NAME(S): Guarana, guarana paste or gum, Brazilian cocoa, Zoom

---

❧❧❧❧ PATIENT INFORMATION ❧❧❧❧

Uses: Guarana is a source of flavoring and caffeine. It has been used as a folk remedy and appetite suppressant.

Side Effects: Severe toxicity has not been reported, but the usual cautions regarding caffeine apply.

BOTANY: Guarana is the dried paste made from the crushed seeds of *P. cupana* or *P. sorbilis*. A fast-growing woody perennial shrub native to Brazil and other regions of the Amazon,[1] guarana bears orange-yellow fruit that contains up to 3 seeds each. The seeds are collected and dry-roasted over fires. The kernels are ground to a paste with cassava, molded into cylindrical sticks, and then sun-dried. The most common forms of guarana include syrups, extracts, and distillates used as a flavoring and source of caffeine by the soft drink industry.

HISTORY: Guarana is often taken during periods of fasting to tolerate dietary restrictions in the Amazon. In certain regions, the extract is believed to be an aphrodisiac and provide protection from malaria and dysentery.[2,3] Guarana is used by the Brazilian Indians in a stimulating beverage, which is sometimes mixed with alcohol to become more intoxicating. It was popular in France at the beginning of the 19th century. Natural diet aids, which rely on daily doses of tablets containing guarana, have been advertised in the lay press. Guarana is occasionally combined with glucomannan in natural weight loss tablets. The advertisements incorrectly indicate that the ingredients in guarana have the same chemical makeup as caffeine and cocaine but can be used for weight reduction without any of the side effects of these drugs.

PHARMACOLOGY: Guarana contains a high level of caffeine, ranging from 3% to > 5% caffeine by dry weight.[2] Coffee beans contain $\approx$ 1% to 2% caffeine and dried tea leaves vary from 1% to 4% caffeine content.[4] Guarana is also high in tannins, present in a concentration of 5% to 6% dry weight; these impart an astringent taste to the product. Guarana does not contain cocaine. The appetite suppressant effect is related to the caffeine content. The increase in energy that guarana tablets are reported to give is also due to caffeine. Guarana extracts also have been shown to inhibit platelet aggregation following either parenteral or oral administration.[5]

TOXICOLOGY: There are no published reports describing severe toxicity from guarana, but people sensitive to caffeine should use guarana with caution. The expected side effects of caffeine should be considered in a person who has ingested guarana.

[1] Angelucci E, et al. *Bol Inst Tech Ailment* 1978;56:183.
[2] Henman AR. *J Ethnopharmacol* 1982;6:311-38.
[3] Lewis WH, et al. *Medical Botany*. John Wiley and Sons, 1977.
[4] DerMarderosian AH, et al. *Natural Product Medicine*. Philadelphia, PA: G.F. Stickley Co., 1988.
[5] Bydlowski SP, et al. *Braz J Med Biol Res* 1988;21(3):535.

Guggul

SCIENTIFIC NAME(S): *Commiphora mukul* Family: Burseracaea

COMMON NAME(S): Guggul, guggal, gum guggal, gum guggulu

❧❧❧ PATIENT INFORMATION ❧❧❧

Uses: Used to treat arthritis, obesity, and other disorders, guggul has been shown to lower cholesterol and triglycerides and to stimulate thyroid activity.

Side Effects: Adverse GI effects have been reported.

BOTANY: The guggul plant is widely distributed throughout India and adjacent regions. It is in the same genus as *C. myrrha*, the myrrh of the Bible.

HISTORY: The plant has been used in traditional Ayurvedic medicine (Asiatic Indian plant medicine) for centuries in the treatment of a variety of disorders,[1] most notably arthritis and as a weight-reducing agent in obesity.[2] More recently, extracts of the plant have been investigated for their ability to reduce serum lipid levels. A commercial product (*Guggulow*) has been introduced in the US touting the cholesterol-lowering properties of the plant. This has raised interest in the activity of the plant.

PHARMACOLOGY: A number of studies have investigated the lipid-lowering activity of guggulsterone and guggul extract. When treated with 500 mg of gugulipid for 12 weeks, a significant lowering of serum cholesterol (24% average) and serum triglycerides (23% average) was observed in 80% of patients.[3] A crossover follow-up to this preliminary investigation compared gugulipid to the antihyperlipidemic drug clofibrate (eg, *Atromid-S*) in 233 patients. With gugulipid, the average fall in serum cholesterol and triglycerides was 11% and 17%, respectively. These modest effects were evident within 3 to 4 weeks of starting therapy. Hypercholesterolemic patients responded better to the gugulipid therapy than did hypertriglyceridemic patients. HDL-cholesterol increased in 60% of responders to gugulipid therapy, but clofibrate had no effect on this parameter.[3]

Furthermore, guggulsterone has been shown to exhibit thyroid-stimulating activity.[4] It also has been shown to exert a protective effect on cardiac enzymes and the cytochrome P450 system against drug-induced myocardial necrosis.[5]

TOXICOLOGY: While the human safety profile of the extract has not been well described, no significant adverse events were reported in clinical studies; the reported events were primarily GI in nature.

---

[1] Antarkar DS, et al. *J Postgrad Med* 1984;30:111.
[2] Satyavati GV. *Indian J Med Res* 1988;87:327.
[3] Niyanand S, et al. *J Assoc Physicians India* 1989;3:323.
[4] Tripathi YB, et al. *Planta Med* 1984;1:78,
[5] Kaul S, et al. *Indian J Med Res* 1989:90:62.

Hawthorn

SCIENTIFIC NAME(S): *Crataegus oxyacantha* L., *C. laevigata*, and *C. monogyna* Jacquin Family: Rosaceae

COMMON NAME(S): Hawthorn, English hawthorn, haw, maybush, whitethorn[1]

❧❧❧ PATIENT INFORMATION ❧❧❧

Uses: Hawthorn has been used to regulate blood pressure and heart rhythm, to treat atherosclerosis and angina pectoris, and as an antispasmodic and sedative.

Side Effects: Hawthorn is reportedly toxic in high doses, which may induce hypotension and sedation.

BOTANY: A spiny bush that grows up to 7.5 m in height, hawthorn has deciduous leaves that are divided into 3 to 5 lobes. The white, strong-smelling flowers grow in large bunches and bloom from April to June. The spherical red fruit contains 1 nut (*C. monogyna*) or 2 to 3 nuts (*C. oxyacantha*).

HISTORY: Hawthorn use dates back to Dioscorides but gained immense popularity in European and American herbal medicine toward the end of the 19th century. The flowers, leaves, and fruits have been used to prepare infusions to treat high or low blood pressure, tachycardia, or arrhythmias.[2] The plant is purported to have antispasmodic and sedative effects and has been used in the treatment of atherosclerosis and angina pectoris.[3,4]

PHARMACOLOGY: Hawthorns have strong cardiac activity. Extracts of hawthorn dilate coronary blood vessels, resulting in reduced peripheral resistance and increased coronary circulation.[5] In vitro increases in coronary circulation ranging from 20% to 140%

have been observed following a dose equal to ≈ 1 mg of the dry extract.[5] These effects have been confirmed in double-blind human trials of hypertensive patients with ischemic heart disease.[6]

Higher doses of the plant result in CNS depression. Hawthorn extracts may increase the intracellular concentrations of cyclic AMP by influencing the activity of the enzyme phosphodiesterase, and they may influence other mechanisms that activate adenylcyclase.[5] Hawthorn may have a further cardioprotective effect that becomes pronounced after prolonged use.[7]

TOXICOLOGY: The acute parenteral LD-50 of Crataegus preparations has been reported to be in the range of 18 to 34 mg/kg, with that of individual constituents ranging from 50 to 2600 mg/kg.[5] Acute oral toxicity has been reported to be in the range of 18.5 to 33.8 mg/kg.[8] Higher doses may induce hypotension and sedation and may affect cardiac rate and blood pressure.

[1] Dobelis IN. *Magic and Medicine of Plants.* Pleasantville, NY: Reader's Digest Association, 1986.
[2] Stepka W, et al. *Lloydia* 1973;36:431.
[3] Duke JA. *Handbook of Medicinal Herbs.* Boca Raton, FL: CRC Press, 1985.
[4] Tyler VE. *The Honest Herbal: a sensible guide to the use of herbs and related remedies.* Binghamton, NY: The Haworth Press, 1993.
[5] Hamon NW. *Can Pharm J* 1988 Nov:708, 724.
[6] Iwamoto M, et al. *Planta Med* 1981;42:1.
[7] He G. *Chung Hsi I Choeh Ho Tsa Chih* 1990;10:361.
[8] Ammon HPT, et al. *Planta Med* 1981;43:105.

Hops

SCIENTIFIC NAME(S): *Humulus lupulus* L. Family: Moraceae or Cannabaceae

COMMON NAME(S): Hops, European hops, common hops, lupulin

✣✣✣ PATIENT INFORMATION ✣✣✣

Uses: Hops have been used as a flavoring, diuretic, sedative, and treatment for intestinal cramping, tuberculosis, cancer, cystitis, menstrual problems, and nervous conditions.

Side Effects: Contact dermatitis has been reported after exposure to hops pollen.

BOTANY: Hops are climbing perennial plants with male and female flowers on separate plants. Hops can attain heights of 7.5 m.[1] Commercially, the female cone-like flowering parts are collected and dried. Lupulin is composed of the separated glandular hairs and contains more resins and volatile oil than hops but may also contain more adulterants.

HISTORY: The major use of hops is in beer production, where oxidation of the bitter principle humulene yields the characteristic flavor.[2] Extracts are used as flavors in foods and beverages. Traditionally, hops had been used as a diuretic and in the treatment of intestinal cramping, tuberculosis, cancer, and cystitis.[1] Brewery sludge baths were used medicinally for their rejuvenating effects and for menstrual problems.[3]

As sedation sometimes occurred in hop pickers, the flowers were used as sedatives and were placed in pillows to relieve nervous conditions.[4] Some extracts are used as emollients in skin preparations.

PHARMACOLOGY: The bitter acids (eg, lupulone, humulone) are reported to have antimicrobial activity,[1] with the more hydrophobic compounds being the most active. In addition the extracts are said to inhibit smooth muscle spasticity. A volatile alcohol, 2-methyl-3-butene-2-ol may account in part for the plant's sedative and hypnotic effects.[4]

Reports have suggested that hops contain compounds that impart estrogenic activity. An early study found a high level of estrogenic activity in the beta-bitter acid fraction of the plant.[3] One poorly designed study, which subsequently became something of a legend, reported that women who participated in hops collection often began menstruating 2 days after starting to reap the hops. However, neither estrogenic nor any other hormonal activity has been observed in a variety of hops extracts tested in several animal models under carefully controlled conditions.[5] Hops are related botanically to marijuana and have been smoked as a mild sedative.[4]

TOXICOLOGY: Extracts can be allergenic, with contact dermatitis having been reported after exposure to hops pollen.[1] However, bronchial hyperresponsiveness among hops packagers occurred with an incidence similar to that in the general population.[6]

[1] Leung AY. *Encyclopedia of Common Natural Ingredients Used in Food, Drugs, and Cosmetics.* New York, NY: John Wiley and Sons, 1980.

[2] Lam KC, et al. *J Agric Food Chem* 1987;35:57.

[3] Zenisek A, et al. *Am Perfumer Arom* 1960;75:61.

[4] Tyler VE. *The New Honest Herbal.* Philadelphia, PA: G.F. Stickley Co., 1987.

[5] Fenselau C, et al. *Food Cosmet Toxicol* 1973;11:597.

[6] Meznar B, et al. *Plucne Bolesti* 1990;42(1-2):27.

SCIENTIFIC NAME(S): *Marrubium vulgare* (Tourn.) L. Family: Labiatae

COMMON NAME(S): Horehound, hoarhound, white horehound

❧❧❧ PATIENT INFORMATION ❧❧❧

Uses: Horehound has been used as a flavoring, expectorant, vasodilator, diaphoretic, diuretic, and treatment for intestinal parasites.

Side Effects: Large doses may induce cardiac irregularities.

BOTANY: Horehound is native to Europe and Asia and has been naturalized to other areas, including the United States.[1] It is a perennial aromatic herb of the mint family. The plant grows to a height of ≈ 0.9 m and has oval leaves covered with white, woolly hairs. Horehound bears small, white flowers in dense whorls, which bloom from June to August.

HISTORY: The leaves and flower tops of the horehound have been used in home remedies as a bitter tonic for the common cold. They are now used primarily as flavorings in liqueurs, candies, and cough drops. In addition, extracts of the plant were used for the treatment of intestinal parasites and as a diaphoretic and diuretic. A different genus, the black horehound (*Ballota nigra*), is a fetid perennial native to the Mediterranean area that is sometimes used as an adulterant of white horehound.

PHARMACOLOGY: Horehound is used in cough lozenges and cold preparations. The volatile oil has been reported to have expectorant and vasodilatory effects. Similarly, marrubiin stimulates secretion by the bronchial mucosa.[2]

TOXICOLOGY: While marrubiin has been reported to have antiarrhythmic properties, it may also induce cardiac irregularities in larger doses.

---

[1] Windholz M, ed. *Merck Index*, 10th ed. Rahway, NJ: Merck and Co., 1983.

[2] Tyler VE. *The New Honest Herbal*. Philadelphia: G.F. Stickley, 1987.

Horse Chestnut

SCIENTIFIC NAME(S): *Aesculus* Family: Hippocastanaceae. The most common member of the genus in the US and Europe is *A. hippocastanum* L.

COMMON NAME(S): Chestnut, horse chestnut

ഇഇഇ PATIENT INFORMATION ഇഇഇ

Uses: Horse chestnuts are potentially useful against edema, inflammation, and venous insufficiency.

Side Effects: All parts of plants in the *Aesculus* family are potentially toxic, especially the seeds. Horse chestnut has been classified by the FDA as an unsafe herb. Horse chestnut components in skin cleansers are potentially carcinogenic.

BOTANY: Members of the genus *Aesculus* grow as trees and shrubs, often attaining heights of 22.5 m. The fruit is a capsule with a thick, leathery husk that contains from 1 to 6 dark seeds (the nuts). As the husk dries, the nuts are released. The pink and white flowers of the plant grow in clusters. The tree is native to the Balkan woods and western Asia but is now cultivated worldwide.[1]

HISTORY: Because of its widespread prevalence, horse chestnut has been used in traditional medicine and for other commercial applications for centuries. Extracts of the bark have been used as a yellow dye, and the wood has been used for furniture and packing cases. In the western US, the crushed unripe seeds of the California buckeye were scattered into streams to stupefy fish, and leaves were steeped as a tea for congestion. The horse chestnut has been used as a traditional remedy for arthritis and rheumatism.[2] Extracts are available commercially for oral, topical, and parenteral administration for the management of varicose veins and hemorrhoids.[2]

Even though the seeds are toxic, several methods were used to reduce their toxicity. Seeds were buried in swampy, cold ground during the winter to free them of toxic bitter components, then eaten in the spring after boiling.[3] Indians roasted the poisonous nuts, peeled, and mashed them, then leached the meal in lime water for several days and used it to make breads.[4]

PHARMACOLOGY: Commerical extracts of horse chestnut have been evaluated in the treatment of several disease states. An extract of the plant (containing 50 mg of triterpene glycosides) decreases venous capillary permeability and appears to have a "tonic" effect on the circulatory system.[5] A commercial horse chestnut extract, which contains 70% aescin, possesses pharmacologic properties in vitro and in vivo, including the ability to contract the canine saphenous isolated vein and to potentiate the contractile response to norepinephrine.[6] The bark yields aesculin, which improves vascular resistance and aids in toning vein walls. This is desirable for such ailments as hemorrhoids, varicose veins, leg ulcers, or frostbite.[1] Triterpene and steroid saponins from horse chestnut are effective in treating or preventing venous insufficiency in another report. Enzyme studies show that elastase (enzymes involved in turnover or perivascular substances) inhibition may be a mechanism involved.[7] Aesculin reduces capillary wall permeability by decreasing fluid retention, by increasing the permeability of capillaries, and allowing reabsorption of excess fluid back into the circulatory system.[1] Anti-inflammatory effects also have been reported.[1,8] One reference reported a dosage of 20 mg/day (max) IV administration of aescin to be effective in preventing or treating postoperative edema.[9] In patients with chronic venous insufficiency, extracts have reduced patient complaints, along with objective measures of edema.[10] In a placebo-controlled study, horse chestnut seed extract improved edema in patients suffering from venous edema of chronic deep-vein incompetence.[11] The bark of the horse chestnut possesses anti-inflammatory activity, primarily because of the presence of the steroids stigmasterol, alpha-spinasterol, and beta-sitosterol.[12]

Other pharmacological effects of horse chestnut preparations include the following: Treatment of whooping cough from a decoction of the leaves,[1] fever reduction,[1,4] absorption the skin-damaging UV-B radiation in suntan products,[13] and antimicrobial actions from recently isolated antifungal proteins.[14]

TOXICOLOGY: The FDA classifies *Aesculus* (horse chestnut) as an unsafe herb;[4] all members of this genus are potentially toxic.[15]

The most important toxic principle is esculin. Poisoning is characterized by muscle twitching, weakness, incoordination, dilated pupils, vomiting, diarrhea, depression, paralysis, and stupor.[16] The nut is the most toxic part of the plant.[17] Children have been poisoned by drinking tea made from the leaves and twigs and by eating the seeds; deaths have followed such ingestion. Gastric lavage and symptomatic treatment have also been suggested.[16]

A potential association between nasal cancer and long-term exposure to wood dusts, including dust from chestnut trees, has been reported.[18] Aflatoxins have been identified in some commercial skin-cleansing products containing horse chestnut. Because aflatoxins are potent carcinogens that can be absorbed through the skin, it is imperative that strict quality control be applied to topical products containing potentially contaminated horse chestnut material.[19]

Horse chestnut pollen is allergenic and often associated with allergic sensitization, particularly in urban children.[20] A case report describes drug-induced hepatic injury to a 37-year-old male induced by venoplant (horse chestnut extract preparation) given for treatment of bone fracture inflammation.[21]

[1] Chevallier A. *Encyclopedia of Medicinal Plants.* New York, NY: DK Publishing, 1996;159.

[2] Tyler V, et al. *Pharmacognosy.* Philadelphia, PA: Lea & Febiger, 1988.

[3] Sweet M. *Common Edible & Useful Plants of the West.* Healdsburg, CA: Naturegraph Publishers, 1976.

[4] Duke J. *Handbook of Medicinal Herbs.* Boca Raton, FL: CRC Press, 1985.

[5] Bisler H, et al. *Dtsch Med Wochenschr* 1986;111(35):1321.

[6] Guillaume M, et al. *Arzneimittelforschung* 1994;44:25.

[7] Facino R, et al. *Arch Pharm* 1995;328(10):720-24.

[8] Tsutsumi S, et al. *Shikwa Gakuho* 1967;67(11):1324-28.

[9] Reynolds J, ed. *Martindale: The Extra Pharmacopoeia,* 31st ed. London, England: Royal Pharmaceutical Society, 1996:1670.

[10] Hitzenberger G. *Wien Med Wochenschr* 1989;139(17):385.

[11] Diehm C, et al. *Vasa* 1992;21:188.

[12] Senatore F, et al. *Boll Soc Ital Biol Sper* 1989;65(2):137.

[13] Bisset N. *Herbal Drugs and Phytopharmaceuticals.* Stuttgart, Germany: CRC Press, 1994;268-72.

[14] Osborn R, et al. *Febs Lett* 1995;368(2):257-62.

[15] Nagy M. *JAMA* (letter) 1973;226(2):213.

[16] Hardin J, et al. *Human Poisoning From Native and Cultivated Plants,* 2nd ed. Durham, NC: Duke University Press, 1974.

[17] Anon. *Vet Hum Toxicol* 1983;25:80.

[18] Battista G, et al. *Scand J Work Environ Health* 1983;9(1):25.

[19] el-Dessouki S. *Food Chem Toxicol* 1992;30:993.

[20] Popp W, et al. *Allergy* 1992;47:380.

[21] Takegoshi K, et al. *Gastroenterol Jpn* 1986;21(1):62-65.

[22] Jaspersen-Schib R, et al. *Schweiz Med Wochenschr* 1996;126(25):1085-98.

Jojoba

SCIENTIFIC NAME(S): *Simmondsia chinensis* (Link) Schneider and *S. californica* Nutall Family: Buxaceae

COMMON NAME(S): Jojoba

ᦸᦸᦸ PATIENT INFORMATION ᦸᦸᦸ

Uses: Jojoba oil has traditionally been used in cosmetics, medicine, and cooking. It appears to alleviate skin irritations and help guard against hair loss.

Side Effects: Do not ingest. Seeds are toxic. One component contributes to myocardial fibrosis. Sensitive individuals may develop contact dermatitis.

BOTANY: *Simmondsia chinensis,* a woody evergreen shrub with thick, leathery, bluish green leaves and dark brown nut-like fruit, is indigenous to Arizona, California, and northern Mexico and grows in deserts worldwide. Male and female flowers are borne on separate plants. It thrives in well-drained, coarse desert soils and coarse mixtures of gravels and clays.[1] The mature plant produces ≈ 2.25 to 4.5 kg of seeds, which range in size between a coffee bean and peanut. It is an important forage plant for desert bighorn sheep and mule deer. It is toxic to humans and most animals.[2]

HISTORY: American indians and Mexicans have for a long time used jojoba oil as a hair conditioner and restorer, and in medicine, cooking, and rituals. In the US, jojoba is considered a viable cash crop for southwestern American Indians.[2,3]

With the banning of the sale of sperm whale oil in 1973, the cosmetic industry turned to jojoba oil for use in shampoos, moisturizers, sunscreens, and conditioners. It has further potential as an industrial lubricant because it does not break down under high temperature or pressure.[4] A major disadvantage to its use is its relatively high cost.

PHARMACOLOGY: Studies with jojoba oil show that the wax may be of value in the management of acne and psoriasis.[5] Other topical irritations such as sunburn and chapped skin respond to topical jojoba therapy.

There has also been success in marketing jojoba preparations promoted to stimulate hair growth and rejuvenation. Jojoba oil penetrates skin and skin oils easily unclogging hair follicles and preventing sebum buildup, which could lead to hair loss.[6] Recent study has shown antioxidant activity of jojoba.[7]

Jojoba oil is used in cosmetic and personal care products. Recommended oil ingredient levels include the following: skin care preparations, 5% to 10%; shampoos and conditioners, 1% to 2%; bar soaps, 0.5% to 3.0%.[6]

TOXICOLOGY: In ocular tests, the oil was only slightly irritating (comparable to olive oil), and its application resulted in less irritation than liquid paraffin. Hypoallergenic sensitivity to the wax has been reported,[8] and cases of contact dermatitis have occurred in people using jojoba oil as shampoo or hair conditioner.[4]

Jojoba oil is 14% erucic acid, a causative factor in myocardial fibrosis.[9] Although no direct relationship has been established between this compound and jojoba toxicity, jojoba should not be ingested in any form. *Lactobacillus acidophilus* and *Lactobacillus bulgari-*

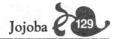

cus grow well on jojoba seed meal, metabolizing toxic simmondsin and other toxicants remaining in the meal after removal of the oil.[10,11]

[1] Wisniak J. *Prog Chem Fats Other Lipids* 1977;15(3):167.

[2] Office of Arid Lands Studies, University of Arizona. Jojoba: What is it? (leaflet). 1979 June.

[3] Majgh TH. *Science* 1977;196:1189.

[4] Scott MJ, et al. *J Am Acad Der* 1982;6(4 Pt 1):545.

[5] Mosovich B. Treatment of acne and psoriasis, Proceedings of the 6th International Jojoba Conference, Ben Gurion University, Israel. 1984 Oct 21-26.

[6] Arndt GJ. *Cosmet Toiletries* 1987;102(6):68.

[7] Mallet JF, et al. *Food Chem* 1994;49(1):61.

[8] Taguchi M, et al. *Cosmet Toiletries* 1977;92(9):53.

[9] Clarke JA, et al. *Biochem Biophys Res Com* 1981;102(4):1409.

[10] Verbiscar AJ, et al. *J Agri Food Chem* 1981;29(2):296.

[11] Perez-Gil F, et al. *Archivos Latinoamericanos de Nutricion* 1989;39(4):591.

Juniper

SCIENTIFIC NAME(S): *Juniperus communis* L. Family: Cupressaceae

COMMON NAME(S): Juniper

♔♔ PATIENT INFORMATION ♔♔

Uses: Juniper berries have long been used as a flavoring for beverages and as a seasoning for cooking. It is also used as a diuretic and in the management of bronchitis and arthritis.

Side Effects: Skin and respiratory allergic reactions, potentially carcinogenic DNA damage and, in large doses, convulsions and renal damage. Use is limited to low concentrations. Juniper should not be ingested by pregnant women.

BOTANY: The genus *Juniperus* includes 60 to 70 species of aromatic evergreens native to Northern Europe, Asia, and North America. The plants bear blue or reddish fruit described as berries or berry-like cones. Junipers are widely used as ornamental trees. The cone is a small green berry during its first year of growth and turns blue-black during the second year. The small flowers bloom from May to June.

HISTORY: Juniper berries (the mature female cone) have long been used as a flavoring in foods and alcoholic beverages such as gin. Production by apothecaries and other historical uses for gin have been reported.[1] The original gin preparation contained juniper for kidney ailments. The berries also serve as seasonings, for pickling meats, and as flavoring for liqueurs and bitters. Other uses include perfumery and cosmetics. Oil of juniper, also known as oil of sabinal, is used for preserving catgut ligatures.[2] In herbal medicine, juniper has been used as a carminative and as a steam inhalant in the management of bronchitis and has been used to control arthritis.

PHARMACOLOGY: Juniper berry oil has been used as a diuretic. This activity most likely is due to the action of terpinen-4-ol, which is known to increase renal glomerular filtration rate.[3] This activity appears to be a local irritant effect. Juniper berries are often found in herbal diuretic products. The effects of juniper berry oil on urinary tract disease have also been reported.[4]

Juniper has been used in phytotherapy and cosmetics in the eastern Mediterranean area.[5] Therapeutic uses of juniper include juniper baths for treatment of neurasthenic neurosis[6] and management of scalp psoriasis in its tar form in combination with other tars.[7]

In traditional Swedish medicine, *Juniperus communis* has been used to treat wounds and inflammatory diseases. A recent study evaluates its inhibitory activity on prostaglandin biosynthesis and platelet activating factor (PAF)-induced exocytosis in vitro.[8]

Berry extracts increase uterine tone and should, therefore, not be ingested by pregnant women. Anti-implantation/anti-fertility activity has been determined in female rats by 3 similar studies, with 1 study reporting 60% to 70% efficacy.[9,10,11]

TOXICOLOGY: Adverse effects in humans are generally of an allergic nature. These include occupational allergy affecting the skin and respiratory tract[12] through a sensitivity to airborne juniper pollen.[13] Two reports note that Chinese, Japanese, and Filipinos tend to be more sensitive to juniper pollens than whites.[14,15] Juniper and other related pollens affect 13% to 36% of patients with pollen allergies.[16]

Epidermal contact with juniper tar (eg, preparation for psoriasis treatment) can

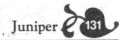

cause potentially carcinogenic DNA damage in human tissue.[17]

Single large doses of juniper berries may cause catharsis, and repeated large doses may be associated with convulsions and renal damage.[2]

Kidney irritation from juniper oil is examined in one report that relates this effect to 1-terpinen-4-ol content.[18]

Because the berries exert their diuretic effect by irritating the renal tissue, juniper products should be used with caution by all and should never be used by those with reduced renal function. Safer and more effective diuretic and carminative drugs exist. The oil can induce gastric irritation and may induce diarrhea. Therefore, its use is limited to low concentrations (< 0.01%) as a beverage flavor.

[1] Clutton DW. *Flavour Ind* 1972 Sep;3:454-56.
[2] Windholz M, et al. *The Merck Index*, 10th ed., Merck and Co., Rahway, 1983.
[3] Janku J, et al. *Experientia* 1957;13:255.
[4] Schilcher H. *Medizinische Monatsschrift Fur Pharmazeuten* 1995;18(7):198-99.
[5] Tammaro F, et al. *J Ethnopharmacol* 1986;16:167.
[6] Jonkov S, et al. *Folia Med* (Plovdiv) 1974;16:291.
[7] Cunliffe WJ, et al. *British Journal of Clinical Practice* 1974 Sep;28:314-16.
[8] Tunon H, et al. *J Ethnopharmacol* 1995;48(2):61-76.
[9] Agrawal OP, et al. *Planta Medica* 1980;(suppl):98-101.
[10] Prakash AO, et al. *ACTA Europaea Fertilitatis.* 1985;16(6):441-48.
[11] Prakash AO. *Int J Crude Drug Res* 1986 Mar;24:16-24.
[12] Rothe A, et al. *Berufsdermatosen* (Germany, West) 1973;21:11.
[13] Anderson JH. *Ann Allergy* 1985;54:390.
[14] Kaufman HS, et al. *Ann Allergy* 1984;53:135.
[15] Kaufman HS, et al. *Ann Allergy* 1988;60(1):53-56.
[16] Bousquet J, et al. *Clin Allergy* 1984;14:249.
[17] Schoket B, et al. *J Invest Dermatol* 1990;94(2):241-46.
[18] Schilcher H, et al. *PZ Wissenschaft* 1993;138(3-4):85-91.

Kava-Kava

SCIENTIFIC NAME(S): *Piper methysticum* Frost Family: Piperaceae

COMMON NAME(S): Awa, kava-kava, kew, tonga

ෲෲ PATIENT INFORMATION ෲෲ

Uses: Kava-kava is used as a sedative and sleep aid.

Drug Interactions: Alcohol consumption increases kava toxicity.

Side Effects: Dry, flaking, discolored skin; scaly rash; red eyes; puffy face; muscle weakness.

BOTANY: Kava is the dried rhizome and roots of *Piper methysticum*, a large shrub widely cultivated in the islands of the South Pacific (eg, Fiji).[1] It has pale yellow-green cordate leaf blades that grow up to 28 cm long. The flower spikes grow up to 9 cm long.[2]

More than 60 varieties of the kava plant have been recognized, the black and white grades having the greatest social and commercial importance. The black grades are preferred by growers because the short growing season yields a quick return on their investment. However, the white grades are generally considered of higher value by the user.[3]

HISTORY: Kava drink is prepared from the rhizome of *P. methysticum*. The pulverized roots are steeped in water; extraction of the root is sometimes hastened by pounding or mastication. The cloudy mixture is then filtered and served at room temperature.[1]

The kava plant is indigenous to the islands of the South Pacific where its most common use has been as a beverage used to induce relaxation.[4,5] The ceremonial preparation and consumption of kava is common to these Pacific Islands.[6] Recently, through mass spectrometry, traces of kava lactones can be found on artifacts in this region, linking the ancient culture of kava drinking to the archeological record.[7] Kava drink has been compared to a Western cocktail, aiding in the establishment of a relaxed, socially cooperative atmosphere.

Folk uses of kava have included the treatment of inflammation of the uterus, headaches, colds, rheumatisms, and venereal diseases; promotion of wound healing; and as a sedative and an aphrodisiac.

PHARMACOLOGY: Seven major and several minor kava lactones have been identified in human urine following kava ingestion. Observed metabolic transformations include reduction and demethylations. Gas chromatography-mass spectroscopy analysis of urine can be used to determine recent kava consumption.[8]

Masticated kava causes numbness of the mouth. Kawain has local anesthetic activity comparable to that of cocaine, with a longer duration of action than benzocaine.[9] Hawaiians have used kava for asthma.[10]

Naloxone inhibits morphine-induced analgesia but is ineffective in reversing kava's antinociceptive activities, showing that the analgesia produced by kava occurs via a non-opiate pathway.[11] Other CNS pharmacologic properties kava may possess are those concerning sleep and anxiety.

Kava reduced non-psychotic type anxiety in patients with minimal adverse effects.[12] A high level of efficacy of kava extract is suggested in neurovegetative and psychosomatic dysfunction in the climacteric.[13]

Kava produces mild euphoric changes characterized by happiness, fluent and lively speech, and increased sensitivity to sounds. High doses may also lead to muscle weakness. Visual or auditory changes occur, as shown by reduced near point of accommodation and convergence, an increase in pupil diameter, and oculomotor balance disturbances.[14] Heavy kava users are more likely to complain of poor health: Twenty percent are underweight, have reduced protein levels, "puffy faces," scaly rashes, increased HDL cholesterol counts, hematuria, blood cell abnormalities (increased red blood cells, decreased platelets and lymphocytes), and some evidence of pulmonary hypertension.[15]

TOXICOLOGY: Two yellow pigments, flavokawain A and B, have been isolated from the kava plant, and their presence provides a possible explanation for the skin discoloration that is observed following the chronic ingestion of kava drink.[16] Chronic ingestion may lead to "kawaism," characterized by dry, flaking, discolored skin and reddened eyes.[17] This scaly eruption is reversible, but the cause is unknown. It may be related to interference with cholesterol metabolism.[18]

Ethanol markedly increases the toxicity of kava. This interaction with alcohol may be of important clinical and social consequence if the two are taken concomitantly (in contrast to the traditional usage).[19] The kava drink may be useful for the management of alcohol abuse.[20]

[1] Tyler VE, et al. *Pharmacognosy*. Philadelphia, PA: Lea & Febiger, 1988.
[2] Cambie R, et al. *Fijian medicinal plants*. Australia: Csiro, 1994.
[3] Getty R. *Econ Bot* 1956;10:241.
[4] Weiner MA. *Econ Bot* 1971;25:423-50.
[5] Nagata Kam *Econ Bot* 1971;25:245-54.
[6] Singh YN. *J Ethnopharm* 1992;37(1):13–45.
[7] Hocart CH, et al. *Rapid Comm in Mass Spectrom* 1993;7(3):219-24.
[8] Duffield AM, et al. *J Chromatogr* 1989;475:273-81.
[9] Meyer HJ. *PHSP* 1967;1645:133.
[10] Hope BE, et al. *Hawaii Med J* 1993;52(6):160-66.
[11] Jamieson DD, et al. *Clin Exp Pharmacol Physiol* 1990;17(7):495-507.
[12] Kinzler E, et al. *Arzneimittlelforschung* 1991;41(6):584-88.
[13] Warnecke G. *Fortschr Med* 1991;109(4):119-22.
[14] Garner LF, et al. *J Ethnopharmacol* 1985 Jul;13:307-11.
[15] Matthews JD, et al. *Med J Austr* 1988;148(11):548-55.
[16] Shulgin AT. *Bull Narc* 1973;25(2):59-74.
[17] Keller F, et al. *Lloydia* 1963;26:1.
[18] Norton SA, et al. *J Am Acad Dermatol* 1994;31(1):89-97.
[19] Jamieson DD, et al. *Clin Exp Pharmacol Physiol* 1990;17(7):509-14.
[20] Cawte J. *Aust NZ J Psychiatry* 1986;20(1):70-76.

Kombucha

SCIENTIFIC NAME(S): Yeast/bacteria fungal mixed culture

COMMON NAME(S): Kombucha tea, kombucha mushroom, Manchurian tea, Combucha tea, Spumonto, Tschambucco, Teekwass, Kwassan, Kargasok tea, "Fungus" Japonicus, Manchurian "fungus," Dr. Sklenar's kombucha mushroom infusion, Champagne of life, T'Chai from the sea

PATIENT INFORMATION

Uses: Kombucha has been used for a variety of illnesses, ranging from memory loss to premenstrual syndrome; there is no good evidence to support the pharmacologic claims for kombucha.

Side Effects: The fermented tea associated with kombucha has been suspected to be fatal in one user. Nausea and allergic responses have been reported.

BOTANY: Kombucha is not a fungus or a mushroom but is a gray, pancake-shaped patty that grows up to 15 cm in diameter. It is fermented in black tea and sugar. The fermentation becomes a mixture of yeast and bacteria.

HISTORY: Kombucha tea has been touted as a miracle cure for illnesses ranging from memory loss to premenstrual syndrome.[1]

The name "kombucha" is derived from the Japanese in that it is brewed in a seaweed (kombu) tea (cha).[2] Users float growing spores on the surface of brewed, sweetened black tea. The mycelium double in mass approximately every week. The mass is then divided, and the new portion is propagated on a new tea media, allowing the mycelium to be propagated at a rapid rate for commercial distribution.[2]

As the growth matures, it slightly ferments the beverage. This fermented tea is drunk for its purported medicinal properties. Drinking fermented teas has long been popular in Eastern countries, and the use of this mycelial growth may date back several centuries.

PHARMACOLOGY: No good evidence supports pharmacologic claims for kombucha. Because the tea is a product of bacterial fermentation, it may contain compounds that affect the bacterial flora of the gut. A report on Dr. Sklenar's kombucha mushroom infusion (1960s) as a cancer therapy showed no solid medical data to support its usefulness.[3] Screening of "Kargasok tea" for anorexia and obesity has also been reported but not validated.[4]

TOXICOLOGY: Nausea and allergic responses have been reported. No kombucha-related deaths have occurred although Iowa health officials have reported the first suspected death linked to the tea.[5] Regulatory agencies are investigating the possibility that kombucha may be a source of bacterial pathogens.[2] In one case, an 83-year-old person with multiple health problems drank 0.5 cup of a kombucha mixture for a 3-week period. Upon examination, laboratory results indicated AST/MLT > 2000 IU/L, lactate dehydrogenase peaking at 4000 IU/L, and a prothrombin time > 25 seconds. The APAP (acetaminophen) level was "trace."[3]

[1] Foster RD. *Natural Health* 1995 Mar/Apr:52.
[2] Marin R, et al. *Newsweek* 1995 Jan 9:64.
[3] Hauser SP. *Schweizerische Rundschau fur Medizin Praxis* 1990;79(9):243.
[4] Kwanashie HO, et al. *Biochem Soc Trans* 1989;17(6):1132.
[5] Hearn W. *Amer Med News* 1995;38(17):16.

SCIENTIFIC NAME(S): *Pueraria lobata* (Willd) Ohwi. Also known as *P. thunbergiana*. Family: Leguminosae

COMMON NAME(S): Japanese arrowroot, kudzu vine[1]

> ### ༺༻ PATIENT INFORMATION ༺༻
>
> *Uses:* Kudzu has been used to treat alcoholism and as fodder.
>
> *Side Effects:* No known toxic effects; safety undefined.

BOTANY: Kudzu is a fast-growing vine native to the tropics, China, and Japan. It has been used as fodder and as a ground cover crop. Because it has long stems, which can attain 20 m in length, and extensive roots, it has been used to control soil erosion. The plant was introduced into the US, where it has taken hold and proliferates, particularly in the moist southern regions, as a noxious weed.

HISTORY: Although kudzu has been widely recognized as a ground cover and fodder crop in the Western world, the plant has a long history of medicinal use in Asian cultures. The plant is cited in botanical herbals from Japan, China, and Fiji.[2] Chinese herbalists have reportedly used extracts of the plant to treat alcoholism.[3]

PHARMACOLOGY: Kudzu has gained attention because the isoflavones contained in the root have been found to be reversible inhibitors of the enzyme alcohol dehydrogenase.[4] Derivatives of these compounds are also potent inhibitors of aldehyde dehydrogenase. Both of these enzymes are required for the normal metabolic degradation of alcohol and its by-products.

In one controlled study, an extract of kudzu significantly reduced alcohol consumption in Syrian Golden hamsters, which are bred for their preference for alcohol. After establishing baseline intakes of water and a 15% ethanol solution, animals were injected with crude kudzu extract, daidzein, or daidzin for 6 days. In each group, the volume of ingested alcohol solution decreased by $\geq$ 50% during the treatment phase. Alcohol consumption returned to pretreatment levels after the study was stopped. This in vivo activity likely is due to the inhibition of enzymes that metabolize alcohol.[5]

TOXICOLOGY: Kudzu has been used as a medicinal herb for centuries without any reported toxic side effects.[4] However, the safety profile of the plant and its extracts are yet to be defined through systematic pharmacologic screens.

[1] Mabberley DJ. *The Plant-Book.* Cambridge, MA: Cambridge University Press, 1987.

[2] Penso G. *Inventory of Medicinal Plants Used in the Different Countries.* World Health Organization. 1982.

[3] Anonymous. *Am J Hosp Pharm* 1994;51:750.

[4] Keung WM. *Alcohol Clin Exp Res* 1993;17:1254.

[5] Keung WM, et al. *Proc Natl Acad Sci USA* 1993;90:10008.

SCIENTIFIC NAME(S): Several *Lavandula* species have been used medicinally, including *L. angustifolia* Mill. (syn. *L. officinalis* Chaix. and *L. spica* L), *L. stoechas, L. dentata, L. latifolia,* and *L. pubescens* Decne. Family: Lamiaceae

COMMON NAME(S): Aspic, lavandin (usually refers to particular hybrids), lavender, spike lavender, true lavender

---

ꙨꙨ PATIENT INFORMATION ꙨꙨ

Uses: Antispasmodic, carminative, antidiabetic agent, treatment of restlessness, insect repellant, and food flavoring agent.

Drug Interactions: May increase or potentiate the CNS-depressant effects of sedative-hypnotics.

Side Effects: Allergic contact dermatitis.

BOTANY: Lavender plants are aromatic evergreen sub-shrubs that grow to ≈ 0.9 m high. The plants are native to the Mediterranean. Fresh flowering tops are collected, and the essential oil is distilled or extracts are obtained by solvent extraction.[1] The plant has small blue or purple flowers. The narrow leaves are fuzzy and gray when young and turn green as they mature.[2]

HISTORY: Lavender has been used as an antispasmodic, carminative, diuretic, and general tonic. Extracts have been used to treat conditions ranging from acne to migraines.[1] Although the plant has increased bile flow output and flow into the intestine, its greatest value is not in the treatment of biliary conditions.[2] Lavender has been used quite extensively as an antidiabetic agent in Spain and is included in some commercial herbal antidiabetic preparations.[3] Fresh leaves and flowers are applied to the forehead to relieve headaches and to joints to treat rheumatic pain. The vapors of steamed flowers are used as a cold remedy.[4] Chileans drink the tea to induce or increase menstrual flow.[5]

Lavender is usually administered as an infusion, decoction, or oil and is taken internally or applied topically for neuralgia. Lavender oil and extracts are used as pharmaceutical fragrances and in cosmetics. Small amounts of the oil are used to flavor food.

PHARMACOLOGY: One report investigated the effects of lavender oil aromatherapy for insomnia and concluded that it is comparable to hypnotics or tranquilizers.[6] Lavender aromatherapy has also been used to increase mental capacity, diminish fatigue,[7] and improve mood and perceived levels of anxiety.[8] Oils of different lavender species yield different results.[9] Lavender electroencephalogram (EEG) studies, which have shown various alpha wave responses to different odors, can be used for psychophysiological response evaluation.[10]

Little evidence supports the use of lavender oil as a choleretic or treatment of GI disorders. A Bulgarian report discusses choleretic and cholagogic action of Bulgarian lavender oil.[11] Many volatile oils also may share these common actions. One of lavender's uses listed in the German Commission E monograph includes helping in functional disorders of the upper abdomen with irritable stomach and intestinal disorders of nervous origin. Its effects are calming and antiflatulent.[12]

A study of percutaneous absorption of lavender oil in massage found that within 5 minutes after application, the

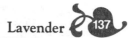

main constituents of the oil were detected in the blood. Most of the lavender oil was excreted within 90 minutes.[13]

Another report evaluated lavender oil as a bath additive to relieve perineal discomfort after childbirth. When compared with placebo and synthetic oil, analysis of daily discomfort scores showed less discomfort between days 3 to 5 with true lavender oil use.[14]

Perillyl alcohol, a compound distilled from lavender but also in cherries, mint, and celery seeds, possesses anticancer activities.[15] This monoterpene is being tested in clinical trials for its role in cancer chemoprevention and therapy.[16,17]

A variety of mechanisms are proposed to explain perillyl alcohol's chemopreventative and chemotherapeutic effects. One such mechanism is that it promotes apoptosis, or programmed cell death, which occurs when its DNA is severely damaged. In cancer, these cells lack this ability, resulting in abnormal cell growth.[14] In one report, liver tumor formation was not promoted by perillyl alcohol, but its growth was inhibited by this apoptosis mechanism by enhancing tumor cell loss.[18] In another report, the rate of apoptosis was > 6-fold higher with perillyl alcohol treated pancreatic adenocarcinoma cells than in untreated cells.[19]

Another proposed mechanism of monoterpenes is inhibition of post-translational isoprenylation of cell growth-regulatory proteins (such as ras).[20] Perillyl alcohol inhibited in vivo prenylation of specific proteins in one report,[21] and altered ras protein synthesis and degradation in another. Interfering with these pathways can regulate malignant cell proliferation.[22]

TOXICOLOGY: Although lavender absolute has been reported to be a skin sensitizer, no human phototoxicity has been reported. Lavender and lavandin oil have been reported to be nonirritating and nonsensitizing to human skin.[1] However, 3 reports discuss allergic contact dermatitis from lavender oil and fragrance.[25,26,27] These examples are few, probably because the oil is used in small quantities in foods and cosmetics and has not been associated with major toxicity during normal use.

[1] Leung AY. *Encyclopedia of Common Natural Ingredients Used in Food, Drugs and Cosmetics.* John Wiley and Sons, 1980.
[2] Weiss RF. *Herbal Medicine.* Hippokrates Verlag, 1988.
[3] Gamez MJ, et al. *Pharmazie* 1987;42:706.
[4] Abulafaith HA. *Econ Bot* 1987;41:354.
[5] San Martin JA. *Econ Bot* 1983;37:216.
[6] Hardy M, et al. *Lancet* 1995 Sept 9;346:701.
[7] Leshchinskaia I, et al. *Kosm Med* 1983;17(2):80-83.
[8] Dunn C, et al. *J Ad Nurs* 1995;21(1):34-40.
[9] Buckle J. *Nurs Times* 1993;89(20):32-35.
[10] Lee CF, et al. *Ann Physiol Anthropol* 1994;13(5):281-91.
[11] Gruncharov V. *Vutr Boles* 1973;12(3):90-96.
[12] Bisset NL. *Herbal Drugs and Phytopharmaceuticals.* Stuttgart, Germany: CRC Press 1994;292-94.
[13] Jager W, et al. *J Soc Cosm Chem* 1992 Jan-Feb;43:49-54.
[14] Dale A, et al. *J Adv Nurs* 1994;19(1):89-96.
[15] Kelloff G, et al. *J Cell Biochem Suppl* 1996;26:1-28.
[16] Jones C. *Herbs for Health* 1998 Jan/Feb:17.
[17] Gould M. *Environ Health Perspect* 1997;105(Suppl)4:977-79.
[18] Mills J, et al. *Cancer Res* 1995;55(5):979-83.
[19] Stayrook K, et al. *Carcinogenesis* 1997;18(8):1655-58.
[20] Crowell P, et al. *Adv Exp Med Biol* 1996;401:131-36
[21] Ren Z, et al. *Biochem Pharmacol* 1997;54(1):113-20.
[22] Hohl R, et al. *Adv Exp Med Biol* 1996;401:137-46.
[23] Brandao FM. *Contact Dermatitis* 1986;15(4):249-50.
[24] Rademaker M. *Contact Dermatitis* 1994;31(1):58-59.
[25] Schaller M, et al. *Clin Exp Dermatol* 1995;20(2):143-45.

Leeches

SCIENTIFIC NAME(S): *Hirudo medicinalis* L. Phylum: Annelida

COMMON NAME(S): Fresh water leech, medicinal leech

⋮⋰⋱⋮ PATIENT INFORMATION ⋮⋰⋱⋮

Uses: Leeches have been used for bloodletting, wound healing, and stimulating blood flow at post-surgical sites.

Side Effects: Allergic reactions, anaphylaxis, and infection, possibly even with hepatitis and HIV, may develop.

HISTORY: Medicinal uses of leeches date back > 2 centuries before Christ. The 19th century heralded the widespread use of leeches for "bloodletting," a practice that grew so quickly that by the 1830s, a leech shortage in France required the importation of > 40 million Mexican leeches.[1] The last 45 years have seen a resurgence in the use of leeches, particularly in post-surgical wound-healing procedures.

THERAPEUTIC USES: Medicinal leeches are used to stimulate blood flow at postoperative surgical sites, a procedure that has been claimed to increase the success of tissue transplants, reduction mammoplasty, and the reattachment of amputated extremities.[2]

The application of leeches to the area immediately surrounding the surgical wound temporarily reestablishes venous blood flow, thereby allowing the nutritive perfusion of the wound site by fresh blood. Blood stasis is a major contributor to unsuccessful reconstructive surgery. It is believed that if sufficient blood flow is maintained at the site until permanent adequate natural perfusion is established, the affected tissue has an improved survival rate.

After attaching to the site, leeches secrete compounds that reduce blood viscosity and draw 20 to 50 ml of blood from each bite. The leeches provide the drainage needed to permit decongestion and to preserve tissue viability until normal venous flow is established ($\approx$ 5 to 7 days after the surgery).[3]

Application method: Leeches from commercial breeders are maintained in a chlorine-free salt solution at 10° to 20°C. Under such conditions, leeches can survive for up to 18 months.

Patients undergoing leech therapy should be administered a broad-spectrum antibiotic such as an aminoglycoside or third-generation cephalosporin to prevent infection by *Aeromonas hydrophilia*, which is in the leech gut.[4,5] Leeches bought in German pharmacies contained up to 11 species of bacteria; viruses and protozoans have survived for months in the gut of the leech and as such, the leech should be considered a vector for infectious diseases.[6]

The area is washed and covered by gauze or transparent dressing with a precut 1 cm hole to reveal the adhesion site. The leech is placed near the site. The biting end of the leech is generally the smaller of the 2 ends and moves in a "searching" fashion.[4] If attachment does not occur readily, the leech can be induced by pricking the skin with a pin to draw blood or the area can be dabbed with a sugar solution. The bite has been described as virtually painless, similar to a mosquito bite. A detailed description of the application technique has been outlined.[7]

One leech is applied 2 to 4 times/day for up to a week.[8] Feeding is complete in $\approx$ 20 minutes, when the leech drops off. Removal of the leech may be hastened by applying solutions of salt, vinegar, a match, or a local anesthetic, but the leech should not be forcibly removed. Bleeding from the attachment site usually continues for several hours.[9] Reuse of leeches is discouraged to minimize cross-infection.

PHARMACOLOGY: Medicinal leeches have an anterior and posterior sucker; within the anterior sucker is a y-shaped mouth with marginal teeth for biting. Following attachment, the leech secretes hirudin, a selective thrombin inhibitor, which enhances bleeding and prevents coagulation.

Recombinant hirudin has been used successfully in the treatment of Kasabach-Merritt syndrome, which leads to loss of circulating platelets and fibrinogen. Paradoxically, low-dose subcutaneous hirudin normalized fibrinogen and platelet activity.[10]

Leeches also secrete a vasodilator, a hyaluronidase, a collagenase, and 2 fibrinases (1 disrupts clots, the other atherosclerotic plaque). The compound calin has also been isolated from leeches. By binding to collagen to interfere with the platelet-collagen interaction, this inhibitor of von Willebrand factor causes an antithrombotic effect in vitro and in hamster models.[11,12] There is conflicting evidence as to whether an anesthetic is secreted.

Studies have confirmed that medicinal leeches improve venous drainage of wound sites in patients who have undergone reattachment surgery after amputation.[13,14] The ability of leeches to improve blood flow across congested surgical flaps has been documented us-

ing Doppler laser perfusion monitoring in pigs. Within 1 hour of applying leeches, blood flow through the surgical area increased 142% at surface probes and 491% at implanted probes. The average change for untreated control flaps was 6%.[1]

However, one study found no changes in ipsilateral activated partial thromboplastin or prothrombin times when leeches were applied to an intact hand,[15] suggesting that significant systemic or local anticoagulation is not likely to occur, and the risk of interference with other therapies may be small.

Salivary extracts of the giant leech (Haementeria) interfere with the metastatic growth of lung tumors.[2]

TOXICOLOGY: Leeches may draw up to 50 ml of blood per feeding. Repeated leeching may decrease hemoglobin levels dramatically. Drops of 1 to 2 gm% during a 5-day course are common. Decreases of up to 7 gm% have been observed following a 6-day course and required tranfusion therapy.[8] Following removal of leeches, the wound site will continue to bleed for up to 4 hours.

Several reports have documented severe wound and systemic infections caused by Aeromonas hydrophila (a gram-negative rod) harbored by leeches, and Providentia has been isolated in transport water.[16]

Local allergic reactions and anaphylaxis have been reported.[9]

[1] Hayden RE, et al. Arch Otolaryngol Head Neck Surg 1988;114:1395.
[2] Lent C. Nature 1986;323:494.
[3] Abrutyn E. Ann Intern Med 1988;109:356.
[4] Kourt B, et al. Am J Hosp Pharm 1994;51:2113.
[5] Bickel KD, et al. J Reconstr Microsurg 1994;10:83.
[6] Nehili M, et al. Parasitol Res 1994;80:277.
[7] Abrutyn. Am J Hosp Pharm 1988;109:356.
[8] Rao P, et al. Practitioner 1985;229:901.
[9] Adams SL. Ann Emerg Med 1989;18:316.
[10] Deckmyn H, et al. Blood 1995;85:712.
[11] Harsfalvi J, et al. Blood 1995;85:705.
[12] Soucacos PN, et al. Int Angiol 1994;13:251.
[13] Soucacos PN, et al. Microsurgery 1994;15:496.
[14] Blackshear JL, et al. Ann Intern Med 1994;121:151.
[15] Dickson P, et al. BMJ 1984;289:1727.

Lemon Balm

SCIENTIFIC NAME(S): *Melissa officinalis* L. Family Lamiaceae (Mints)

COMMON NAME(S): Lemon balm, balm, melissa, sweet balm

☙☙☙ PATIENT INFORMATION ☙☙☙

Uses: Lemon balm has been used for Graves' disease as a sedative, antispasmodic, and a topical agent for cold sores.

Side Effects: No side effects have been reported.

BOTANY: Lemon balm is a low perennial herb with ovate- or heart-shaped leaves that have a lemon odor when bruised. The small yellow or white flowers are attractive to bees and other insects. It is indigenous to the Mediterranean region and western Asia, and widely naturalized in Europe, Asia, and North America. The leaves are harvested before flowering and used medicinally.

HISTORY: Lemon balm has been used in herbal medicine since the times of Pliny, Dioscorides, Paracelsus, and Gerard. The name "melissa" corresponds to the Greek word for bee, while "balm" is a contraction of balsam. The plant had culinary and medicinal uses, with the principal historical medicinal uses being carminative, diaphoretic, and antipyretic.

PHARMACOLOGY: Lemon balm's traditional medicinal use was as a sedative and antispasmodic. This extract also was active in an acetic acid writhing analgesia assay but not in the hot plate test. The volatile oil of the plant had much weaker activity or was inactive in the same assays.

Lemon balm has antiviral activity against a variety of viruses, including herpes simplex virus (HSV) and HIV-1. The activity has been attributed to caffeic acid and its di- and trimeric derivatives as well as to tannins.[1,2] A clinical trial of a cream formulation of melissa extract demonstrated evidence of activity against HSV cold sores.[3]

Another use of melissa has been in Graves' disease, in which the thyroid is abnormally activated by thyroid-stimulating immunoglobulin (TSI). Freeze-dried extracts of melissa bound thyrotropin and prevented it and the Graves' TSI from activating its receptor[4-7] although with less potency than the extracts of *Lithospermum officinales*, *Lycopus virginicus*, and *Lycopus europaeus*. In all cases, the activity was traced to caffeic acid oligomers such as rosmarinic acid and lithospermic acid. Auto-oxidation of the caffeic acid derivatives to ortho-quinones was postulated to be important for the biological activity.

Rosmarinic acid has also been found to inhibit the C3 and C5 convertase steps in the complement cascade.[8-10]

Lemon balm is approved in the German Commission E monographs for nervous sleeping disorders and functional GI complaints. It is also monographed in ESCOP F-2, WHO vol. 2, and BHP vol. 2.[11]

TOXICOLOGY: The antithyroid activity of melissa extract mentioned above is weak enough that it does not present a serious safety concern in patients without Graves' disease. The topical use for herpes cold sores has not produced any reports of dermal toxicity. Melissa extract was not found to be genotoxic in a screen of several medicinal plants.[12]

[1] Kucera LS, et al. *Proc Soc Exp Biol Med* 1967;124(3):865.

[2] Herrmann EC Jr, et al. *Proc Soc Exp Biol Med* 1967;124(3):869.

[3] Wöbling RH, et al. *Phytomedicine* 1994;125.

[4] Auf'mkolk M, et al. *Endocrinology* 1984;115(2):527.

[5] Auf'mkolk M, et al. *Endocrinology* 1985;116(5):1687.

[6] Auf'mkolk M, et al. *Endocrinology* 1985;116(5):1677.

[7] Sourgens H, et al. *Planta Med* 1982;45:78.

[8] Rampart M, et al. *Biochem Pharmacol* 1986;35(8):1397.

[9] Engelberger W, et al. *Int J Immunopharmacol* 1988;10(6):729.

[10] Peake PW, et al. *Int J Immunopharmacol* 1991;13(7):853.

[11] Barrett, M. *CRN: Reference on Evaluating Botanicals* Washington, D.C.: Council for Responsible Nutrition, 1998.

[12] Ramos Ruiz A, et al. *J Ethnopharmacol* 1996;52(3):123.

Lemongrass

SCIENTIFIC NAME(S): *Cymbopogon citratus* (DC) Stapf. Synon. with *Andropogon citratus* DC. The related plant *C. flexuosus* W. Wats. is also used medicinally. Family: Gramineae

COMMON NAME(S): Lemongrass. *C. citratus* is known as capim-cidrao, Guatemala or Madagascar lemongrass. *C. flexuosus* is known as cochin lemongrass or British Indian lemongrass.

❧❧❧ PATIENT INFORMATION ❧❧❧

Uses: Lemongrass is used as a fragrance and flavoring and in folk medicine as an antispasmodic, hypotensive, anticonvulsive, analgesic, antiemetic, antitussive, antirheumatic, antiseptic, and treatment for nervous and GI disorders and fevers. There is little evidence to support its effectiveness in oral dosage.

Side Effects: Lemongrass is considered to be of low toxicity.

BOTANY: *Cymbopogon* is a perennial grass native to tropical Asia. *C. citratus* is cultivated in the West Indies, Central and South America, and tropical regions, whereas *C. flexuosus* is grown mainly in western India. The freshly cut and partially dried leaves are used medicinally and are the source of the essential oil.

HISTORY: Lemongrass is one of the most widely used plants in South American folk medicine. It is used as an antispasmodic, analgesic, for the management of nervous and GI disorders, to treat fevers, and as an antiemetic. In India, it is used as an antitussive, antirheumatic, and antiseptic. It is usually taken by infusion made by pouring boiling water on fresh or dried leaves.

PHARMACOLOGY: Comprehensive studies have been conducted in South America to attempt to define the pharmacologic profile of this plant.

The general lack of pharmacologic activity of oral doses of lemongrass have been substantiated in humans. Volunteers who took a single oral dose or 2 weeks of oral intake of the tea showed no changes in any hematologic or urinary tests, as well as electroencephalogram (EEG) or electrocardiogram (ECG) tracings. Some subjects showed mild elevations of direct bilirubin and amylase levels, but none were accompanied by any clinical manifestations. The hypnotic effect was further investigated in 50 volunteers who ingested a tea prepared under double-blind conditions 3 different nights 3 to 5 days apart. The parameters tested (sleep induction time, sleep quality, dream recall, reawakening) did not show any effect of lemongrass compared with placebo. Furthermore, 18 patients with documented anxiety traits showed no differences in their anxiety scores after taking a single 150 ml dose of lemongrass tea under double-blind conditions.[1]

These data indicate that despite its widespread popularity, there is little substantive evidence that oral doses of lemongrass tea exert any beneficial pharmacologic effect in humans.

TOXICOLOGY: The lack of toxicity and pharmacologic activity make lemongrass a valuable placebo.[2]

---

[1] Leite JR, et al. *J Ethnopharmacol* 1986;17:75.

[2] Formigoni MLOS, et al. *J Ethnopharmacol* 1986;17:65.

SCIENTIFIC NAME(S): *Aloysia triphylla* (L'Her.) Britt. Formerly described as *A. citriodora* (Cav.) Ort., *Verbena citriodora* Cav., *V. triphylla, Lippia citriodora* (Ort.) HBK Family: Verbenaceae

COMMON NAME(S): Lemon verbena, louisa

~~~ PATIENT INFORMATION ~~~

Uses: Lemon verbena is used in teas, flavorings, fragrances, antispasmodics, carminatives, sedatives, and stomachics.

Side Effects: Some individuals may experience contact hypersensitivity.

BOTANY: Lemon verbena is an aromatic plant native to Argentina and Chile.[1] It is a deciduous plant that is commonly cultivated in the tropics and Europe. It is grown commercially in France and North Africa. The plant grows to 3 m and is characterized by fragrant, lemon-scented narrow leaves. It bears small white flowers in terminal panicles.[1]

HISTORY: Lemon verbena has been used medicinally for centuries, having been touted for use as an antispasmodic, antipyretic, carminative, sedative, and stomachic. The leaves and flowering tops are used in teas and as beverage flavors. Its fragrance is used in perfumery. Although the plant is grown as an ornamental, it requires shelter during cold periods.[1]

PHARMACOLOGY: The essential oil is said to be acaricidal and bactericidal. An alcoholic leaf extract has been reported to have antibiotic activity in vitro against *Escherichia coli, Mycobacterium tuberculosis*, and *Staphylococcus aureus,* although it had no antimalarial activity. A 2% emulsion of the oil has been reported to kill mites and aphids.[2]

A component of the related plant, *Verbena officinalis,* has been reported by Chinese investigators to have antitussive activity.[3]

TOXICOLOGY: Lemon verbena generally is recognized as safe for human consumption and for use as a flavoring in alcoholic beverages. Contact hypersensitivity has been associated with members of the related *Verbena genus.*

[1] Simon JE, et al. *Herbs: an indexed bibliography, 1971-1980.* Hamden, CT: The Shoe String Press, 1984.

[2] Duke JA. *Handbook of Medicinal Herbs.* Boca Raton, FL: CRC Press, 1985.

[3] Gui CH. *Chung Yao Tung Pao* 1985;10:35.

SCIENTIFIC NAME(S): *Lentinula edodes* (Berk.) Pegler, syn. with *Tricholomopsis edodes* Sing., *Lentinus edodes* (Berk.) Singer

COMMON NAME(S): Shiitake, snake butter, pasania fungus, forest mushroom, hua gu

---

≈≈≈ PATIENT INFORMATION ≈≈≈

Uses: Lentinan is proving to be a valuable component in cancer and infection treatments. It has also demonstrated cholesterol-lowering and immune-regulatory properties.

Side Effects: Lentinan is derived from the Shiitake mushroom, which is edible and is not generally associated with side effects. Reports of lentinan side effects are rare.

BOTANY: Lentinan is a polysaccharide derived from the vegetative parts of the edible Japanese shiitake mushroom. It is the cell wall constituent extracted from the fruiting bodies or mycelium of *L. edodes*.[1] The light, amber fungi are found on fallen broadleaf trees, such as chestnut, beech, or mulberry. They have decurrent, even or ragged gills, a stem, and are covered with delicate, white flocking.[2] Shiitake mushrooms are commonly sold in food markets in the Orient and are now widely available in the United States, Canada, and Europe.

HISTORY: Lentinan is a complex polysaccharide that possesses immuno-stimulating antitumor properties. Lentinan was isolated from edible shiitake mushrooms that have been used in traditional Asian cooking and herbal medicine. Shiitake has been renowned in Japan and China as a food and medicine for thousands of years and is now commonplace throughout the world. Extracts of these mushrooms are being incorporated into *otc* dietary supplements designed to improve the status of the immune system.

PHARMACOLOGY: The antitumor activity of lentinan has been recognized for almost 30 years. Because a number of naturally occurring polysaccharides had previously been found to have antitumor activity, lentinan was considered for detailed evaluation. In addition to antitumor activity, lentinan also possesses immune-regulatory effects, antiviral activity, antimicrobial properties and cholesterol-lowering effects. The following is a brief outline of key aspects of lentinan pharmacology.

Antitumor activity: Therapeutic effects of lentinan in cancers of the GI tract have been noted. Lentinan used as an agent for postoperative adjuvant therapy was investigated in patients with stages II to IV GI cancer. Stage IV patients had higher lymphocyte counts than control patients, suggesting lentinan's immuno-potentiating efficacy in advanced GI cancer.[3] Another study reports lifespan prolongation in stomach cancer patients, using lentinan combination therapy.[4] Other successful chemotherapies using lentinan include: CDDP and 5-FU,[5] mitomycin and 5-FU,[6] cisplatin with radiation,[7] and interleukin–2.[8] Another study involving gastric cancer describes how lentinan causes marked development of reticular fibers related to antitumor effect and enhanced interstitial response.[9] Intracavitary injection of lentinan is useful for malignant effusions in gastric carcinoma patients.[10] Resistance to lentinan chemoimmunotherapy is also reported.[11]

Lentinan's effects in other cancers have also been reported. In prostatic cancer,

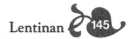

lentinan 2 mg weekly in combination with *Tegafur* was evaluated. A 5-year average survival rate of treated patients was 43% compared with 29% in the control group.[12] Another report referred to the safety and efficacy of lentinan post-treatment with surgical therapy in 33 breast cancer patients.[13] Lentinan has also been evaluated in cervical cancer patients.[14-16]

Survival rates using lentinan therapies have increased. One study reports 129 days vs 49 days in malignant ascites and pleural effusion patients given lentinan 4 mg/week for 4 weeks.[17] A 4-year follow-up survey of stomach cancer patients reports increased survival at 1, 2, and 3 years, with few reported side effects.[4]

Immune system effects: Although not directly cytotoxic, beta-1,3 glucan has been shown to enhance natural immunity. When administered IP to mice with implanted tumors, lentinan effectively increased the activity of cytotoxic peritoneal exudate cells.[18] Direct action of lentinan on tumor cells in mice by scanning electron microscopy has been reported. Lentinan contributes to antitumor immunity enhancement, but not to direct killing activity against tumor cells.[19] Evidence suggests that lentinan preferentially acts on T-cells and may enhance T-helper cell function. Furthermore, lentinan augments natural killer cell activity and activates macrophages.[20] Lentinan also triggers production of interleukin–1 by a direct action on macrophages or indirectly by augmenting colony-stimulating factor.[21] Many other studies are available where lentinan is found to improve immune function by stimulating T-cell/killer cell/monocyte produc-

tion,[3,8,10,22-27] increasing natural cell-mediated cytotoxicity,[28] stimulating production of acute-phase transport proteins,[29] affecting lymphocyte and enzyme concentrations,[30] and activating complement.[31]

Anti-viral activity: Lentinan has anti-viral activity and has been found to protect against encephalitis caused by the intranasally infected vesicular stomatitis virus in mice.[32] Lentinan enhances AZT's effects when used in combination against HIV for in vitro studies.[33]

Antimicrobial properties. Rabbits with induced septic insult without lentinan treatment were reported to have low platelet counts, and elevated bilirubin and creatinine. In lentinan-treated septic animals, platelet counts did not decrease, and elevation of plasma bilirubin and creatinine levels were less prominent. Findings suggest a modified septic process by administration of lentinan.[34] Host resistance against microbial infection by lentinan is reviewed in another report.[35]

Cholesterol-lowering effects: The compound lentinacin has been shown to reduce cholesterol levels in rats by 25% after 7 days of oral administration in a dose as low as 0.005% of feed intake.[36] Other compounds isolated from Shiitake have also been shown to lower blood cholesterol and lipids as well.[37]

TOXICOLOGY: The shiitake mushroom is edible and has not been associated with toxicity. In animals, lentinan shows little toxicity. In mice, the LD-50 is > 1500 mg/kg IP. In a phase I study conducted in 50 patients with advanced cancer, minor side effects were observed in 3 patients; in a study of 185 patients, 17 experienced minor adverse reactions.[6] Few toxic effects are mentioned in 2 reports of lentinan use.[38,39]

[1] Chihara G, et al. *Cancer Res* 1970;30:2776.
[2] Hobbs C. *Medicinal Mushrooms* Santa Cruz, CA: Botanica Press, 1995;125.
[3] Tanabe H, et al. *Nippon Gan Chiryo Gakki Shi* 1990;25(80):1657-67.
[4] Tagachi T. *Cancer Detect Prev* 1987;1(Suppl):333-49.
[5] Mio H, et al. *Gan To Kagaku Ryoho* 1994;21(4):531-34.
[6] Jeannin JF, et al. *Int J Immunopharm* 1988;10:855.
[7] Egawa S, et al. *Nippon Hinyokika Gakki Zasshi* 1989;8(2):249-55.
[8] Suzuki M, et al. *Int J Immunopharm* 1990;12(6):613-23.
[9] Ogawa K, et al. *Gan To Kagaku Ryoho* 1994;21(13):2101-4.
[10] Hazama S, et al. *Gan To Kagaku Ryoho* 1995;22(11):1595-97.
[11] Hamuro J, et al. *Br J Cancer* 1996;73(4):465-71.
[12] Tari K, et al. *Hinyokika Kiyo-Acta Urologica Japonica* 1994;40(2):199-23.
[13] Kosaka A, et al. *Gan To Kagaku Ryoho* 1987;14(2):516-22.
[14] Shimizu H, et al. *Nippon Sanka Fujinka Gakkai Zasshi* 1988;40(12):1899-900.
[15] Shimizu Y, et al. *Nippon Sanka Fujinka Gakkai Zasshi* 1988;40(10):1557-58.
[16] Shimizu Y, et al. *Nippon Sanka Fujinka Gakkai Zasshi* 1990;42(1):37-44.
[17] Oka M, et al. *Biotherapy* 1992;5(2):107-12.
[18] Hamuro J et al, *Immunology* 1980;39:551.
[19] Kurokawa T, et al. *Nippon Gan Chiryo Gakki Shi* 1990;25(12):2822-27.
[20] Reed FC, et al. *Int J Immunopharm* 1982;4:264.
[21] Hamuro J, et al. *Int J Immunopharm* 1982;4:267.
[22] Hanaue H, et al. *Nippon Gan Chiryo Gakki Shi* 1989;24(8):1566-71.
[23] Hanaue H, et al. *Clin Ther* 1989;11(5):614-22.
[24] Tani M, et al. *Anticancer Res* 1993;13(5C):1773-76.
[25] Tani M, et al. *Eur J Clin Pharmacol* 1992;42(6):623-27.
[26] Arinaga S, et al. *Int J Immunopharm* 1992;14(4):535-39.
[27] Arinaga S, et al. *Int J Immunopharm* 1992;14(1):43-47.
[28] Peter G, et al. *Immunopharm Immunotox* 1988;10(2):157-63.
[29] Suga T, et al. *Int J Immunopharm* 1986;8(7):691-99.
[30] Feher J, et al. *Immunopharm Immunotox* 1989;11(1):55-62.
[31] Takeshita K, et al. *Nippon Geka Gakkai Zasshi* 1991;92(1):5-11.
[32] Chang KSS, *Int J Immunopharm* 1982;4:267.
[33] Tochikura T, et al. *Jpn J Cancer Res* 1987;78(6):583-89.
[34] Tsujinaka T, et al. *Eur Surg Res* 1990;22(6):340-46.
[35] Kaneko Y, et al. *Adv Exp Med Biol* 1992;319:201-15.
[36] Chibata I et al, *Experientia* 1969;25:1237.
[37] Hobbs C. *Medicinal Mushrooms*, Santa Cruz, CA: Botanica Press, 1995;p. 133-34.
[38] Chihara G, et al. *Cancer Detect Prev* 1987;1:423-43.
[39] Chihara G. *Dev Biol Stand* 1992;77:191-97.

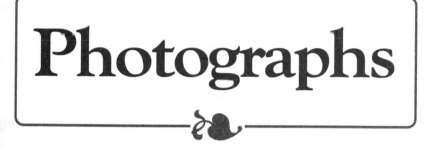

Photographs

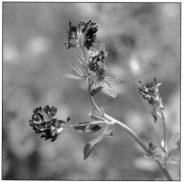

Alfalfa

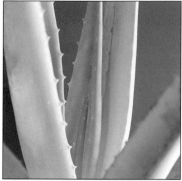

Aloe Vera

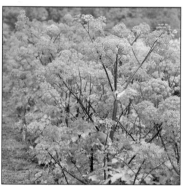

Angelica

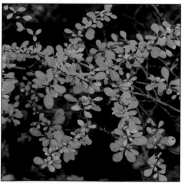

Barberry

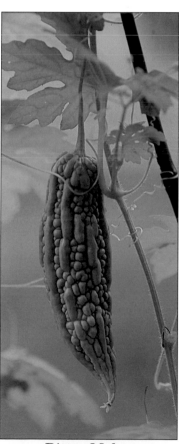

Bitter Melon

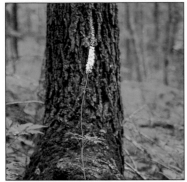

Black Cohosh (flower)

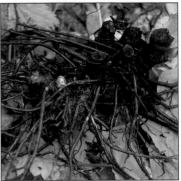

Black Cohosh (root & leaf)

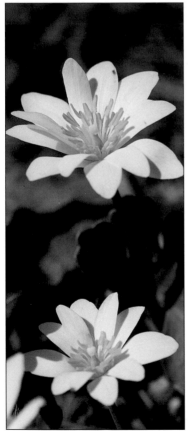

Bloodroot (flower)

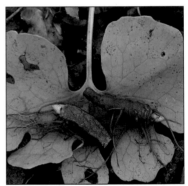

Blood Root (root & leaf)

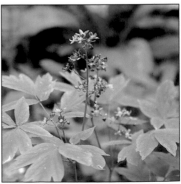

Blue Cohosh

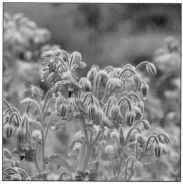

Borage

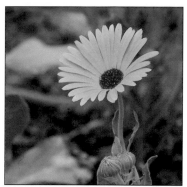

Calendula

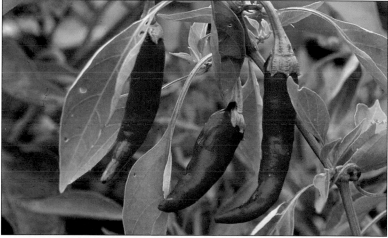

Capsicum Peppers

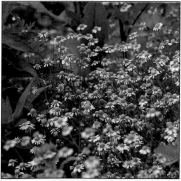

Chamomile

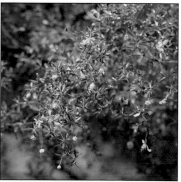

Chaparral

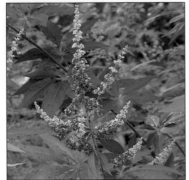

Chaste Tree

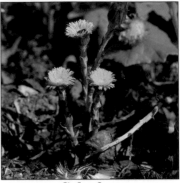

Coltsfoot

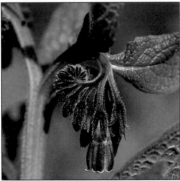

Comfrey

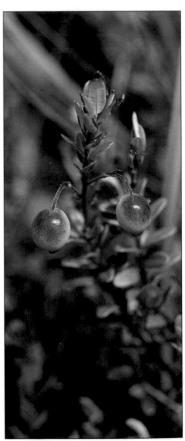

Cranberry

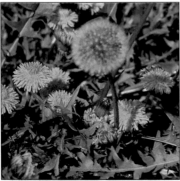

Dandelion

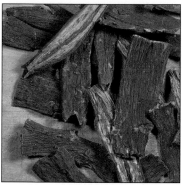

Danshen

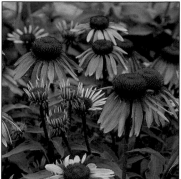

Echinacea

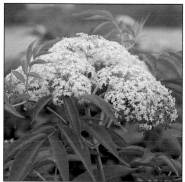

Elderberry

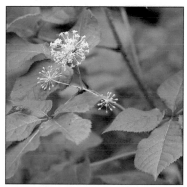

Eleutherococcus

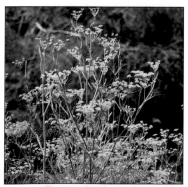

Fennel (flower)

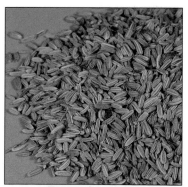

Fennel (seeds)

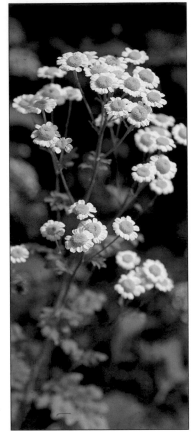

Feverfew

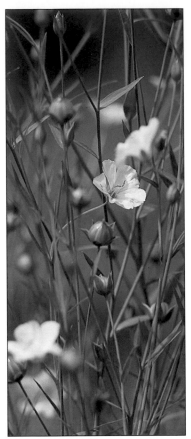

Flax

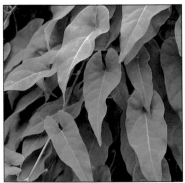

Fo-Ti (plant)

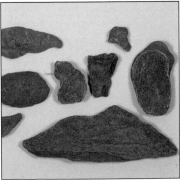

Fo-Ti (root)

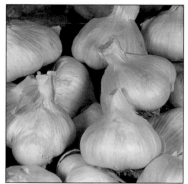

Garlic (bulb)

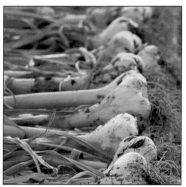

Garlic (bulb & root)

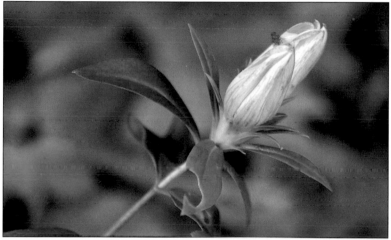

Gentian

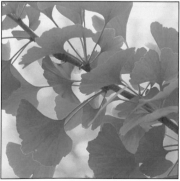

Ginkgo

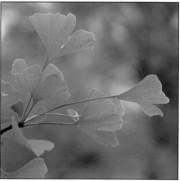

Ginkgo

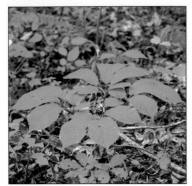

Ginseng (American)

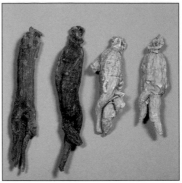

Ginseng (Asian)

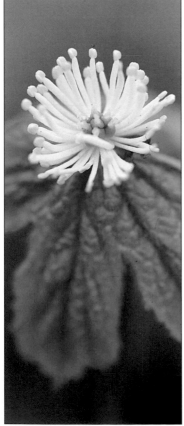

Goldenseal (flower)

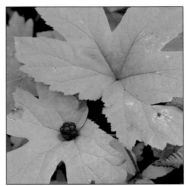

Goldenseal (leaf)

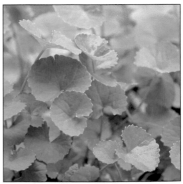

Gotu Kola

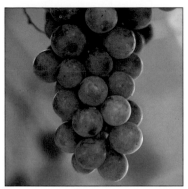

Grape

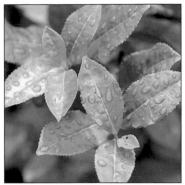

Green Tea

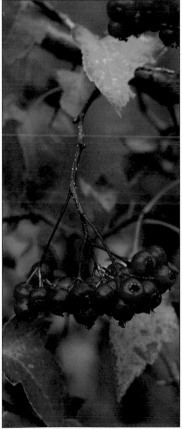

Hawthorn

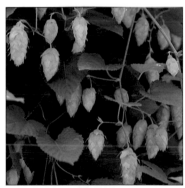

Hops

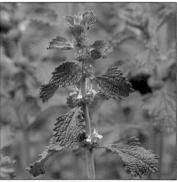

Horehound

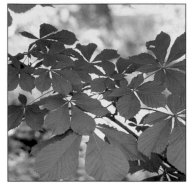

Horse Chestnut

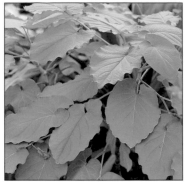

Kava Kava

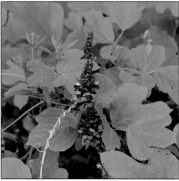

Kudzu

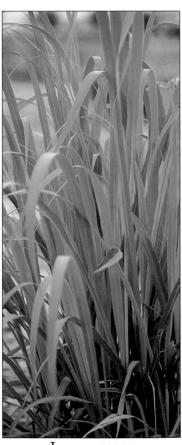

Lemongrass

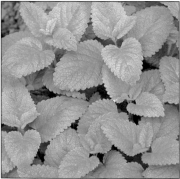

Lemon Balm

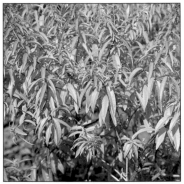

Lemon Verbena

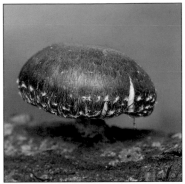

Lentinan

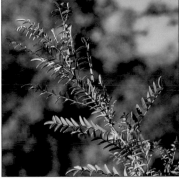

Licorice

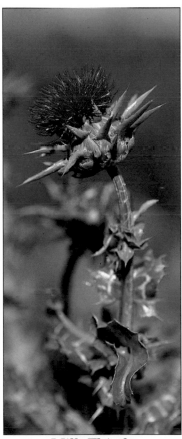

Milk Thistle

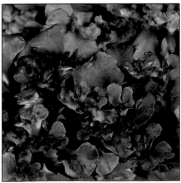

Maitake

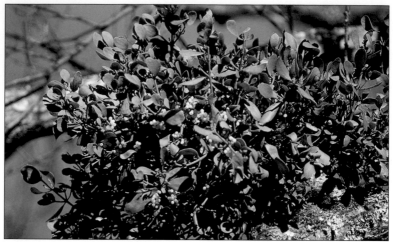

Mistletoe (American)

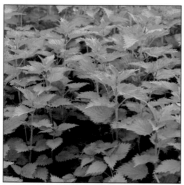

Nettles

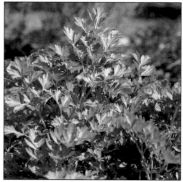

Parsley

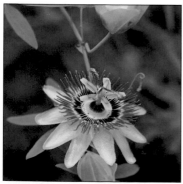

Passion Flower

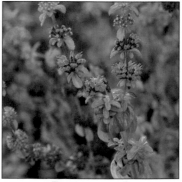

Pennyroyal

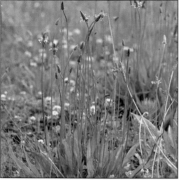

Plantain

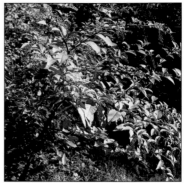

Pokeweed (flower)

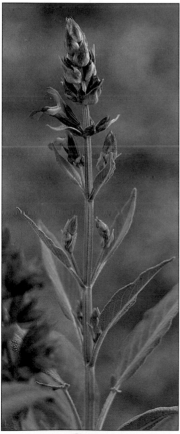

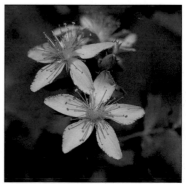

Pokeweed (root)

Sage

St. John's Wort

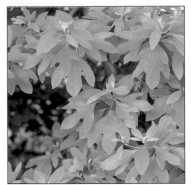

Sassafras

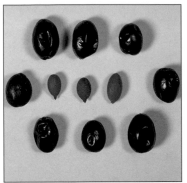

Saw Palmetto (berries)

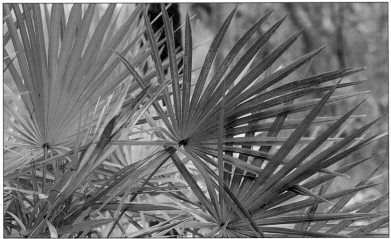

Saw Palmetto (leaves)

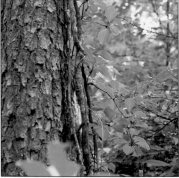

Schisandra (vine)

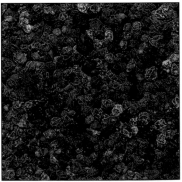

Schisandra (fruit)

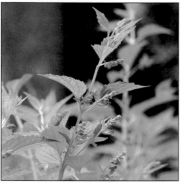

Scullcap

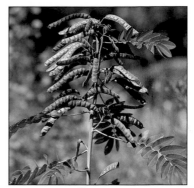

Senna

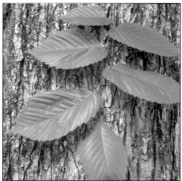

Slippery Elm

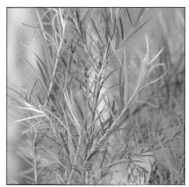

Tea Tree

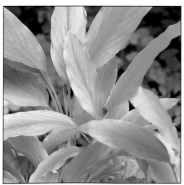

Turmeric (leaves)

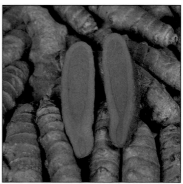

Turmeric (root)

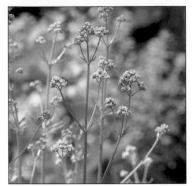

Valerian

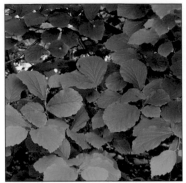

Witch Hazel

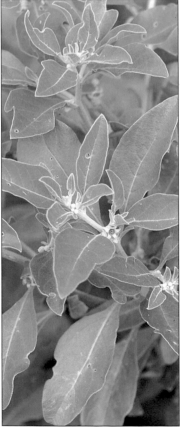

Withania

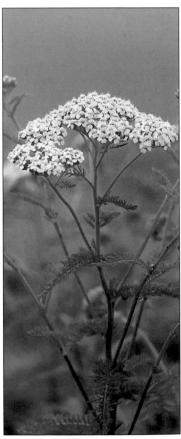

Yarrow

SCIENTIFIC NAME(S): *Glycyrrhiza glabra* L, *G. uralensis* Fisch. ex DC, *G. pallidiflora* Maxim Family: Leguminosae

COMMON NAME(S): Licorice, Spanish licorice, Russian licorice

ᕽᕽ PATIENT INFORMATION ᕽᕽ

Uses: Used historically for GI complaints, licorice is used today as a flavoring and in shampoos.

Side Effects: Large amounts of licorice taken daily for a long time can cause a range of side effects from lethargy to quadriplegia (body paralysis). Do not over-consume licorice.

BOTANY: *Glycyrrhiza glabra* is a 1.2 to 1.5 m shrub that grows in subtropical climates with rich soil. The name "glycyrrhiza" is derived from Greek words meaning "sweet roots." The roots are harvested to produce licorice. Most commercial licorice is extracted from varieties of *G. glabra*. The most common variety, *G. glabra* var. *typica* (Spanish licorice), has blue flowers, and *G. glabra* var. *glandulifera* (Russian licorice) has violet blossoms. Turkey, Greece, and Asia Minor supply most commercial licorice.

HISTORY: Therapeutic use of licorice dates back to the Roman Empire. Hippocrates and Theophratus extolled its uses, and Pliny the Elder (A.D. 23) recommended it as an expectorant and carminative. Licorice also figures prominently in Chinese herbal medicine as a "drug of first class" — an agent that exerts godly influence on the body and lengthens life. Licorice is used in modern medicinals chiefly as a flavoring agent that masks bitter agents, such as quinine, and in cough and cold preparations for its expectorant activity. Most recently, a sample of historic licorice from A.D. 756 was analyzed and was found to still contain active principles even after 1200 years.[1]

PHARMACOLOGY: As a result of licorice's extensive folk history for gastric irritation, it has undergone extensive research for use as an anti-ulcerogenic agent. While the specific mechanism of action is unknown, carbenoxolone, a semisynthetic succinic acid ester of 18β glycyrrhetic acid, a compound combined in licorice, acts to enhance mucous secretions, increase the lifespan of gastric epithelial cells, inhibit back diffusion of hydrogen ions induced by bile, and possibly inhibit peptic activity.

Controlled trials show carbenoxolone is less effective than cimetidine in treating gastric and duodenal disease. In one study, 78% of patients receiving cimetidine demonstrated ulcer improvement by gastroscopy compared with 52% of those receiving carbenoxolone. Additionally, carbenoxolone patients experienced more side effects including edema, hypertension, and hypokalemia. These side effects are more pronounced in elderly patients and those with underlying renal, hepatic, or cardiovascular disease. A proposed mechanism of action for these side effects involves carbenoxolone's action on the renin-aldosterone-angiotensin axis. Spironolactone relieves the side effects but also attenuates the therapeutic effects.

Another licorice product tested as an anti-ulcer agent is deglycyrrhizinated licorice (DGL), which consists of licorice that has had virtually all of its glycyrrhizin removed. Several studies have evaluated the efficacy of DGL, but all have been inconclusive. These agents have not shown consistent results nor the serious side effects exhibited by carbenoxolone.

Another use for glycyrrhizins is suppression of scalp sebum secretion. A 10% glycyrrhizin shampoo prevented sebum secretion for 1 week compared with citric acid shampoo, which delayed oil accumulation by 1 day.

Alcohol extracts of *G. glabra* have in vitro antibacterial activity and weak in vivo antiviral activity.

Prepared Chinese licorice, *Zhigancao*, was found to have antiarrhythmic effects, such as prolonging P-R and Q-T intervals.[2]

TOXICOLOGY: The toxic manifestations of excess licorice ingestion are well documented. One case documented the ingestion of 30 to 40 g of licorice/day for 9 months as a diet food. The subject became increasingly lethargic with flaccid weakness and dulled reflexes. She also suffered from hypokalemia and myoglobinuria. Treatment with potassium supplements reversed her symptoms. Excessive licorice intake can result in sodium and fluid retention, hypertension, and inhibition of the renin-angiotensin system.[3]

After consuming large amounts of licorice, human intoxication with aldosterone-like effects was found.[4]

A 70-year-old patient with hypertension and hypokalemia caused by chronic licorice intoxication in excess of $\approx$ 80 candies (2.5 g each having 0.3 glycyrrhizic acid)/day over 4 to 5 years, discontinued use 1 week before hospital admission. After discontinuing licorice and monitoring a treatment plan including licorice, the activity of 11-β-hydroxysteroid dehydrogenase was suppressed when the patient had been without licorice, but the 11-β-hydroxysteroid dehydrogenase increased as the levels of urinary glycyrrhetic acid decreased.[5]

Other documented complications include paraparesis, hypertensive encephalopathy, and one case of quadriplegia. Products that contain licorice as a flavoring, such as chewing tobacco, have also been implicated in cases of toxicity. Hypersensitivity reactions to glycyrrhiza-containing products have also been noted.

[1] Shibata S. *Int J Pharmacog* 1994;32(1):75-89.
[2] Chen RX, et al. *Chung Kuo Chung Yao Tsa Chih* 1991;16(10):617-19.
[3] Sigurjonsdottir HA, et al. *J Human Hyperten* 1995;9(5):345-48.
[4] Bielenberg J. *Pharmazeutische Zeitung* 1989;134(12):9-12.
[5] Farese RV, et al. *N Engl J Med* 1991;325(10):1223-27.

SCIENTIFIC NAME(S): *Grifola frondosa* (Dickson ex Fr.) S.F. Gray (Polyporaceae)

COMMON NAME(S): Maitake, "king of mushrooms," dancing mushroom, "monkey's bench," shelf fungi

---

❧❧❧ PATIENT INFORMATION ❧❧❧

Uses: Maitake has been used for cancer, diabetes, high blood pressure, cholesterol, and obesity.

Side Effects: Most studies report no side effects.

BOTANY: The maitake mushroom is from northeastern Japan. It grows in clusters at the foot of oak trees and can reach 50 cm in base diameter. One bunch can weigh up to 45 kg. Maitake has no cap but has a rippling, flowery appearance, resembling "dancing butterflies" (hence, one of its common names "dancing mushroom").[1]

HISTORY: In China and Japan, maitake mushrooms have been consumed for 3000 years. Years ago in Japan, the maitake had monetary value and was worth its weight in silver. This mushroom was offered to Shogun, the national leader, by local lords. In the late 1980s, Japanese scientists identified the maitake to be more potent than lentinan, shiitake, suehirotake, and kawaratake mushrooms, all used in traditional Asian medicine for immune function enhancement.

PHARMACOLOGY: Immunostimulant activity is characteristic of many of the medicinal mushrooms, including shiitake, enokitake, or kawaratake. Maitake exerts its effects by activation of natural killer cells, cytotoxic T-cells, interleukin-1, and superoxide anions, all of which aid in anticancer activity.[2] It has also been determined that the large molecular weight of the polysaccharide molecule and branched structure are necessary for its antitumor effect or immunological enhancement.[3-5]

Maitake extract has been studied in *Escherichia coli*;[6] it has activated macrophages, enhancing cytokine production in vivo.[7]

There is a small number of clinical trials investigating maitake's effects in cancer therapy. Additional controlled studies are needed. In a 165-patient study, quality of life indicators improved, including cancer symptoms (eg, nausea, hair loss) and pain reduction.[8] Cancers that were improved by maitake in clinical cases include liver, lung, breast, brain, and prostate.[1]

Maitake may control blood glucose levels by possible reduction of insulin resistance and enhancement of insulin sensitivity.[1]

Studies are available concerning maitake's antiobesity activity.[9] In an observatory trial, 30 patients lost between 7 and 26 pounds from administration of 20 to 500 mg tablets of maitake powder per day for 2 months.[10]

TOXICOLOGY: Little or no information regarding maitake toxicity is available. Most studies report no side effects.[1] Because potential toxicity exists from mistaken mushroom identity, use caution when obtaining this particular natural product.

[1] Lieberman S, et al. *Maitake King of Mushrooms*. New Canaan, CT: Keats Publishing, Inc. 1997;7-48.

[2] Adachi K, et al. *Chem Pharm Bull* 1987;35(1):262-70.

[3] Adachi K, et al. *Chem Pharm Bull* 1989;37(7):1838-43.

[4] Adachi K, et al. *Chem Pharm Bull* 1990;38(2):477-81.

[5] Ohno N, et al. *Biol Pharm Bull* 1995;18(1):126-33.

[6] Jin Z, et al. *Chung Hua Yu Fang I Hsueh Tsa Chih* 1994;28(3):147-50.

[7] Adachi Y, et al. *Biol Pharm Bull* 1994;17(12):1554-60.

[8] Nanba H. *Townsend Letter for Doctors and Patients* 1996;84-85.

[9] Ohtsuru M. *Anshin* 1992 Jul:188-200.

[10] Yokota M. *Anshin* 1992 Jul:202-4.

SCIENTIFIC NAME(S): Melatonin, N-acetyl-5-methoxytryptamine

COMMON NAME(S): Melatonin, MEL

✷✷✷ PATIENT INFORMATION ✷✷✷

Uses: Melatonin is used to regulate sleep, protect against cancer, and provide a variety of other benefits.

Side Effects: Possible adverse effects include headache and depression.

HISTORY: Melatonin (MEL) is a hormone of the pineal gland that is also produced by extrapineal tissues.[1,2]

Melatonin secretion is inhibited by environmental light and stimulated by darkness, with secretion starting at 9 pm and peaking between 2 and 4 am. Nocturnal secretion of melatonin is highest in children and decreases with age.[3,4] Studies in the past decade have widely expanded melatonin use for easing insomnia, combatting jet lag, preventing pregnancy, protecting cells from free-radical damage, boosting the immune system, preventing cancer, and extending life.[5]

Although melatonin is not approved by the FDA as a drug product, it has been classified as an orphan drug since November 1993 (Sponsor: Dr. Robert Sack, Oregon Health Sciences University)[4] for the treatment of circadian rhythm sleep disorders in blind people with no light perception. It is commercially available as a nutritional supplement either as a synthetic product or derived from animal pineal tissue. Use of the nonsynthetic product is discouraged because of an increased risk of contamination or viral transmission.

PHARMACOLOGY: The FDA does not control melatonin and warns that users are taking it "without any assurance that it is safe or that it will have any beneficial effect."

Blind entrainment: The sleep-wake cycle in humans without light-dark cues is ≈ 25 hours, shifting the sleep cycle by 1 hour each day. Blind people with little or no perception of light often develop *free-running* circadian rhythms > 24 hours and subsequently develop sleep disturbances characterized by chronic fatigue and involuntary napping during the day. In case reports and small controlled studies, oral melatonin (dosage range: 0.5 to 10 mg) has been used to entrain free-running activity rhythms in the blind by advancing and stabilizing the phase of endogenous melatonin secretion.[4,6,7] Although success has varied, the importance of melatonin administration time is recognized. For example, the administration of melatonin (5 or 10 mg for 2 to 4 weeks at bedtime) to an 18-year-old blind man with chronic sleep disturbances produced slightly improved sleep onset but did not reduce daytime fatigue or hypersomnolence.[4,7] However, the administration of melatonin (5 mg for 3 weeks) at 2 to 3 hours prior to habitual bedtime decreased sleep onset (≈ 1.4 hours), slightly increased sleep duration (34 minutes), and improved sleep quality and daytime alertness. The authors suggest that there is a phase response curve (PRC) for the exogenous administration of melatonin; the maximum phase-advancing effects occur when melatonin is administered ≈ 6 hours prior to onset of endogenous melatonin secretion.[4,8] The average cumulative phase advancement (CPA) of melatonin rhythms after 3 weeks of treatment with 5 mg and 0.5 mg daily was 8.41 and 7 hours, respectively.[4,6]

Jet lag: Melatonin's ability to modulate circadian rhythms has prompted several studies on its use in preventing jet lag.[4,9-11] Although the effects have been variable, most patients have reported general improvement in daytime fatigue, disturbed sleep cycles, mood, and recovery times. These studies are limited by the small number of participants and a focus on subjective ratings of effects with little or no evidence of actual changes in circadian shift (ie, changes in oral temperature or cortisol levels). As with entrainment studies in the blind, it appears that timing of administration and the development of optimal regimens require further study. Several melatonin regimens have been examined (5 to 10 mg daily) for various durations. In one study, 52 aircraft personnel were randomized to placebo, early, or late melatonin groups. The early group started melatonin (5 mg daily) 3 days before departure until 5 days after arrival.[4,10] The late group received melatonin upon arrival and for 4 additional days. When compared to placebo, the late melatonin group reported significantly less jet lag, fewer overall sleep disturbances, and faster recovery of energy and alertness. However, the early group (receiving melatonin for 8 days) reported jet lag symptoms similar to the placebo group and a worsened overall recovery. Additional data from uncontrolled studies suggest that benefits were also experienced by international travelers when melatonin was given on the day or night of departure and for 2 to 3 nights after arrival.[4,9,11] (Note: Because driving skills may be affected, one may experience drowsiness within 30 minutes after taking melatonin and then for ≈ 1 hour.)

Insomnia: Although melatonin has been shown to shift melatonin secretion and circadian rhythm patterns, its direct hypnotic effect has not been clearly established. Decreased circulating melatonin serum levels have been demonstrated in insomniacs of all ages and in the healthy elderly.[3,4] In small studies of healthy volunteers or chronic insomniacs, large melatonin doses (75 to 100 mg) administered at night (9 pm to 10 pm) produced serum melatonin levels exceeding normal nocturnal ranges and hypnotic effects.[4,12,13] Midday administration of large doses increased serum melatonin levels beyond normal nocturnal ranges, increased subjective fatigue, and decreased cognitive function and vigor.[4,14] Administration of smaller doses (0.3 to 5 mg) has produced inconsistent hypnotic results, possibly due to the inclusion of different sleep disorders, drug formulations, and administration times.[4,15-20] The time to reach peak hypnotic effect was significantly longer when melatonin (5 mg) was administered at 12 noon vs 9 pm (3.66 hrs vs 1 hr).[4,21] Delayed latency with daytime administration may be related to the already low circulating melatonin levels during the day. Low doses (0.3 mg or 1 mg) administered to healthy volunteers at 6 pm, 8 pm, or 9 pm decreased onset latency and latency to Stage 2 sleep but did not suppress rapid eye movement (REM) sleep nor induce hangover effects.

In patients with difficulty falling asleep, low melatonin doses should be sufficient in promoting sleep onset. However, in patients with difficulty maintaining sleep, low melatonin doses may not produce sufficient blood concentrations to maintain slumber. A 2 mg oral melatonin dose produced peak levels ≈ 10 times higher than physiological levels, but it remained elevated for only 3 to 4 hours.[4,22] To maintain effective serum concentrations of melatonin throughout the night, a high dose, repeated low doses, or a controlled-release formulation may be needed. When compared to placebo in a trial of 12 elderly chronic insomniacs, melatonin significantly increased sleep efficiency (75% vs 83%) and decreased wake time after sleep onset (73 vs 49 minutes).[4,19] There were no significant differences between the groups for total sleep time (365 vs 360 minutes) or sleep onset (33 vs 19 minutes). Sleep onset and sleep maintenance were improved in elderly insomniacs after 1 week of immediate (1 mg) and sustained-release (2 mg) melatonin preparations. Sleep onset improved further when the sustained-release form was continued for 2 months.[4,20]

Cancer protection: Melatonin has demonstrated inhibitory effects on tumor growth in animal models and in vitro cancerous breast cell lines.[3] Proposed oncoprotective mechanisms of melatonin include stimulatory effects on circulating natural killer cells and potent antioxidant activity. Preliminary studies have examined the use of melatonin in patients with solid tumors unresponsive to standard therapies, melanoma, and as adjunctive amplifier therapy with interleukin in various metastatic tumors (ie, endocrine, colorectal).[4,21-25] European studies on B-Oval (containing melatonin) are ongoing, but it appears to slow the growth rate of human tumor cells. A nightly supplement (10 mg melatonin) has improved 1-year survival rates with metastatic lung cancer patients.[3] Well-controlled trials are needed before the role of melatonin as an oncostatic agent can be confirmed.

Oral contraceptive: Because melatonin plays a role in the endocrine-reproductive system and reduces circulating LH, its use as a contraceptive has been studied.[4,26] Melatonin, in various dosage combinations with a synthetic progestin, in 32 women for 4 months produced anovulatory effects.

TOXICOLOGY: Most studies note the absence of adverse events with melatonin. Minor side effects with doses < 8 mg have included heavy head, headache, and transient depression.[4,10,11] In psychiatric patients, melatonin has aggravated depressive symptoms.[3,4,27] Toxicological studies have shown that an LD-50 could not be obtained even at extremely high doses. Researchers gave human volunteers 6 g melatonin each night for a month and found no major problems, except for stomach discomfort or residual sleepiness.[5]

[1] Windholz M, et al. *Merck Index*, 11th ed. Rahway, NJ: Merck and Co., 1989.
[2] Bowman WC, et al. *Textbook of Pharmacology*, 2nd ed. St. Louis, MO: Blackwell Scientific Publications, 1980.
[3] Webb SM, et al. *Clin Endocrinol* 1995;42(3):221.
[4] Generali JA. *Drug Newsletter* 1996;15(1):3.
[5] Cowley G. *Newsweek* 1995 Aug 7:46.
[6] Sack RL, et al. *J Biol Rhythms* 1991;6(3):249.
[7] Tzichinsky O, et al. *J Pineal Res* 1992;12:105.
[8] Lewy AJ, et al. *Chronobiol Int* 1992;9(5):380.
[9] Lino A, et al. *Biol Psychiatry* 1993;34:587.
[10] Petrie K, et al. *Biol Psychiatry* 1993;33:526.
[11] Claustrat B, et al. *Biol Psychiatry* 1992;32:705.
[12] Waldhauser F, et al. *Psychopharmacol* 1990;100:222.
[13] MacFarlane JG, et al. *Biol Psychiatry* 1991;30:371.
[14] Dollins AB, et al. *Psychopharmacol* 1993;112:490.
[15] James SP, et al. *Neuropsychopharmacol* 1989;3:19.
[16] Tzichinsky O, et al. *Sleep* 1994;17(7):638.
[17] Aldhous M, et al. *Br J Clin Pharmacol* 1985;19:517.
[18] Nave R, et al. *Eur J Pharmacol* 1995;275:213.
[19] Zhdanova IV, et al. *Clin Pharmacol & Ther* 1995;57:552.
[20] Garfinkel D, et al. *Lancet* 1995;346:541.
[21] Haimov I, et al. *Sleep* 1995;18(7):598.
[22] Jan JE, et al. *Dev Med and Child Neurol* 1994;36:97.
[23] Lissoni P, et al. *Oncology* 1991;48:448.
[24] Zumoff B. *Obstet Gynecol Clin North Am* 1994;21(4):751.
[25] Lissoni P, et al. *Oncology* 1995;52:163.
[26] Lissoni P, et al. *Oncology* 1995;52:360.
[27] Barni S, et al. *Oncology* 1995;52:243.
[28] Voordouw BCG, et al. *J Clin Endocrinol Metab* 1992;74:108.
[29] Arendt J. *Clin Endocrinol* 1988;29:205.

Milk Thistle

SCIENTIFIC NAME(S): *Silybum marianum* (L.) Gaertn. Family: Compositae referred to in older texts as *Carduus marianus*. Recently changed to *Carduus marianum*.

COMMON NAME(S): Holy thistle, lady's thistle, marian thistle, Mary thistle, Milk thistle, St. Mary thistle, silybum

---

⋟⋞⋟ PATIENT INFORMATION ⋟⋞⋟

Uses: Treatment or protection against liver damage, as in cirrhosis, Amanita mushroom poisoning, and hepatitis.

Side Effects: Few adverse effects have been seen other than brief GI disturbances and mild allergic reactions; possible urticaria in one patient.

BOTANY: This plant is indigenous to Kashmir, but is found in North America from Canada to Mexico. Milk thistle grows from ≈ 1.5 to 3 m and has large prickly leaves. When broken, the leaves and stems exude a milky sap. The reddish purple flowers are ridged with sharp spines. The drug consists of the shiny mottled black or grey-toned seeds (fruit). These make up the "thistle" portion, along with its silvery pappus, which readily falls off.[1]

HISTORY: Milk thistle was once grown in Europe as a vegetable. The de-spined leaves were used in salads; the stalks and root parts were also consumed, even the flower portion was eaten "artichoke-style." The roasted seeds were used as a coffee substitute. Various preparations of milk thistle have been used medicinally for more than 2000 years. Its use as a liver protectant can be traced back to Greek references. Pliny the Elder, a first century Roman writer, (A.D. 23 to 79) noted that the plant's juice was excellent for "carrying off bile."[2] Culpeper (England's premier herbalist) noted milk thistle to be of use in removing obstructions of liver and spleen, and to be good against jaundice. The Eclectics (19th to 20th century) used milk thistle for varicose veins, menstrual difficulty, and congestion in liver, spleen, and kidneys.[3]

In homeopathy, a tincture of the seeds has been used to treat liver disorders, jaundice, gall stones, peritonitis, hemorrhage, bronchitis, and varicose veins.[4]

PHARMACOLOGY: Milk thistle's primary use is as a hepatoprotectant and antioxidant. The properties of silymarin (the extract from milk thistle seeds) are due mainly to its flavonolignans content.[5] Medicinal value may also be attributed in part to the presence of trace metals in the plant.[6]

Hepatoprotection: Silymarin protects liver cells against many hepatotoxins in humans and animals. Some Amanitas (eg, *A. phalloides*, the death cup fungus) contain two toxins: Phalloidin, which destroys the hepatocyte cell membrane, and alpha-amanatin, which reaches the cell nucleus and inhibits polymerase-b activity, thereby blocking protein synthesis. Silymarin is capable of negating both of these effects by blocking the toxin's binding sites, increasing the regenerative capacity of liver cells, and blocking enterohepatic circulation of the toxin.[3] In one study, 60 patients with severe Amanita poisoning were treated with infusions of 20 mg/kg of silybin (one of sylimarin's 3 flavonolignans) with good results. Although the death rate following this type of mushroom poisoning can exceed 50%, none of the patients treated in this series died.[7] In a clinical trial of

205 patients with Amanita toxicity, 46 patients died; however, all 16 patients who received silybin survived.[8] Administration of silybin within 48 hours of ingestion at a dose of 20 to 50 mg/kg/day was an effective prophylactic measure against severe liver damage.[9] A multicenter trial performed in European hospitals between 1979 and 1982 was conducted using silybin in supportive treatment of 220 Amanita poisoning cases. A 12.8% mortality rate was reported.[10] The death rate using other modern supportive measures such as activated charcoal can be 40%.[3] Silymarin alone or in combination with penicillin reduced death rates from ingestion of death cup fungus to 10%.[11] In addition to mushroom toxin protection, silymarin also offers liver protection against tetracycline-induced lesions in rats,[12] d-galactosamine-induced toxicity,[13] thallium-induced liver damage,[14] and erythromycin estolate, amitriptyline, nortriptyline, and tert-butylhydroperoxide hepatotoxin exposure of neonatal hepatocyte cell cultures.[15] In a later Italian double-blind, placebo-controlled report, silymarin was elevated in 60 women on long-term phenothiazine or butyrophenone therapy. Results suggested that silymarin treatment can reduce lipoperoxidative hepatic damage caused by chronic use of these psychotropic drugs.[16]

Cirrhosis: Use of milk thistle is inadvisable in decompensated cirrhosis.[17] In two 1-month, double-blind studies performed on an average of 50 patients with alcoholic cirrhosis treated with silymarin, elevated liver enzyme levels (AST, ALT) and serum bilirubin levels were normalized. It also reduced high levels of gamma-glutamyl transferase, increased lectin-induced lymphoblast transformation and produced other changes not seen in the placebo group.[18-20] A 41–month double-blind study performed in 170 patients with alcoholic cirrhosis indicated silymarin to be effective in treatment as well.[21] Silymarin ameliorated indices of cytolysis in a study also using ursodeoxycholic acid in active cirrhosis patients.[22] However, one study suggested no change in evolution or mortality of alcoholic liver disease as compared with placebo in a controlled trial of 72 patients using 280 mg/day of silymarin.[23]

Hepatitis: In patients with acute viral hepatitis, silymarin shortened treatment time and showed improvement in serum levels of bilirubin, AST, and ALT.[24,25] Biochemical values returned to normal sooner in silymarin-treated patients.[26] Histological improvement was seen in patients with chronic hepatitis vs placebo in another controlled trial.[27]

In a 116-patient double-blind study of silymarin vs placebo, silymarin 420 mg/day given to histologically proven alcoholic hepatitis patients was shown not to be clinically useful in treating this disease.[28] A later report suggests stable remission in a 6- to 12–month Russian study evaluating treatment of chronic persistent hepatitis.[17] In 20 chronic active hepatitis patients given 240 mg silybin twice daily vs placebo, improved liver function tests related to hepatocellular necrosis were reported.[29]

Blood and immunomodulation: Silymarin's immunomodulatory activity in liver disease patients may also be involved in its hepatoprotective action.[30] Silybin can increase activity of superoxide dismutase and glutathione peroxidase, which may also explain its protective effects against free radicals.[31] Silymarin had an anti-inflammatory effect on human blood platelets.[32] Silybin may have antiallergic activity. Its effect on histamine release from human basophils was reversed and may be due to membrane-stabilizing activity.[33] Silybin inhibition of human T-lymphocyte activation is also reported.[34]

Lipid and biliary effects: Administration of silymarin 420 mg/day for 3 months to 14 type II hyperlipidemic patients resulted in slightly decreased total cholesterol and HDL-cholesterol levels.[35] Silybin-induced reduction of biliary cholesterol may be due in part to decreased liver cholesterol synthesis.[36] Biliary excretion of silybin was evaluated by high performance liquid chromatography (HPLC). Bioavailability of silybin is greater after silipide (a lipophilic silybin-phosphatidylcholine complex) administration than after silymarin administration; therefore, increased delivery of silipide to the liver results.[37] Use of silymarin prevents disturbance of bile secretion, thereby increasing bile secretion, cholate excretion, and bilirubin excretion.[17]

Various other effects: Silybin and silymarin have also been evaluated (including case reports) in diabetes patients for possible value in prophylaxis of diabetic complications[38] and in combination therapy to treat aged skin.[39] Traditional uses of milk thistle include stimulation of milk production in nursing mothers and antidepressant therapy.[5] Other uses include steroid secretory modulation[40] and as therapy of acute promyelocytic leukemia.[41]

Extracts, tablets, or capsules (35 to 70 mg) standardized to 70% silymarin are available as commercial preparations in average daily doses of 200 to 400 mg.[42]

TOXICOLOGY: Human studies of silymarin have shown few adverse effects.[5] Tolerability of silymarin is good; only brief disturbances of GI function and mild allergic reactions have been observed, but rarely enough to discontinue treatment.[17] Mild laxative effects in isolated cases have been reported.[43] A case of urticaria with a foreign commercial milk thistle preparation has been noted.[44]

[1] Bisset N. *Herbal Drugs and Phytopharmaceuticals* London, England: CRC Press, 1994;121-23.

[2] Foster S. *Botanical Series No. 305* Austin, TX: American Botanical Council, 1991;3-7.

[3] Hobbs C. *Milk Thistle: The Liver Herb*, 2nd ed., Capitola, CA: Botanica Press, 1992;1-32.

[4] Schauenberg P, et al. *Guide to Medicinal Plants* New Canaan, CT: Keats Publishing, 1974.

[5] Awang D. *Can Pharm J* 1993 Oct:403-4.

[6] Parmar V, et al. *Int J Pharmacognosy* 1993;31(4):324-26.

[7] Vogel G, Proceeding of the International Bioflavonoid Symposium, Munich 1981.

[8] Floersheim GL, et al. *Schweiz med Wochenschr* 1982;112:1164.

[9] Hruby, et al. *Hum Toxicol* 1983;2:183.

[10] Hruby K. *Forum* 1984;6:23-26.

[11] Hruby K. *Intensivmed* 1987;24:269-74.

[12] Skakun N, et al. *Antibiot Meditsin Biotekh* 1986;31(10):781-84.

[13] Tyutyulkova N, et al. *Methods Find Exp Clin Pharmacol* 1981;3:71.

[14] Mourelle M, et al. *J Appl Toxicol* 1988;8(5):351-54.

[15] Davila J, et al *Toxicology* 1989;57(3):267-86.

[16] Palasciano G, et al. *Curr Ther Res* 1994;55(5):537-45.

[17] Rumyantseva Z. *Vrach Delo* 1991;(5):15-19.

[18] Lang I, et al. *Acta Med Hung* 1988;45(3-4):287-95.

[19] Lang I, et al. *Tokai J Exp Clin Med* 1990;15(2-3):123-27.

[20] Lang I, et al. *Ital J Gastroenterol* 1990;22(5):283-87.

[21] Ferneci P, et al. *J Hepatol* 1989;9(1):105-13.

[22] Lirussi F, et al. *Acta Physiol Hung* 1992;80(1-4):363-67.

[23] Bunout D, et al. *Rev Med Chil* 1992;120(12):1370-75.

[24] Magliulo E, et al. *Med Klin* 1978;73:1060-65.

[25] Cavalieri S. *Gazz Med Ital* 1974;133:628.

[26] Wilhelm H, et al. *Wien Med Wochenschr* 1973;123:302.

[27] Kriesewetter E, et al. *Leber Magen Darm* 1977;7:318-23.

[28] Trinchet J, et al. *Gastroenterol Clin Biol* 1989;13(2):120-4.

[29] Buzzelli G, et al. *Int J Clin Pharmacol Ther Toxicol* 1993;31(9):456-60.

[30] Deak G, et al. *Orv Hetil* 1990;131(24):1291-92, 1295-96.

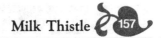

[31] Altorjay I, et al. *Acta Physiol Hung* 1992;80(1-4):375-80.

[32] Max B. *Trends Pharmacol Sci* 1986 Nov;7:435-37.

[33] Miadonna A, et al. *Br J Clin Pharmacol* 1987;24(6):747-52.

[34] Meroni P, et al. *Int J Tissue React* 1988;10(3):177-81.

[35] Somogyi A, et al. *Acta Med Hung* 1989;46(4):289-95.

[36] Nassuato G, et al. *J Hepatol* 1991;12(3):290-95.

[37] Schandalik R, et al. *Arzneimittel-Forschung* 1992;42(7):964-68.

[38] Zhang J, et al. *Chung-Kuo Chung Hsi I Chieh Ho Tsa Chih* 1993;13(12):725-26, 708.

[39] Esteve M, et al. *Parfuemerie und Kosmetik* 1991 Dec;72:920, 822, 824, 826, 828-29.

[40] Racz K, et al. *J Endocrinol* 1990;124(2):341-45.

[41] Invernizzi R, et al. *Haematologica* 1993;78(5):340-41.

[42] Leung A, et al. *Encyclopedia of Common Natural Ingredients Used in Food, Drugs and Cosmetics* New York, NY: John Wiley and Sons, Inc., 1996;366-68.

[43] Brown D. *Drug Store News for the Pharmacist* 1994 Nov;4:58, 60.

[44] Mironets V, et al. *Vrach Delo* 1990;(7):86-87.

Mistletoe

SCIENTIFIC NAME(S): *Viscum album* L. Family: Loranthaceae, *Phoradendron serotinum* (Raf.) M.C. Johnston, *P. flavescens* (Pursh) Nuttal, *P. tomentosum* (DC) Englem

COMMON NAME(S): Mistletoe, bird lime, all heal, devil's fuge, golden bough[1,2]

⋙⋙ PATIENT INFORMATION ⋙⋙

Uses: Mistletoe has been used in traditional medicine and as a cancer treatment. It has been shown to be hyper- and hypotensive and to increase uterine and intestinal motility.

Side Effects: Mistletoe is acutely toxic and may cause cardiac arrest.

BOTANY: American mistletoe comprises the *Phoradendron* species and European mistletoes *V. album*, *V. abietis* and *V. austriacum*. Mistletoes are semiparasitic woody perennials commonly found on oaks and other deciduous trees. These evergreen plants produce small white berries and are used as Christmas ornaments. These plants should not be confused with the New Zealand mistletoe *(Ileostylus micranthus),* which contains cytotoxic compounds that may be derived from the host tree (*Podocarpus totara*).[3]

HISTORY: An early pagan custom required hanging mistletoe to inspire passion during the pagan holiday of "Hoeul." Today's custom of kissing under the plant is a simpler version of this event. European mistletoe has been used for centuries in traditional medicine and gained wide popularity in the early 1900s as a cancer treatment.[4]

PHARMACOLOGY: Despite the popular knowledge that the two types of mistletoe have opposite pharmacologic effects (ie, American mistletoe: Stimulates smooth muscle, raises blood pressure, increases uterine and intestinal motility; European mistletoe: Reduces blood pressure, antispasmodic, calming agent), investigations have shown that the stems and leaves of these plants contain the proteinaceous phoratoxins and viscotoxins and thus exert similar pharmacologic effects. These compounds produce dose-dependent hypertension or hypotension,[5] bradycardia, and increased uterine and intestinal motility.[6] The irreversible depolarization observed in experimental isolated muscle preparations appears to be reversible with calcium.[7]

A proteinaceous component of *V. album* had been shown to possess antineoplastic activity in vitro.[8] The phoratoxins and viscotoxins are cytotoxic and, along with several other lectins, account for the anticancer activity of the plant.[9] Lectins increase the secretion of tumor necrosis factor, interleukin-1, and interleukin-6 in vitro and in humans.[10]

TOXICOLOGY: All parts of mistletoe, including the berries and leaves, should be regarded as toxic, and symptomatic treatment should be instituted rapidly. Symptoms of toxicity include nausea, bradycardia, gastroenteritis, hypertension, delirium, and hallucinations. Diarrhea and vomiting may lead to serious dehydration. Vasoconstriction and cardiac arrest may occur. Rapid gastric emptying has been suggested even if as few as 1 or 2 berries have been ingested.[6] However, a comprehensive analysis of > 300 reported cases of mistletoe ingestion in the US found that the majority of patients remained asymptomatic, and no deaths occurred. These data lead to the conclusion that ingestion of up to 3 berries or 2 leaves is unlikely to produce serious toxicity.[11]

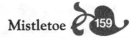

Hepatitis following the ingestion of an herbal compound containing mistletoe has been reported,[12] but other investigators have suggested that, based on the lack of documented hepatic toxicity of the components of mistletoe, the reported toxic effect was more likely due to an adulterant.[13] Death has been reported following the ingestion of teas brewed from these plants for use as a tonic or abortifacient.[14,15] Allergic rhinitis has been reported in a subject handling commercial mistletoe tea (*V. album*).[16]

[1] Dobelis IN, ed. *The Magic and Medicine of Plants*. Pleasantville, NY: Readers Digest Association, 1986.

[2] Meyer JE. *The Herbalist*. Hammond, IN: Hammond Book Co., 1934.

[3] Bloor SJ, et al. *J Nat Prod* 1991;54:1326.

[4] Lecompte JTJ, et al. *Biochemistry* 1987;26:1187.

[5] Fukunaga T, et al. *J Pharm Soc Japan* 1989;109:600.

[6] Mack RB. *North Carolina Med J* 1984;45:791.

[7] Sauviat MP. *Toxicon* 1990;28:83.

[8] Vester F, et al. *Experientia* 1965;21:197.

[9] Jung ML, et al. *Cancer Lett* 1990;51:103.

[10] Hajto T, et al. *Cancer Res* 1990;50:3322.

[11] Hall AH, et al. *Ann Emerg Med* 1986;15:1320.

[12] Harvey J, et al. *BMJ* 1981;282:186.

[13] Farnsworth N, et al. *BMJ* 1981;283:1058.

[14] Cann HM, et al. *Nat Clearinghouse for Poison Control Centers Bulletin* Dec. 1, 1959.

[15] Moore HW. *South Carolina Med Assn* 1963;59:269.

[16] Seidemann W. *Allergologie* 1984;7:461.

SCIENTIFIC NAME(S): *Morinda citrifolia*

COMMON NAME(S): Morinda, noni, hog apple, Indian mulberry, mengkoedoe, mora de la India, pain killer, ruibarbo caribe, wild pine

---

⁂ PATIENT INFORMATION ⁂

Uses: Morinda has been used for heart remedies, arthritis, headache, and digestive and liver ailments.

Side Effects: No information is available on the side effects of morinda.

BOTANY: The *Morinda* plant, native to Asia, Australia, and Polynesia, is a 3 to 8 m high tree or shrub. Its evergreen leaves are oblong and 10 to 45 cm in length. The plant's white flowers are tubular, with cone-like heads. The fruit is yellow-white, oval, and about the size of a potato and with a "bumpy" surface. The ripened fruit has a cheese-like, offensive odor. Each fruit contains 4 seeds, 3 mm in length.[1]

HISTORY: It is believed that Polynesian healers have used morinda fruits for thousands of years to help treat a variety of health problems such as diabetes, high blood pressure, arthritis, and aging. Ancient healing manuscripts cite the fruit as a primary ingredient in natural healing formulations. Today, morinda is sold as juice, dried fruit, and capsules of dry extract. US patents can also be found, such as for processing morinda fruit into powder,[2] and for xeronine, an alkaloid isolated for medical, food, and industrial use.[3]

PHARMACOLOGY: Morinda has been used for heart remedies, arthritis (by wrapping the leaves around affected joints), headache (local application of leaves on forehead), and GI and liver ailments.[1]

It has been theorized that xeronine works at a molecular level to repair damaged cells, regulating their function. It is claimed that all body cells and systems, including digestive, respiratory, bone, and skin can benefit.[2]

Alcoholic extracts of morinda leaves displayed good anthelmintic activity in vitro against human *Ascaris lumbricoides*.[4] Lyophilized aqueous root extracts of the plant showed central analgesic activity, among other effects, suggesting sedative properties of the plant as well.[5]

The fruit is eaten layered in sugar, and leaves are consumed raw or cooked. The roots yield a red dye; the bark, a yellow dye.[1]

TOXICOLOGY: No information is available about the toxicity of morinda or its constituents. The fruit has long been reported as edible.

---

[1] Morton J. *Atlas of Medicinal Plants of Middle America.* Springfield, IL: Charles C. Thomas Publ., 1981;868-69.

[2] US patent # 5,288,491, Feb. 22, 1994.

[3] US patent # 4,409,144, Oct. 11,1983.

[4] Raj R. *Indian J Physiol Pharmacol* 1975;19(1):47-49.

[5] Younos C, et al. *Planta Med* 1990;56(5):430-34.

SCIENTIFIC NAME(S): *Commiphora molmol* Engl. Synonymous with *C. myrrha*, *C. abyssinica*, and other *Commiphora* species are used in commerce. Family: Burseraceae

COMMON NAME(S): African myrrh, Somali myrrh (*C. molmol*), Arabian and Yemen myrrh (*C. abyssinica*), myrrha, gum myrrh,[1] bola, bal, bol, heerabol[2]

❧❧❧ PATIENT INFORMATION ❧❧❧

Uses: Myrrh has been used as a fragrance, flavoring, astringent, antiseptic, emmenagogue, antispasmodic, and treatment for cancer and infectious diseases.

Side Effects: It has reportedly been associated with dermatitis.

BOTANY: The Commiphora species are trees that grow to heights of 9 m. They are native to Africa and are found in the Red Sea region. A pale yellow-white viscous liquid exudes from natural cracks in the bark or from fissures cut to harvest the material.[2] This exudate hardens into yellow-brown tears that weigh up to 250 g that form myrrh resin.[1,2]

HISTORY: Myrrh has been used for centuries[2] as an astringent, antiseptic, emmenagogue, and antispasmodic. It also has been used to treat a variety of infectious diseases (including leprosy and syphilis) and cancers.[1] Myrrh played a key role in ancient Egyptian religious ceremonies.[3] It finds use in African, Middle Eastern, and Chinese traditional medicine. Today, myrrh is used in fragrances, mouthwashes, and gargles.[1,4] It is sometimes used to flavor beverages and foods.

PHARMACOLOGY: Myrrh has mild astringent properties[5] and has antimicrobial activity in vitro.[1]

Myrrh has a locally stimulating action on smooth muscle tissue and may stimulate peristalsis.[6,7]

TOXICOLOGY: Although myrrh is generally considered to be nonirritating, nonsensitizing, and nonphototoxic to skin,[1] dermatitis due to myrrh has been reported.[8]

[1] Leung AY. *Encyclopedia of Common Natural Ingredients Used in Food, Drugs and Cosmetics.* New York, NY: John Wiley and Sons, 1980.

[2] Evans, WC. *Trease and Evans' Pharmacognosy.* 13th ed. London: Balliere Tindall, 1989.

[3] Dobelis IN. *Magic and Medicine of Plants.* Pleasantville, NY: Reader's Digest Association, 1986.

[4] Michie CA, et al. *J R Soc Med* 1991;84:602.

[5] Tyler VE. *The Honest Herbal: a sensible guide to the use of herbs and related remedies.* Binghamton, NY: The Haworth Press, 1993.

[6] Spoerke DG. *Herbal Medications.* Santa Barbara, CA: Woodbridge Press, 1980.

[7] Morton JF. *Major Medicinal Plants.* Springfield, IL: Charles C. Thomas, 1977.

[8] Lee TY, et al. *Contact Dermatitis* 1993;28:89.

Nettles

SCIENTIFIC NAME(S): *Urtica dioica* L. Family: Urticaceae

COMMON NAME(S): Stinging nettle, nettle

❧❧❧ PATIENT INFORMATION ❧❧❧

Uses: Proven as a diuretic, nettles are also being investigated as treatment for hay fever and irrigation of the urinary tract.

Side Effects: External side effects result from skin contact and take the form of burning and stinging that persist for ≥ 12 hours. Internal side effects are rare and are allergic in nature.

BOTANY: Nettles are perennial plants native to Europe and found throughout the US and parts of Canada. This plant has an erect stalk and stands up to 0.9 m. It has dark green serrated leaves that grow opposite each other along the stalk. The plant flowers from June to September. The leaves contain bristles that transmit irritating principles upon contact. The nettle fruit is a small, oval, yellow-brown seed ≈ 1 mm wide.[1]

HISTORY: This plant is known for its stinging properties. However, it has been used in traditional medicine as a diuretic, antispasmodic, expectorant, and treatment for asthma. The juice has been purported to stimulate hair growth when applied to the scalp. Extracts of the leaves have been used topically for the treatment of rheumatic disorders. The tender tips of young nettles have been used as a cooked pot herb in salads.

PHARMACOLOGY: Nettles mainly have diuretic actions. Treatment over 14 days increases urine volume and decreases systolic blood pressure.[1] Nettle's claims against diabetes, cancer, eczema, rheumatism, hair loss, and aging have been reported[2,3] but are unsubstantiated. Other folk medicine applications include wound healing, treatment of scalp seborrhea and greasy hair, and gastric juice secretion.[1] A combination product includes nettle to treat hyposecretory gastritis.[4]

Nettle in a combination product containing several other herbs has been tested in 22 patients for bladder irrigation. Postoperative blood loss, bacteriuria, and inflammation were reduced following prostatic adenomectomy.[5] The German Commission E Monograph supports this indication by its similar listing for "irrigation in inflammation of the urinary tract and in the prevention and treatment of kidney gravel."[1] Nettles' use in expelling bile has been studied.[6]

Nettles in a combined extract with pygeum (*Pygeum africanum*, see page 189) was studied as a treatment of benign prostatic hyperplasia (BPH) in 134 patients. It was effective in reducing urine flow, nocturia, and residual urine. A 300 mg dose of the plant extract was as effective as 150 mg.[7] A possible mechanism may be a hydrophobic constituent (eg, steroidal), which inhibits the sodium-potassium ATP-ase activity of the prostate, leading to suppressed cell growth in this area.[8] Another report posits a different mechanism but suggests the aqueous extract is the active component in BPH therapy to inhibit the sex hormone-binding globulin to its receptor.[9]

Freeze-dried nettles have been evaluated for allergic rhinitis. In a double-blind trial, 57% of 69 hay fever sufferers who completed the trial judged the nettles preparations to be moderately to highly effective in treatment vs placebo.[10]

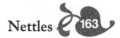
A study concerning a lectin present in nettles suggests a potent and selective inhibitor of HIV and cytomegalovirus replication in vitro. When evaluated for its antidiabetic effect, nettles slightly increased glycemia, aggravating the condition in 2 reports.[11,12]

TOXICOLOGY: Nettles are known primarily for their ability to induce topical irritation following contact with exposed skin, accompanied by a stinging sensation lasting $\geq$ 12 hours. A report closely associates mast cells and dermal dendritic cells. Immediate reaction to nettle stings is caused by histamine content, while the persistence of the sting may be caused by other substances directly toxic to nerves.[13]

The stinging hairs of the nettle plant comprise a fine capillary tube, a bladder-like base filled with the chemical irritant, and a minute spherical tip, which breaks off on contact, leaving a sharp point that penetrates the skin. The irritants are forced into the skin as the hair bends and constricts the bladder at the base.

Topical irritation is treated by gently washing the affected area with mild soapy water. Treatment with systemic antihistamines and topical steroids may be of benefit. Other side effects of nettle are rare but include allergic effects such as edema, oliguria, and gastric irritation.[1]

[1] Bisset N. *Herbal Drugs and Phytopharmaceuticals*, Stuttgart, Germany: CRC Press. 1994;502-7.

[2] Atasu E, et al. *Farmasotik Bilimler Dergisi* 1984;9(2):73-81.

[3] Wichtl M. *Deutsche Apotheker Zeitung* 1992 Jul 23;132:1569-76.

[4] Krivenko V, et al. *Vrachebnoe Delo* 1989;(3):76-78.

[5] Davidov M, et al. *Urologiia I Nefrologiia* 1995;(5):19-20.

[6] Rossiiskaya G, et al. *Farmatsiia* 1985;34(1):38-41.

[7] Krzeski T, et al. *Clin Ther* 1993;15(6):1011-20.

[8] Hirano T, et al. *Planta Med* 1994;60(1):30-33.

[9] Hryb D, et al. *Planta Med* 1995;61(1):31-32.

[10] Mittman P. *Planta Med* 1990;56(1):44-47.

[11] Swanston-Flatt S, et al. *Diabetes Res* 1989;10(2):69-73.

[12] Roman R, et al. *Arch Med Res* 1992;23(1):59-64.

[13] Oliver F, et al. *Clin Exp Dermatol* 1991;16(1):1-7.

Nutmeg

SCIENTIFIC NAME(S): *Myristica fragrans* Houtt. Family: Myristicaceae

COMMON NAME(S): Nutmeg, mace, nux moschata

❧❧❧ PATIENT INFORMATION ❧❧❧

Uses: Nutmeg is used as a flavoring agent and a fragrance. It has also been used as a larvicidal, a hallucinogen, and treatment for diarrhea, mouth sores, and insomnia.

Side Effects: Side effects after ingestion of large quantities include weak pulse, hypothermia, disorientation, giddiness, nausea, vomiting, a feeling of pressure in the chest or lower abdomen, a sensation of loss of limbs, a fear of impending death, and, after a very large dose, death.

BOTANY: The nutmeg tree is the source of nutmeg and mace. This evergreen grows to > 18 m. It is found in India, Ceylon, Malaysia, and Granada. This slow-growing tree produces a fruit called a nutmeg apple, which looks like a peach or apricot. When the fruit ripens, it splits to expose a bright-red, net-like aril wrapped around a shell, which contains the nut. The nut is removed and dried to produce nutmeg. The dried aril yields the spice mace, which tastes similar to nutmeg.[1,2]

HISTORY: Nutmeg is a widely used spice that has received attention as an alternative hallucinogen. Nutmeg and mace have been used in Indian cooking and folk medicine. Folk uses of nutmeg included treatment of gastric disorders and rheumatism, and it has been used as a hypnotic[3] and an aphrodisiac.[4]

Pliny, in the 1st century, described a "comacum" tree with a fragrant nut and 2 perfumes. During the 6th century, nutmeg and mace were imported by Arab traders. By the 12th century, these spices were well known in Europe. Chaucer writes of "nutmeg in ale" in *The Canterbury Tales* during the 14th century.[5]

At the turn of the 19th century, interest developed in the use of nutmeg as an abortifacient and menstrual stimulant. These properties have been largely discounted but remain a persistent cause of nutmeg intoxication in women with delayed menses.[6,7]

PHARMACOLOGY: Nutmeg was known for its psychoactive properties as early as the year 1525 and has gained a reputation among inmates and drug cultists as a hallucinogen.[8] Doses of 5 to 20 g appear to be required for pharmacologic activity to occur. This is equivalent to 1 to 3 whole nuts; 2 tablespoons of commercial ground nutmeg weight, ≈ 14 g; or 2 grated nuts.[9]

Debate surrounds the issue of whether myristicin is the psychoactive component of nutmeg. It does not appear that myristicin alone can induce hallucinations.[10] Because synthetic myristicin does not imitate nutmeg intoxication, it has been suggested that the presence of other compounds (eugenol, geraniol) may be needed for the characteristic pharmacologic effect.[11] The structural similarities of the allyl benzene components of nutmeg to those of amphetamine-like compounds may be responsible for the CNS activity of the spice.[12] A similarity exists among the metabolites of nutmeg, amphetamine and mescaline.

The effects of nutmeg intoxication are variable, and the loss of the volatile oil from the ground spice results, in part, in the variability of the experience. Generally, nutmeg for intoxication is

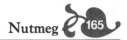

Nutmeg 165

chewed or the powdered nut is suspended in a liquid and consumed. Geraniol, another constituent, is ≈ 3 times as potent as ipecac in inducing emesis; hence, users may combine ground nutmeg with cola syrup to avoid emesis. This mixture is appropriately referred to as "brown slime."[13]

Nutmeg has been used in the treatment of human diarrhea secondary to thyroid medullary carcinoma[14] and in the treatment of human diarrhea in doses of 4 to 6 tablespoons of nutmeg/day. A fall in serum calcium levels was also noted, improving chronic hypercalcemia possibly related to this therapy.[15] Inhibition of the synthesis and activity of prostaglandins appears to be responsible for this effect.[16] In human colon resections, nutmeg reduced prostaglandin-like activity in doses from 0.1 to 500 mcg/ml (however, at 5 mcg/ml, an increase, not understood, was noted).[17] Eugenol appears to be the most potent antiprostaglandin component of nutmeg oil.[18] A report on 2 subjects found no differences in aggregation using 1.5 to 4 g of freshly ground nutmeg 3 to 4 times a day for a 2-day period.[19] Other uses of nutmeg include as a larvicidal agent, a flavoring agent in many foods, and a fragrance component in soaps and perfumes.[1]

Nutmeg has also been used for mouth sores and insomnia.[20]

TOXICOLOGY: Symptoms appear 3 to 8 hours after ingestion of large amounts. The episodes are characterized by weak pulse, hypothermia, disorientation, giddiness, nausea and vomiting, and a feeling of pressure in the chest or lower abdomen. For up to 24 hours, an extended period of alternating delirium and stupor persists, ending in a heavy sleep. There is often a sensation of loss of limbs and a fear of impending death. Death has been reported following the ingestion of a very large dose.[21] A 25-year-old male showed psychotic symptoms upon ingestion of 120 to 650 mg nutmeg. Haloperidol therapy was necessary to stabilize the patient.[22] Another case report discusses similar findings in a 23-year-old with acute psychotic break and anticholinergic toxic episode symptoms, such as hallucinations and palpitations.[23] In a similar case, an acute anticholinergic hyperstimulation occurred in a pregnant woman after excessive nutmeg ingestion.[24] Gastric lavage and supportive therapy have been recommended for nutmeg toxicity.[25] Recovery usually occurs within 24 hours but may take several days.[26]

[1] Leung A, et al. *Encyclopedia of Common Natural Ingredients.* New York, NY: John Wiley and Sons, Inc., 1996;385-88.

[2] Dermarderosian A, et al. *Natural Product Medicine.* Philadelphia, PA: G. F. Stickley Co., 1988;329-31.

[3] Forrest JE, et al. *Lloydia* 1972;35:440.

[4] Weil AF. *J Psyc Drugs* 1971;3:72.

[5] Rosengarten F. *The Book of Spices.* Wynnewood, PA: Livingston Publishing Co., 1969;308-15.

[6] Green RC. *JAMA* 1959;171:1342.

[7] Painter JC, et al. *Clin Toxicol* 1971;4:1.

[8] Faguet RA, et al. *Am J Psychiatry* 1978;135:860.

[9] Mack RB. *N Carolina Med J* 1982 Jun;439.

[10] Farnsworth NR. *Am J Psychiatry* 1979;136:858.

[11] Truitt EB, et al. *J Neuropsych* 1961;2:205.

[12] Weil AT. *Economic Botany* 1965;19:194.

[13] Giannini AJ, et al. *Am Fam Physician* 1986;33:207.

[14] Barrowman J, et al. *BMJ* 1975 Jul 5;3:11-12.

[15] Shafran I, et al. *N Engl J Med* 1975 Dec 11;293:1266.

[16] Fawell W, et al. *N Engl J Med* 1973 Jul 12;289:108-9.

[17] Bennett A, et al. *N Engl J Med* 1974 Jan 10;290:110-11.

[18] Rasheed A, et al. *N Engl J Med* 1984;310:50.

[19] Dietz W, et al. *N Engl J Med* 1976 Feb 26;294:503.

[20] Van Gils C. *J Ethnopharmacol* 1994;42(2):117-24.

[21] Updyke DLT. *Food Cosmet Toxicol* 1976;14:631.

[22] Brenner N, et al. *J R Soc Med* 1993 Mar;86:179-80.

23 Abernethy N, et al. *Am J Emerg Med* 1992;10(5):429-30.

24 Lavy G. *J Reprod Med* 1987;32(1):63-64.

25 Hardin JW, et al. *Human Poisoning from Native and Cultivated Plants.* Duke University Press, 1974.

26 Brown JK, et al. *Pacific Information Service on Street Drugs* 1977;5:20.

SCIENTIFIC NAME(S): *Nerium oleander* L. Synonymous with *N. indicum* Mill. Family: Apocyanaceae

COMMON NAME(S): Oleander, adelfa, laurier rose, rosa laurel, rose bay, rosa francesa[1]

❦❦❦❦ PATIENT INFORMATION ❦❦❦❦

Uses: Oleander has been used in traditional medicine for treatment of cardiac illness, asthma, corns, cancer, and epilepsy.

Side Effects: Extreme, digitalis-like toxicity precludes oleander use in any form. Toxicity signs include pain in the oral cavity, nausea, emesis, abdominal pain, cramping, and diarrhea.

BOTANY: The oleander is a shrub that grows to ≈ 6 m in height. It has long narrow leaves that attain almost 30 cm in length and are typically grouped in 3s around the stem. The red, pink, or white fluffy flowers form in small clusters. Cultivated plants rarely produce fruits.[1] Although native to the Mediterranean, the oleander is widely cultivated throughout warm climates.

HISTORY: Despite its toxic potential, the oleander has been used in traditional medicine for centuries for the management of cardiac illnesses, asthma, corns, cancer, and epilepsy.[2]

PHARMACOLOGY: All parts of the plant contain the cardiac glycosides oleandrin, neriin, gentiobiosyloleandrin, and odoroside A[2] and other pharmacologically active compounds, including folinerin, rosagenin, rutin, and oleandomycin.[2]

The flavonol glycosides influence vascular permeability and possess diuretic properties. Cornerine has been effective in the treatment of cardiac ailments, improving heart muscle function.[2]

TOXICOLOGY: The entire oleander plant is toxic. Smoke from the plant and water in which the plant has been immersed also can be toxic.[1] Deaths have been reported in children who ingested a handful of flowers and in adults who used the fresh twigs as meat skewers; the nectar makes honey toxic.[2,3]

Symptoms of toxicity include oral cavity pain, nausea, emesis, abdominal pain, cramping, and diarrhea. Special attention must be given to cardiac function. The cardioactive glycosides may induce conduction defects such as sinus bradycardia, and systemic hyperkalemia induced by the plant may worsen cardiac function.[1]

Oleander toxicity should be managed aggressively. Gastric lavage or induced emesis should be done, and activated charcoal may be administered orally. Saline cathartics have been of use. ECG monitoring for cardiac impairment and monitoring of serum potassium levels should be done frequently, and the conduction defects should be managed with atropine, phenytoin, transvenous pacing or other appropriate antiarrhythmic treatment, depending on the characteristics of the impairment.[1]

Assays for serum digoxin levels were conducted in a patient who ingested oleander; the levels of the glycoside were high (4.4 ng/ml) and were associated with bradyarrhythmias and tachyarrhythmias, which decreased as the serum concentration of the toxin decreased.[4]

Digoxin-specific Fab has been used successfully to treat human oleander toxicity.[5,6]

[1] Lampe KE. *AMA Handbook of Poisonous and Injurious Plants*. Chicago, IL: Chicago Review Press, 1985.

[2] Duke JA. *Handbook of Medicinal Herbs*. Boca Raton, FL: CRC Press, 1985.

[3] Osol A, et al, eds. *The Dispensatory of the United States of America*, 25th ed. Philadelphia, PA: JB Lippincott, 1955.

[4] Mesa MD, et al. *Rev Esp Cardiol* 1991;44:347.

[5] Romano GA, et al. *Schweiz Med Wochenschr* 1990;120:596.

[6] Bayer MJ. *Am J Emerg Med* 1991;9(2 Suppl 1):29.

SCIENTIFIC NAME(S): *Petroselinum crispum* (Mill.) Mansfield, *P. hortense* Hoffman, and *P. sativum* Family: Umbelliferae

COMMON NAME(S): Parsley, rock parsley, garden parsley

ᕮᕮᕮ PATIENT INFORMATION ᕮᕮᕮ

Uses: Parsley, in addition to being a source of vitamins and minerals, has been used in the treatment of prostate, liver, and spleen diseases, anemia, arthritis, and cancer.

Side Effects: Adverse effects from the ingestion of parsley oil include headache, giddiness, loss of balance, convulsions, and renal damage. Pregnant women should not take parsley because of its potential uterotonic effects.

BOTANY: Parsley is an herb indigenous to the Mediterranean but is now cultivated world-wide. It is deep green, with much-divided, curled leaves.

HISTORY: Parsley leaves and roots are popular as condiments and garnish. In Lebanon, parsley is a major ingredient in a national dish called tabbouleh. An average adult may consume as much as 50 g parsley per meal.[1]

Parsley seeds were used traditionally as a carminative to decrease flatulence and colic pain. The root was used as a diuretic and the juice to treat kidney ailments. Parsley oil has also been used to regulate menstrual flow in the treatment of amenorrhea and dysmenorrhea, and is purported to be an abortifacient. Bruised leaves have been used to treat tumors, insect bites, lice and skin parasites, and contusions.[2,3] Parsley tea once was used to treat dysentery and gallstones.[2] Other traditional uses include the treatment of diseases of the prostate, liver, and spleen, anemia, and arthritis; as an expectorant, antimicrobial, aphrodisiac, hypotensive, laxative; and as a scalp lotion to stimulate hair growth.[2,4]

PHARMACOLOGY: Parsley is a good natural source of vitamins and minerals including calcium, iron, carotene, ascorbic acid, and vitamin A.[2,5]

Myristicin, a component of parsley oil, has been thought to be in part responsible for the hallucinogenic effect of nutmeg. It is not known whether parsley oil induces hallucinations, but smoking parsley as a cannabis substitute was common during the 1960s. Parsley may have been smoked for a euphoric effect or as a carrier for potent drugs such as phencyclidine.[6]

Apiol, another parsley component, is an antipyretic and, like myristicin, is a uterine stimulant. Apiol was once available in capsules for use as an abortifacient. Although the effectiveness of this compound as a uterotonic has not been quantitated, a Russian product called "Supetin" (which contains about 85% parsley juice) is used to stimulate uterine contractions during labor.[7] Data regarding the safety and efficacy of this drug are not readily available.

Apiol and myristicin may be responsible for the mild diuretic effect of the seeds and oil.[8] Parsley extracts have shown slight antibacterial and antifungal activity when tested in vitro,[9] but it is not known to what extent this activity is retained in vivo.

TOXICOLOGY: Adverse effects from parsley are uncommon. People allergic to other members of the Umbelliferae family (carrot, fennel, celery) may be sensitive to the constituents (especially in the flowers) of parsley. Because of the potential uterotonic effects, parsley oil, juice, and seeds should not be taken by pregnant women. Adverse effects from the ingestion of the oil have included headache, giddiness, loss of balance, convulsions, and renal damage.

The psoralen compounds found in parsley have been linked to a photoderma-titis reaction found among parsley cutters. This skin reaction is usually only evident if the areas that have contacted the juice are exposed to very strong sunlight; it can be minimized by the use of protective clothing and sunscreens.[10]

[1] Zaynoun S, et al. *Clin Exp Dermatol* 1985;10:328.

[2] Duke JA. *Handbook of Medicinal Herbs*. Boca Raton, FL: CRC Press, 1985.

[3] Meyer J. *The Herbalist*. Hammond, IN: Hammond Book Co., 1934.

[4] Hoffman D. *The Herbal Handbook*. Rochester, VT: Healing Arts Press, 1988.

[5] Tyler VE, et al. *Pharmacognosy*, 9th ed. Philadelphia, PA: Lea & Febiger, 1988.

[6] Cook CE, et al. *Clin Pharm Ther* 1982;31:635.

[7] Chemical Abstracts 90:115465, 1979.

[8] Marczal G, et al. *Acta Agron Acad Sci Hung* 1977;26:7.

[9] Ross SA, et al. *Fitotherapia* 1980;51:303.

[10] Smith DA. *Practitioner* 1985;229:673.

SCIENTIFIC NAME(S): *Passiflora incarnata* L. Family: Passifloraceae

COMMON NAME(S): Passion flower; Maypop, apricot vine, wild passion flower

---

ꙥꙥ PATIENT INFORMATION ꙥꙥ

Uses: Passion flower has been used to treat sleep disorders and, historically, in homeopathic medicine to treat pain, insomnia related to neurasthenia or hysteria, and nervous exhaustion.

Side Effects: Although no adverse side effects of the passion flower have been reported, large doses may result in CNS depression.

BOTANY: The term "passion flower" connotes many of the roughly 400 species of the genus *Passiflora*, which includes primarily vines. Some of the species are noted for their showy flowers, others for their edible fruit. *Passiflora* species are native to tropical and subtropical areas of the Americas. In the US, passion flower is found from Virginia to Florida and as far west as Missouri and Texas. The flowers of *Passiflora* have 5 petals, sepals, and stamens, 3 stigmas, and a crown of filaments. The fruit is egg-shaped, with a pulpy consistency, and includes many small seeds.

HISTORY: The passion flower was discovered in 1569 by Spanish explorers in Peru, who saw the flowers as symbolic of the passion of Christ and hence a sign of Christ's approval of their efforts.[2] The folklore surrounding this plant may date further in the past, with the floral parts representing the elements of the crucifixion (3 styles represent 3 nails, the ovary looks like a hammer, the corona is the crown of thorns, the petals represent the 10 true apostles).[3]

In Europe it has been used in homeopathic medicine to treat pain, insomnia related to neurasthenia or hysteria, and nervous exhaustion. Other indications have included bronchial disorders (particularly asthma), in compresses for burns and against inflammation, inflamed hemorrhoids, climacteric complaints, pediatric attention disorders, and pediatric nervousness and excitability.[4]

PHARMACOLOGY: Animal studies have shown that *Passiflora* extracts have a complex activity on the CNS, inducing dose-dependent stimulation and depression.[5] There is disagreement as to which components contribute most to the pharmacologic effect.

The neurodepressive effects of the extracts have been used to treat sleep disorders; however, few clinical trials exist to support this therapeutic effect. The pharmacologic activity of *Passiflora* is attributed chiefly to the alkaloids and flavonoids, which are present in low concentrations. At low doses (3 to 6 mg), harman alkaloids have produced CNS effects similar to those of coffee or tea. Doses of 15 to 35 mg have caused strong motor unrest, followed by drowsiness. Higher doses have produced hallucinations, very severe motor unrest, and vomiting. The harmala alkaloids in passion flower have been found to inhibit monoamine oxidase, and this may account for part of their pharmacologic effect.[6]

Harmala alkaloids have a spasmolytic effect on smooth muscle, lower blood pressure, and dilate coronary vessels. Systemic clearance is rapid: Less than 10% of an injected dose of 0.5 mg/kg can be found in the blood after 2 minutes, and only 1% is found after 4 hours. The entire dose is excreted in the urine within 24 hours.

Recent studies have demonstrated that the sedative effect of passion flower may occur only when complexes of alkaloids and flavonoids are present.[7] In dry extract of passion flower, an acid-soluble fraction was found to contain 0.05% maltol. Maltol and ethyl maltol may mask the stimulant effects of passion flower's harmala alkaloids.[6]

In vitro experiments have demonstrated that passicol, a passion flower constituent, kills a wide variety of molds, yeasts, and bacteria. Group A hemolytic streptococci are much more susceptible than *Staphylococcus aureus,* with *Candida albicans* being intermediate in susceptibility. The antimicrobial activity of passicol disappears rapidly from dried plant residues and fades gradually in aqueous extracts. Addition of dextran, milk, or milk products has a stabilizing effect on dry passicol.[8]

TOXICOLOGY: Little information is available on the clinical toxicity of passion flower.[9] Although no significant human toxicity has been reported, the pharmacologic profile of passion flower extracts suggests that large doses may result in CNS depression.

[1] Seymour ELD. *The Garden Encyclopedia*. New York, NY: Wm. H. Wise, 1940.

[2] *Encyclopedia Americana*. Danbury, CT: Grolier, 1987.

[3] Tyler, VE. *The New Honest Herbal*, Philadelphia, PA: G.F. Stickley Co., 1987.

[4] Lutomski J, et al. *Pharm Unserer Zeit* 1981;10:45.

[5] Speroni E, et al. *Planta Med* 1988;54:488.

[6] Aoyagi N, et al. *Chem Pharm Bull* 1974;22:1008.

[7] Lutomski J, et al. *Planta Med* 1975;27:381.

[8] Nicolls JM, et al. *Antimicrob Agents Chemother* 1973;3:110.

SCIENTIFIC NAME(S): *Lapacho colorado,* L. *morado.* References to *Tabebuia avellanedae* Lorentz ex Griseb are more accurately described as *T. impetiginosa* (Mart.) Standl. and references to *T. altissima* cannot be validated because this is not an acknowledged species.[1] Family: Bignoniaceae

COMMON NAME(S): Pau D'Arco, lapacho, ipes, trumpet bush, taheebo

---

﹩﹩﹩ PATIENT INFORMATION ﹩﹩﹩

Uses: The bark and extracts of taheebo have been used as herbal teas with no known curative properties.

Side Effects: Some side effects reported with taheebo have been nausea, dizziness, and rarely, diarrhea.

BOTANY: The inner bark of *L. colorado* and *L. morado* (purple lapacho) are used in the preparation of Taheebo. *L. colorado* or red lapacho, so called because of its scarlet flowers, grows in Northern Argentina, Brazil, and Paraguay and has been used for centuries by the medicine men of the native Indian tribes. Another name for Lapacho is Ipes, a name used in Brazil. Red Lapacho is called Ipe roxo. Still another name for the tree is Pau D'Arco, which means "bow stick;" the natives use the wood to make archery bows.

HISTORY: According to reports in the Brazilian and American lay press, teas prepared from the inner bark of these trees have been used successfully to treat various diseases including leukemia, diabetes, and cancer. Folk uses have included the treatment of boils, chlorosis, syphilis, and external wounds. Extracts of the plant have recently been used topically for the management of *Candida albicans* infections.

PHARMACOLOGY: Lapachol and the related compound xyloidone, found in taheebo, have been assessed for antimicrobial activity; lapachol was active against gram-positive and acid-fast bacilli but inactive toward yeasts and fungi, while xyloidone was active against *Brucella* and *Candida.* Lapachol is an active antimalarial and antitrypanosome.[2] Aqueous extracts of taheebo have been shown to be inactive against *Candida* cultures. Aqueous extracts of taheebo bark inhibited the growth of an animal tumor system (Walker 256 carcinoma) by 44% following doses of 200 mg/kg IP in rats. Lapachol inhibited Yoshida sarcoma and Walker 256 carcinoma by 82% and 50%, respectively; β-lapachone showed somewhat less antitumor activity.[3] The Natural Products Branch of the National Cancer Institute (NCI) has tested taheebo extensively for antineoplastic activity. Screening of Tabebuia found that the antitumor activity observed in aqueous extracts could not reasonably be attributed to lapachol or related lapachones, but may be due to unidentified compounds or a "prodrug" compound. Because of its activity in the Walker 256 system, lapachol was approved for human testing by the NCI. No antineoplastic effects were observed, presumably because absorption of oral lapachol was incomplete (blood levels never reached 30 mcg/ml, the critical antitumor concentration, despite doses of 50 mg/kg).[2] The drug was subsequently eliminated from the testing program.

Since the first Brazilian reports in the early 1960s describing the antineoplastic properties of taheebo tea, anecdotal stories have continued to praise its curative properties. Brazilian researchers have reported encouraging results based on very limited patient observations. Although it is still used by some South American physicians, the Brazilian Cancer Society strongly disputes the claims made for taheebo. When evaluated in concentrations ranging from 0.01 to 1 mg/ml, lapachol was found to cause a cytotoxic or immunosuppressive effect on human granulocytes and lymphocytes; in the lower doses, however, the compound showed immunostimulant properties.[4]

TOXICOLOGY: The LD–50 of lapachol and β-lapachone administered IP to rats were 1600 mg/kg and 80 mg/kg, respectively. Oral administration of multiple doses of lapachol 500 mg/kg to rats caused death with severe histopathologic changes in most organs. At 9 mg/kg, β-lapachone caused death after 6 doses with anorexia, weight loss, and diarrhea.[5] In clinical trials, oral lapachol caused nausea, vomiting, and anticoagulant effects.[6] These latter effects were reversible with vitamin K. Brazilian researchers reported nausea, dizziness, and rarely, diarrhea.

[1] Tyler VE, Ph.D., written communication, October, 1983.

[2] Awang DVC. *Can Pharm J* 1988;5:323.

[3] Rao KV, et al. *Cancer Res* 1968;28:1952.

[4] Wagner H, et al. *Planta Med* 1986;52:550.

[5] Ferreira de Santana C, et al. *Chem Abstract* 74:40989.

[6] Block JB, et al. *Cancer Chemother Reports* 1974;24:27.

SCIENTIFIC NAME(S): *Hedeoma pulegeoides* (L.) Persoon and *Mentha pulegium* L. Family: Labiatae

COMMON NAME(S): Pennyroyal, squawmint, mosquito plant, pudding grass

---

❧❧❧ PATIENT INFORMATION ❧❧❧

Uses: Pennyroyal may be used as an insect repellent, antiseptic, fragrance, flavoring, emmenagogue, carminative, stimulant, or antispasmodic, and for bowel disorders, skin eruptions, and pneumonia.

Side Effects: Pennyroyal can cause abdominal pain, nausea, vomiting, lethargy, increased blood pressure, increased pulse rate, and dermatitis, and, in large quantities, abortion, irreversible renal damage, severe liver damage, and death. A teaspoon of oil can produce delirium, unconsciousness, shock, seizures, and auditory and visual hallucinations.

BOTANY: *H. pulegeoides* (American pennyroyal) grows in woods through most of the northern and eastern US and Canada, while *M. pulegium* is found in parts of Europe. Both plants are members of the mint family and both are referred to as pennyroyal. Pennyroyal is a perennial, creeping herb that possesses small, lilac flowers at the stem ends. It can grow to 30 to 50 cm in height. The leaves are grayish green and, like those of other mint family members, are very aromatic.[1,2]

HISTORY: Pennyroyal has been recorded in history as far back as the 1st century, where it was mentioned by Roman naturalist Pliny and Greek physician Dioscorides. In the 17th century, English herbalist Nicholas Culpeper wrote about uses for the plant including its role in women's ailments, venomous bites, and digestion. European settlers used the plant for respiratory ailments, mouth sores, and female disorders.[1] The plant's oil has been used as a flea-killing bath, hence the name *pulegeoides* (from the Latin word meaning flea), and has been used externally as a rubefacient. In addition, the oil has been used frequently among natural health advocates as an abortifacient and as a means of inducing delayed menses.

The oil and infusions of the leaves have been used in the treatment of weakness and stomach pains.[3]

PHARMACOLOGY: Pennyroyal has been used as an insect repellent and antiseptic.[1,2,4,5] It has been employed as a flavoring agent for food and spice[5] and also as a fragrance in detergents, perfumes, and soaps.[2,5]

The plant has been reported to be of use for female problems as an emmenagogue (to induce menstruation). It has also been used as a carminative, stimulant, and antispasmodic, and for bowel disorders, skin eruptions, pneumonia, and other uses.[1,2,4,5]

TOXICOLOGY: Pennyroyal herb teas are generally used without reported side effects (presumably because of low concentration of the oil),[4] but toxicity for pennyroyal oil is well recognized, with many reports of adverse events and fatalities.

American or European pennyroyal can cause dermatitis and, in large doses, abortion, irreversible renal damage, severe liver damage, and death. A teaspoonful of the oil can produce delirium, unconsciousness, and shock.[5]

One case of pennyroyal oil ingestion resulted in generalized seizures and auditory and visual hallucinations following the ingestion of < 5 ml of the oil; the patient recovered uneventfully.[6] Other symptoms of plant ingestion may also include abdominal pain, nausea, vomiting, lethargy, increased blood pressure, and increased pulse rate.[4]

The major component, pulegone, is oxidized by hepatic cytochrome P450 to the hepatotoxic compound menthofuran.[7] Pulegone, or a metabolite, is also responsible for neurotoxicity and destruction of bronchiolar epithelial cells.[8,9]

Pulegone extensively depletes glutathione in the liver, and its metabolites are detoxified by the presence of glutathione in the liver. Hepatic toxicity has been prevented by the early administration of acetylcysteine following ingestion of pennyroyal oil.[10] Various metabolite studies are available regarding hepatotoxicity.[11,12]

One woman who ingested up to 30 ml of the oil experienced abdominal cramps, nausea, vomiting, and alternating lethargy and agitation. She later exhibited loss of renal function, hepatotoxicity, and evidence of disseminated intravascular coagulation. She died 7 days after ingesting the oil. Another woman ingested 10 ml of the oil and only experienced dizziness.[13] Two infants (8 weeks of age and 6 months of age) who ingested mint tea containing pennyroyal oil developed hepatic and neurologic injury. One infant died; the other suffered hepatic dysfunction and severe epileptic encephalopathy.[14] A review of 18 previous cases reported moderate-to-severe toxicity in patients exposed to ≥ 10 ml of the oil, concluding that pennyroyal continues to be an herbal toxin of concern to public health.[15] Another review also concluded that pennyroyal oil is toxic.[16]

Pennyroyal is contraindicated in pregnancy. It possesses abortifacient actions and irritates the GU tract.[4] The abortifacient effect of the oil is thought to be caused by irritation of the uterus with subsequent uterine contraction. Its action is unpredictable and dangerous.[17] The dose at which the herb induces abortion is close to lethal, and in some cases it is lethal.[2,5] However, one letter does report a pregnancy unaffected by pennyroyal use.[18]

[1] Low T, et al. eds. *Magic and Medicine of Plants*. Sydney, Australia: Reader's Digest, 1994;278.

[2] Lawless J. *The Illustrated Encyclopedia of Essential Oils*. Rockport, MA: Element Books, Inc., 1995;176.

[3] Da Legnano LP. *The Medicinal Plants*. Rome, Italy: Edizioni Mediterranee, 1973.

[4] Newall C, et al. *Herbal Medicines*. London, England: Pharmaceutical Press, 1996;208.

[5] Duke J. *CRC Handbook of Medicinal Herbs*. Boca Raton, FL: CRC Press Inc., 1989;223,307-8.

[6] Early DF. *Lancet* 1961;2:580.

[7] Gordon WP, et al. *Drug Metab Disp* 1987;15(5):589.

[8] Thomassen D, et al. *J Pharmacol Exp Ther* 1990;253(2):567.

[9] Gordon WP, et al. *Toxicol Appl Pharmacol* 1982;65:413.

[10] Buechel DW, et al. *J Am Osteopath Assn* 1983;2:793.

[11] Thomassen D, et al. *J Pharmacol Exp Ther* 1988;244(3):825-29.

[12] Carmichael P. *Ann Intern Med* 1997;126(3):250-51.

[13] Sullivan JB Jr., et al. *JAMA* 1979;242:2873.

[14] Bakerink J, et al. *Pediatrics* 1996 Nov;98:944-47.

[15] Anderson I, et al. *Ann Intern Med* 1996;124(8):726-34.

[16] Mack R. *NC Med J* 1997;58(6):456-57.

[17] Allen WT. *Lancet* 1897;2:1022.

[18] Black D. *J Am Osteopath Assoc* 1985;85(5):282.

Peppermint

SCIENTIFIC NAME(S): *Mentha* x *piperita* L. Peppermint is a hybrid of *M. spicata* L. (spearmint) and *M. aquatica* L. Family: Labiatae

COMMON NAME(S): Peppermint

❧❧❧ PATIENT INFORMATION ❧❧❧

Uses: In addition to being recognized as a seasoning and flavoring, peppermint has been used to treat irritable bowel and abdominal pain.

Side Effects: Peppermint oil may cause allergic reactions characterized by contact dermatitis, flushing, and headache and worsen the symptoms of hiatal hernias.

BOTANY: This perennial is a classic member of the mint family. It has a squarish purple-green stem with dark green or purple leaves and lilac flowers. The plant is generally sterile and spreads by means of stolons (basal branches). A variety of peppermints exist and are cultivated worldwide.

HISTORY: Peppermint and its oil have been used in Eastern and Western traditional medicine as an aromatic, antispasmodic, and antiseptic in treating indigestion, nausea, sore throat, colds, toothaches, cramps, and cancers. Today, the oil is used as a flavoring and as an ingredient in cough and cold preparations. It is also in many antiseptic and local anesthetic preparations.

PHARMACOLOGY: As is observed with other volatile oils, peppermint oil possesses antibacterial activity in vitro. However, this has not been of significant clinical benefit. Peppermint extracts have been reported to have antiviral activity against Newcastle disease, herpes simplex, vaccinia, and other viruses in culture.[1]

Peppermint oil has exhibited spasmolytic activity on smooth muscles. Commercial preparations are available for the treatment of irritable bowel, abdominal pain, and related symptoms.[2] Generally administered as enteric-coated capsules, these preparations release their contents in the large intestine and colon; peppermint, therefore, appears to act directly on smooth muscle. The spasmolytic activity is related to menthol content, and it has been demonstrated that this activity is due to the calcium antagonist effect of menthol.[3]

TOXICOLOGY: Peppermint is generally recognized as safe for human consumption as a seasoning or flavoring, as are other mints from which menthol is derived as a plant extract.

Menthol, the major component of peppermint oil, may cause allergic reactions (characterized by contact dermatitis, flushing, and headache).[1] Application of menthol-containing ointment to the nostrils of an infant for the treatment of cold symptoms was reported to cause instant collapse.[2]

Because of the oil's ability to relax GI smooth muscle, people with hiatal hernias may experience worsening of symptoms while ingesting peppermint-containing preparations.

[1] Leung AY. *Encyclopedia of Common Natural Ingredients Used in Food, Drugs, and Cosmetics.* Wiley Interscience, 1980.

[2] Rees WDW, et al. *BMJ* 1979;2:835.
[3] Taylor BA, et al. Proceedings of the British Pharmacol Soc. April, 1985.

SCIENTIFIC NAME(S): *Plantago lanceolata* L., P. major L., *P. psyllium* L., *P. arenaria* Waldst. & Kit. (*P. ramosa* Asch.) (Spanish or French psyllium seed), *P. ovata* Forsk. (Blond or Indian plantago seed) Family: Plantaginaceae. (Not to be confused with *Musa paradisiaca*, or edible plantain.)

COMMON NAME(S): Plantain, Spanish psyllium, French psyllium, blond plantago, Indian plantago, psyllium seed, flea seed, black psyllium.

ꙮꙮꙮ PATIENT INFORMATION ꙮꙮꙮ

Uses: The psyllium in plantain has been used as GI therapy, to treat hyperlipidemia, as a topical agent to treat some skin problems, as an anti-inflammatory and diuretic, for anticancer effects, and for respiratory treatment.

Drug Interactions: Plantain may interact with lithium and carbamazepine, decreasing their plasma concentrations and effectiveness.

Side Effects: Adverse events include anaphylaxis, chest congestion, sneezing, watery eyes, occupational asthma, and a situation involving the occurence of a giant phytobezoar composed of psyllium seed husks.

BOTANY: Plantain is a perennial weed with almost worldwide distribution. There are ≈ 250 species, of which 20 have wide geographic ranges, 9 have discontinuous ranges, 200 are limited to 1 region, and 9 have very narrow ranges. *P. lanceolata* and *P. major* are among the most widely distributed.[1] Plantain species are herbs and shrubby plants characterized by basal leaves and inconspicuous flowers in heads or spikes. They grow aggressively. Plantain is wind-pollinated, facilitating its growth where there are no bees and few other plantain plants. It is very tolerant to viral infections. *P. major* produces 13,000 to 15,000 seeds per plant, and the seeds have been reported to remain viable in soil for up to 60 years. *P. lanceolata* produces 2500 to 10,000 seeds per plant and has a somewhat shorter seed viability. Plantain seeds can survive passage through the gut of birds and other animals, facilitating their distribution further.[1] Plantain, or psyllium seeds, are small (1.5 to 3.5 mm), oval, boat-shaped, dark reddish brown, odorless, and nearly taste-less. They are coated with mucilage, which aids in their transportation by allowing adhesion to various surfaces.[1,2]

HISTORY: Certain plantain species have been spread by European colonization. As such, North American Indians and New Zealand Maori refer to plantain as "Englishman's foot." *P. lanceolata* and *P. major* have been used in herbal remedies and were sometimes carried to colonies for that purpose. Psyllium seed has been found in malt refuse (formerly used as fertilizer) and in wool imported to England. It commonly has been used in birdseed.[1] Pulverized seeds are mixed with oil and applied topically to inflamed sites; decoctions have been mixed with honey for sore throats. The seeds and refined colloid are used in commercial bulk laxative preparations.[1,3]

PHARMACOLOGY: Plantain's pharmacology involves GI tract therapy, hyperlipidemia treatment, anticancer effects, respiratory effects, and other actions.

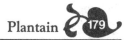

GI: Psyllium seed is classified as a bulk laxative. Mixed with water, it produces a mucilaginous mass. The indigestible seeds provide bulk for treatment of chronic constipation, while the mucilage serves as a mild laxative comparable to agar or mineral oil. The usual dose is 0.5 to 2 g of husk (5 to 15 g of seeds) mixed in 8 oz of water. A study of 10 healthy volunteers examined the effects of a 3 g ispaghula mixture (dried psyllium seed husks) given 3 times daily. It decreased intestinal transit time.[4] Effectiveness of psyllium seed on 78 subjects with irritable bowel syndrome (IBS) has been reported.[5] *P. ovata* fiber is also effective in regulating colon motility in similar patients.[6] When a postcholecystectomy patient with chronic diarrhea was given a 6.5 g dose of a 50% psyllium preparation, symptoms resolved in 2 days.[7,8] Plantago seed as a cellulose/pectin mixture was as effective as a bulk laxative in 50 adult subjects.[9] Gastroprotective action from plantago extract (polyholozidic substances) has also been reported.[10]

In a triple-blind, crossover study of 17 female patients, *P. ovata* seed preparation was investigated on appetite variables. The preparation was useful in weight-control diets where a feeling of fullness was desired. Total fat intake was also decreased, suggesting the product to be a beneficial weight-control diet supplement.[11]

A trial involving 393 patients with anal fissures found conservative treatment with psyllium effective. After 5 years of follow-up, 44% of the patients were cured without surgery within 4 to 8 weeks. There were complications (abscesses and fistulas requiring surgery) in 8% of the cases. The recurrence rate was 27%, but about one-third of these were fistulas that responded to further conservative management.[12]

A double-blind study of 51 patients with symptomatic hemorrhoids showed *Vi-Siblin*, a psyllium-containing preparation, to be effective in reducing bleeding and pain during defecation: 84% of the patients receiving the preparation reported improvement or elimination of symptoms, compared with 52% taking placebo.[13]

Hyperlipidemia: Many reports on psyllium have concluded that it can be helpful in treating various hyperlipidemias.[14,15]

Attention has been focused on the cholesterol-lowering effects of psyllium preparations in human trials. Psyllium hydrophilic mucilloid (*Metamucil*, Procter & Gamble) lowered serum cholesterol in a study of 28 patients who took 3 doses (3.4 g/dose)/day compared with placebo for 8 weeks. After 4 weeks, the psyllium-treated patients showed decreases in total serum cholesterol levels compared with the placebo group. Decreases were also seen in LDL cholesterol and the LDL/HDL ratio. At the end of 8 weeks, values for total cholesterol, LDL cholesterol and the LDL/HDL ratio were 14%, 20%, and 15%, respectively, below baseline (all, $p < 0.01$). This study suggested that high cholesterol levels could be managed safely and easily by including psyllium preparations in the diet.[16]

Similar results of cholesterol reduction have been reported, including: Psyllium colloid administration for 2 to 29 months, reducing cholesterol levels by 16.9% and triglycerides by 52%,[17] a trial of 75 hypercholesterolemic patients, evaluating adjunct therapy of psyllium seed to a low cholesterol diet,[18] a 16-week, double-blind trial, proving plantago seed improved total and LDL cholesterol in 37 patients,[19] and increased tolerance of psyllium seed in combination with colestipol (rather than monotherapy alone) in 105 hyperlipidemic patients.[20]

Psyllium seed was found to be more effective than *P. ovata* husk in reducing serum cholesterol in healthy and ileostomy patients.[21] A report on 20 hypercholesterolemic pediatric patients on low-fat diets, however, found psyllium seed to be ineffective in lowering cholesterol or LDL levels.[22]

Issues of cereal companies including plantago seed in their products and claims of "cholesterol reduction" have been addressed.[23]

A polyphenolic compound from *P. major* leaves exhibited hypocholesterolemic activity,[24] but in addition, the mechanism by which plantago reduces cholesterol may also include enhancement of cholesterol elimination as fecal bile acids.[25]

Anticancer: Immunotropic activity of *P. lanceolata* extract on murine and human lymphatic cells in vivo and in vitro has been demonstrated.[26]

Respiratory: In human studies, plantain has been effective for chronic bronchitis,[27] asthma, cough, and cold.[3]

Other actions: A physician reported using crushed plantain leaves topically to treat poison ivy in 10 people. Although the trial was not conducted scientifically, the treatment eliminated itching and prevented spread of dermatitis in all cases, 1 to 4 applications being required.[28] Fresh leaves of the plant have been poulticed onto herpes, sores, ulcers, boils, and infections. Plantain has been used for insect bites and gout.[3] Aqueous extracts of plantain leaves possess antimicrobial activity.[2]

Aerial parts of plantago have been used as an anti-inflammatory and as a diuretic in folk medicine.[29]

TOXICOLOGY: Plantain pollen contains at least 16 antigens, of which 6 are potentially allergenic. The pollen contains allergenic glycoproteins that react with concanavalin A, as well as components that bind IgE.[30] Antigenic and allergenic analysis have been performed on psyllium seed. All 3 fractions, husk, endosperm, and embryo, contained similar antigens.[31] Formation of IgE antibodies to psyllium laxative has been demonstrated.[32] In addition, IgE-mediated sensitization to plantain pollen has been performed, contributing to seasonal allergy.[33]

There are many reported incidences of varying degrees of psyllium allergy including the following: Nurses experiencing symptoms such as anaphylactoid reaction, chest congestion, sneezing, and watery eyes, some of these reactions taking several years to acquire;[34,35] a case report describing severe anaphylactic shock following psyllium laxative ingestion, linked occupational respiratory allergies in pharmaceutical workers exposed to the substance;[36] consumption of plantago seed in cereal, responsible for anaphylaxis in a 60-year-old female (immunoglobulin E-mediated sensitization was documented, and patient was successfully treated with oral diphenhydramine);[37] and a report on workers in a psyllium processing plant evaluated for occupational asthma and IgE sensitization to psyllium.[38]

Another unusual adverse situation involves the occurrence of a giant phytobezoar composed of psyllium seed husks. The bezoar, located in the right colon, resulted in complete blockage of gastric emptying.[39] All psyllium preparations must be taken with adequate volumes of fluid. The seeds contain a pigment that may be toxic to the kidneys,[40] but this has been removed from most commercial preparations.[41]

Drug interactions reported with psyllium involve lithium and carbamazepine. Psyllium may inhibit absorption of lithium in the GI tract, decreasing blood levels of lithium, as seen in a

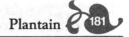

47-year-old woman with schizo-affective disorder.[42] Plantago seed also has decreased the bioavailability of carbamazepine in 4 male subjects.[43]

[1] Hammond J. *Adv Vir Res* 1982;27:103.

[2] Bisset N. *Herbal Drugs and Phytopharmaceuticals*. Stuttgart, Germany: CRC Press, Inc., 1994;378-83.

[3] Duke J. *CRC Handbook of Medicinal Herbs*. Boca Raton, FL: CRC Press, Inc. 1989;386.

[4] Connaughton J, et al. *Ir Med J* 1982;75:93.

[5] Arthurs Y, et al. *Ir Med J* 1983;76:253.

[6] Soifer L, et al. *Acta Gastroenterol Latinoam* 1987;17(4):317-23.

[7] Dorworth T, et al. *ASHP Annual Meeting* 1989 Jun;46:P-57D.

[8] Strommen G, et al. *Clin Pharm* 1990 Mar;9:206-8.

[9] Spiller G, et al. *J Clin Pharmacol* 1979 May-Jun;19:313-20.

[10] Hriscu A, et al. *Rev Med Chir Soc Med Nat Iasi* 1990;94(1):165-70.

[11] Turnbull W, et al. *Int J Obes Rel Metab Dis* 1995;19(5):338-42.

[12] Shub HA, et al. *Dis Colon Rectum* 1978;21:582.

[13] Moesgaard F, et al. *Dis Colon Rectum* 1982;25:454.

[14] Generali J. *US Pharmacist* 1989 Feb;14:16, 20-21.

[15] Chan E, et al. *Ann Pharmacother* 1995 Jun;29:625-27.

[16] Anderson J, et al. *Arch Intern Med* 1988 Feb;148:292-96.

[17] Danielsson A, et al. *Acta Hepatogastroenterol* 1979;26:148.

[18] Bell L, et al. *JAMA* 1989 Jun 16;261:3419-23.

[19] Sprecher D, et al. *Ann Intern Med* 1993 Oct 1;119:545-54.

[20] Spence J, et al. *Ann Intern Med* 1995 Oct 1;123:493-99.

[21] Gelissen I, et al. *Am J Clin Nutr* 1994;59(2):395-400.

[22] Dennison B, et al. *J Pediatr* 1993 Jul;123:24-29.

[23] Gannon K. *Drug Topics* 1989 Oct 2;133:24.

[24] Maksyutina N, et al. *Farmat Zhurnal* 1978;33(4):56-61.

[25] Miettinen T, et al. *Clin Chim Acta* 1989;183(3):253-62.

[26] Strzelecka H, et al. *Herba Polonica* 1995;41(1):23-32.

[27] Newall C, et al. *Herbal Medicines*. London, England: Pharmaceutical Press., 1996;210-11.

[28] Duckett S. *N Engl J Med* 1980;303:583.

[29] Tosun F. *Hacettepe U Eczacilik Fakultesi Dergisi* 1995;15(1):23-32.

[30] Baldo BA, et al. *Int Arch Allergy Appl Immunol* 1982;68:295.

[31] Arlian L, et al. *J Allergy Clin Immunol* 1992;89(4):866-76.

[32] Rosenberg S, et al. *Ann Allergy* 1982;48:294.

[33] Mehta V, et al. *Int Arch Allergy Appl Immunol* 1991;96(3):211-17.

[34] Wray M. ASHP Midyear Clinical Meeting. 1989 Dec;24:P-90D.

[35] Ford M, et al. *Hosp Pharm* 1992 Dec;27:1061-62.

[36] Suhonen R, et al. *Allergy* 1983;38:363.

[37] Lantner R, et al. *JAMA* 1990;264:2534-36.

[38] Bardy J, et al. *Am Rev Respir Dis* 1987;135(5):1033-38.

[39] Agha FP, et al. *Am J Gastroenterol* 1984;79:319.

[40] Kamoda Y, et al. *Tokyo Ika Shika Daigaku Iyo Kizai Kenkyusho Hokoku* 1989;23:81-85.

[41] Morton JF. *Major Medicinal Plants*. Springfield IL: C.C. Thomas, 1977.

[42] Perlman B. *Lancet* 1990 Feb 17;335:416.

[43] Etman M. *Drug Devel Indus Pharm* 1995;21(16):1901-6.

Pokeweed

SCIENTIFIC NAME(S): *P. americana* L., *P. decandra* L., *P. rigida*. Family: Phytolaccaceae

COMMON NAME(S): American nightshade, cancer jalap, cancerroot, chongras, coakum, pokeberry, crowberry, garget, inkberry, pigeonberry, poke, red ink plant, scoke, poke salad

---

❧❧❧ PATIENT INFORMATION ❧❧❧

Uses: Young pokeweed leaves may be eaten and the berries used for food, only after being cooked properly.

Side Effects: Ingestion of poisonous parts of the plant causes severe stomach cramping, nausea with persistent diarrhea and vomiting, slow and difficult breathing, weakness, spasms, hypotension, severe convulsions, and death.

BOTANY: Pokeweed is a ubiquitous plant found in fields, along fences, in damp woods, and in other undisturbed areas. This vigorous shrub-like perennial can grow to 3.6 m. The reddish stem has large pointed leaves, which taper at both ends.[1] The flowers are numerous, small, and greenish white and develop into juicy purple berries that mature from July to September.

HISTORY: Folk uses of pokeweed leaves have included the treatment of chronic rheumatism and arthritis and use as an emetic and purgative.[2] The plant has been used to treat edema,[3] skin cancers, rheumatism, catarrh, dysmenorrhea, mumps, ringworm, scabies, tonsillitis and syphilis. Poke greens, the young immature leaves, are canned and sold under the name "poke salet." Berry juice has been used as an ink, dye, and coloring in wine.[4]

PHARMACOLOGY: The plant's pharmacologic activity has not been well defined. Small doses of all parts of the plant can cause adverse reactions (see Toxicology), but the mechanisms of these actions are generally unknown.[5] Several anti-inflammatory saponins have been isolated from the root;[6] the root, however, has no known medicinal value.

TOXICOLOGY: Pokeweed poisonings were common in eastern North America during the 19th century, especially from the use of tinctures as antirheumatic preparations, and from eating berries and roots collected in error for parsnip, Jerusalem artichoke, or horseradish.[7]

All parts of pokeweed are toxic except the above-ground leaves that grow in the early spring. The poisonous principles are in highest concentration in the rootstock, less in the mature leaves and stems, and least in the fruits. Young leaves collected before acquiring a red color are edible if boiled for 5 minutes, rinsed, and reboiled. Berries are toxic when raw but are edible when cooked.

Ingestion of poisonous parts of the plant causes severe stomach cramping, nausea with persistent diarrhea and vomiting, slow and difficult breathing, weakness, spasms, hypotension, severe convulsions, and death.[8] Fewer than 10 uncooked berries are generally harmless to adults. Several investigators have reported deaths in children following the ingestion of uncooked berries or pokeberry juice.[8,9]

Severe poisonings have been reported in adults who ingested mature pokeweed leaves[10] and following the ingestion of a cup of tea brewed from ½ teaspoonful of powdered pokeroot.[7]

In addition, the CDC reported a case of toxicity in campers who ingested *prop-*

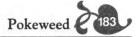

erly cooked young shoots. Sixteen of the 51 cases exhibited case-definitive symptoms (vomiting followed by any 3 of the following: Nausea, diarrhea, stomach cramps, dizziness, headache). These symptoms persisted for up to 48 hours (mean, 24 hours).[11]

Poisoning may also occur when the toxic components enter the circulatory system through cuts and abrasions in the skin.

Symptoms of mild poisoning generally last 24 hours. In severe cases, gastric lavage, emesis, and symptomatic and supportive treatment have been suggested.[8]

In an attempt to curb potential poisonings from the use of this commercially available plant, the Herb Trade Association (HTA) formulated a policy stressing that the poke root is toxic and "should not be sold as an herbal beverage or food, or in any other form which could threaten the health of the uninformed consumer." Further, the HTA recommended that products containing pokeroot be labeled clearly as to their toxicity.[12]

The FDA classifies pokeweed as an herb of undefined safety that has demonstrated narcotic effects.

[1] Dobelis I, ed. *Magic and Medicine of Plants.* Pleasantville, NY: Reader's Digest Association, Inc., 1986.

[2] Bianchini F, et al. *Health Plants of the World.* New York, NY: Newsweek Books, 1975.

[3] Kang S, et al. *J Nat Prod* 1980;43:510.

[4] Duke J. *CRC Handbook of Medicinal Herbs.* Boca Raton, FL: CRC Press, 1985.

[5] Barker BE, et al. *Pediatrics* 1966;38:490.

[6] Woo WS, et al. *Planta Med* 1978;34:87.

[7] Lewis WH, et al. *JAMA* 1975;242:2759.

[8] Hardin JW, et al. *Human Poisoning from Native and Cultivated Plants*, 2nd ed. Durham, NC: Duke University Press, 1974.

[9] Toxic reactions to plant products sold in health food stores. *Med Lett Drugs Ther* 1979;21:29.

[10] Stein ZLG. *Am J Hosp Pharm* 1979;36:1303.

[11] Plant poisonings - New Jersey. *MMWR* 1981;30:65.

[12] Herb Trade Association Policy Statement #2. May 1979.

SCIENTIFIC NAME(S): Although members of the genus *Papaver* are called poppies, *P. somniferum* L. and *P. bracteatum* Lindl. are important medicinally.[1] Family: Papaveraceae

COMMON NAME(S): *P. somniferum*: Opium poppy, poppyseed poppy. *P. bracteatum:* Thebaine poppy, great scarlet poppy

---

❧❧❧ PATIENT INFORMATION ❧❧❧

Uses: Codeine and morphine have been used to relax smooth muscle tone, making them useful in the treatment of diarrhea and abdominal cramping, and have been used as sedative analgesics and antitussives.

Side Effects: Opium is known for its highly addictive qualities and has been associated with poisoning and symptoms of sedation, sluggishness, and abdominal contractions.

BOTANY: The opium poppy is a small annual. The bright showy flowers of the genus *Papaver* range in color from white to deep reds and purples. The seeds of the plants vary in color from light cream to blue-black.

HISTORY: The earliest accounts of the use of poppy derivatives date to the Sumerians in Mesopotamia, where the plant was used medicinally and was known as *hul gil* (the plant of joy).[2] The medicinal uses of poppy were described by the Ancient Greeks, and opium was described as an addictive agent by the Arabs more than 900 years ago. Because of the wide distribution of the opium poppy, its use has been recognized by most major cultures. Opium has been used in the US since its birth and was used widely during the Civil War. Morphine was isolated from crude opium in 1803, and in 1874, morphine was boiled with acetic anhydride to yield diacetylmorphine (heroin). This compound was developed by Bayer for cough, chest pain, and pneumonia. It was later recognized as having a high addiction potential. Opium derivatives continue to play a major role as antitussives, antidiarrheals, and analgesics. Their abuse potential remains high; strict efforts to curtail the illicit cultiva-

tion of the opium poppy have met with limited success. Poppy seeds are used in the preparation of confections and breads.

PHARMACOLOGY: Codeine and morphine are sedative analgesics and can relax smooth muscle tone, making them useful in the treatment of diarrhea and abdominal cramping. Codeine and its derivatives are antitussives. Papaverine relaxes involuntary smooth muscle and increases cerebral blood flow. Although large doses of thebaine can induce convulsions, no case of thebaine abuse has been reported.[3] The addictive characteristics of the opium alkaloids have been recognized for millenia.

TOXICOLOGY: The abuse potential of opium has had an enormous impact on most societies. Deaths due to respiratory depression have been reported and heroin-induced deaths are common. As little as 300 mg opium can be fatal to humans, although addicts tolerate 2000 mg over 4 hours. Death from circulatory and respiratory collapse is accompanied by cold, clammy skin, pulmonary edema, cyanosis, and pupillary constriction.[4]

Attention has been focused on the fact that morphine and codeine can be de-

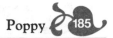
tected in significant amounts in urine following the ingestion of foods prepared with poppy seeds. After the ingestion of 3 poppy-seed bagels, urinary codeine and morphine levels were 214 ng/ml and 2797 ng/ml, respectively after 3 hours. Analysis of poppy seeds indicated that an individual consuming a single poppy-seed bagel could ingest up to 1.5 mg of morphine and 0.1 mg of codeine.[5] Opiates have been detected in urine more than 48 hours after the ingestion of culinary poppy seeds.[6] These results confirm that a positive finding of morphine or codeine in urine may not always be due to the ingestion of drugs of abuse.

[1] Duke JA. *Economic Botany* 1973;27:390.
[2] Hoffmann JP. *J Psychoactive Drugs* 1990;22:53.
[3] Theuns HG, et al. *Economic Botany* 1986;40:485.
[4] Duke JA. *Handbook of Medicinal Herbs*. Boca Raton, FL: CRC Press, 1985.
[5] Struempler RE. *J Analytical Toxicol* 1987;11:97.
[6] Hayes LW, et al. *Clin Chem* 1987;33:806.

Propolis

SCIENTIFIC NAME(S): Propolis balsam, propolis resin, propolis wax

COMMON NAME(S): Propolis, bee glue, hive dross

❧❧❧ PATIENT INFORMATION ❧❧❧

Uses: Studies have shown that propolis has anti-inflammatory, antitumor, and antioxidant effects.

Side Effects: Propolis has been reported to cause propolis-induced dermatitis and acute oral mucositis with ulceration.

BOTANY: Propolis is a natural resinous product collected from conifer buds and used by honeybees to fill cracks in their hives.[1] It is a greenish brown sticky mass with a slight aromatic odor and is important in defending the hive.[2]

HISTORY: Propolis displays strong antimicrobial activity and has been used as a chemotherapeutic agent since ancient times.[3] Its use was found in folk medicine as early as 300 B.C. for medical and cosmetic purposes and as an anti-inflammatory drug and wound-healing agent.[4–6] More recently, it has been reported to possess versatile biologic activity as an antibacterial, antiviral, fungicidal, local anesthetic, anti-ulcer, anti-inflammatory, immunostimulant, and hypotensive and has cytostatic properties in vitro.[7,8] Proponents of the use of propolis suggest that it stimulates the immune system, thereby raising the body's natural resistance to infection.[1] It has been advocated for internal and external use.

PHARMACOLOGY: Researchers have published numerous reports of clinical trials in which propolis was given to aid wound healing and to treat tuberculosis and fungal and bacterial infections.[9] More recently, researchers have investigated the antibacterial properties of this material. Propolis was active in vitro against some gram-positive bacterial and tubercle bacillus; it also demonstrated limited activity against gram-negative bacilli. Some propolis flavonoids have demonstrated antiviral activity in vitro.[10] Propolis inhibits bacterial growth of *Streptococcus agalactiae* by preventing cell division and disorganizing the cytoplasm, cytoplasmic membrane, and cell wall. It also causes a partial bacteriolysis and inhibits protein synthesis.[11] None of the chemical constituents, however, are as effective as anti-infective agents in vitro as streptomycin, chloramphenicol, oxytetracycline, nystatin, and griseofulvin.[12,13]

Ethanolic and aqueous extracts of propolis demonstrate anti-inflammatory and antibiotic activities in vitro and in vivo. The exact mechanism for these effects is not clear. An aqueous extract of propolis has inhibited the enzyme dihydrofolate reductase. This activity may be partially due to the caffeic acid content in propolis. This may explain some of the protective functions of propolis, similar to those shown for several nonsteroidal anti-inflammatory drugs (NSAIDs).[14]

Diethyl ether extracts of propolis possessed cytostatic activity against cultured human KB (nasopharynx carcinoma) and HeLa (carcinoma cervicis uteri) cells in vitro.[7] Ethanolic extracts have been shown to accelerate bone formation, regenerate tissue, and induce some enzyme systems in vitro.[1]

The effect of the active component of propolis, caffeic acid phenethyl ester (CAPE), was studied on the growth and antigenic phenotype of a human melanoma cell line (HO-1) and a human glioblastoma multiforme cell line

(GBM-18). The growth of both cell lines was suppressed by CAPE in a dose-dependent way, with HO-1 cells being more sensitive than GBM-1 cells. The results suggest a potential role for CAPE as an antitumor agent.[15]

Ethanolic extracts of 2 propolis types showed a similar scavenging action against the different species of oxygen radicals. The antioxidative properties of propolis may be attributed to their free radical scavenging activity against alkoxy radicals.[16]

Activity tests prove the high antioxidative and inhibitory capacities of propolis in vitro. Experiments documented the photodynamic quenching properties of propolis extracts.[4] Topical application of propolis extract to dental sockets have been shown to enhance epithelial growth.[17] Propolis, prepared as a mouth rinse, aids repair of intrabuccal surgical wounds and exerts a small pain-killing and anti-inflammatory effect in patients who underwent sulcoplasty.[18]

TOXICOLOGY: While reports of toxicity are rare, propolis has long been recognized by apiary workers as being a potent skin sensitizer. Several cases of propolis-induced dermatitis have been reported. These have occurred after the topical use of cosmetics containing propolis and, in 1 case, after the application of a 10% alcoholic propolis solution for the treatment of genital herpes.[19] Acute oral mucositis with ulceration following the use of propolis-containing lozenges has also been reported.[20]

[1] Tyler VE. The New Honest Herbal. Philadelphia, PA: G.F. Stickley Co., 1987.

[2] Ikeno K, et al. Caries Res 1991;25(5):347.

[3] Higashi KO, et al. J Ethnopharmacol 1994;43(2):149.

[4] Volpert R, et al. Z Naturforsch 1993;48(11-12):858.

[5] Volpert R, et al. Z Naturforsch 1993;48(11-12):851.

[6] Frenkel K, et al. Cancer Res 1993;53(6):1255.

[7] Hladon B, et al. Arzneimettelforschung 1980;30(11):1847.

[8] Bankova VS, et al. J Nat Prod 1983;46(4):471.

[9] New Research in Apitherapy. Second International Symposium of Apitherapy. September 2-7, 1976; Bucharest, Romania. Bucharest, Romania: Apimondia Press, 1976.

[10] Debiaggi M, et al. Microbiologica 1990;13(3):207.

[11] Takaisi-Kikuni NB, et al. Planta Med 1994;60(3):222.

[12] Metzner J, et al. Pharmazie 1979;34:97.

[13] Brumfitt W, et al. Microbios 1990;62(250):19.

[14] Strehl E, et al. Z Naturforsch 1994;49(1-2):39.

[15] Guarini L, et al. Cell Mol Biol 1992;38(5):513.

[16] Pascual C, et al. J Ethnopharmacol 1994;41(1-2):9.

[17] Magro-Filho O, et al. J Nihon Univ Sch Dent 1990;32(1):4.

[18] Magro-Filho O, et al. J Nihon Univ Sch Dent 1994;36(2):102.

[19] Pincelli C, et al. Contact Dermatitis 1984;11(1):49.

[20] Hay KD, et al. Oral Surg Oral Med Oral Pathol 1990;70(5):584.

Pycnogenol

✒✒✒ PATIENT INFORMATION ✒✒✒

Uses: Pycnogenol is said to assist in the treatment of hypoxia following atherosclerosis, cardiac or cerebral infarction, reduce tumor promotion, inflammation, ischemia, alteration of synovial fluid, and collagen degradation.

Side Effects: There are no reported side effects.

SOURCE: The name "pycnogenol" is a source of confusion. In product literature, this term is a trademark of a British company for a proprietary mixture of water-soluble bioflavonoids, allegedly derived from the bark of the European coastal pine, *Pinus maritima* (also known as *P. nigra* var. *maritima*, a widely planted variety of pine in Europe).

However, pycnogenol has also been assigned to a group of flavonoids termed the flavan-3-ol derivatives.[1] Numerous plants have been found to be sources for the class of compounds generally termed the flavonoids, and the chemical condensation of flavonoid precursors results in the formation of compounds known as condensed tannins. The broader term, bioflavonoid, has been used to designate those flavonoids with biologic activity.

HISTORY: Pycnogenol is available commercially in the US in health-food stores and pharmacies. Product literature indicates that pycnogenol, when taken as a dietary supplement, is a free radical scavenger. The compound may improve circulation, reduce inflammation, and protect collagen from natural degradation. Pycnogenol has been available in Europe for some time, where it is taken as a supplement or incorporated into topical "anti-aging" creams.

PHARMACOLOGY: A US patent for this material describes a mixture of proanthocyanidins that are effective in combating the deleterious effects of free radicals. The compound is said to assist in the treatment of hypoxia following atherosclerosis, cardiac or cerebral infarction, and to reduce tumor promotion, inflammation, ischemia, alterations of synovial fluid, and collagen degradation.

Several studies have been conducted in Europe to evaluate the pharmacologic activity of pycnogenol. In one study, daily oral doses of pycnogenol were given for 30 days to patients with a variety of peripheral circulatory disorders. Pain, limb heaviness, and feeling of swelling decreased during therapy in most patients.[2] Other investigators reported similar results.[3]

TOXICOLOGY: No reports of adverse effects from pycnogenol have been published.

[1] Masquelier J, et al. *Int J Vitam Nutr Res* 1979;49:307.
[2] Sarrat L. *Bordeaux Medical* 1981;14:685.
[3] Mollmann H, et al. *Therapiewoche* 1983;33:4967.

SCIENTIFIC NAME(S): *Pygeum africanum* Hook. f., or *Prunus africana* (Hook. f.) Kalkm. (Rosaceae)

COMMON NAME(S): Pygeum, African plum tree

ᴤᴤᴤᴤ PATIENT INFORMATION ᴤᴤᴤᴤ

Uses: Pygeum has been used to improve symptoms of benign prostatic hypertrophy and to improve sexual function. Usual dosage is 100 mg/day in 6- to 8-week cycles.

Side Effects: GI irritation has been reported with pygeum.

BOTANY: Pygeum is an evergreen tree native to African forests. It can grow to 45 m in height. The thick leaves are oblong; the flowers are small and white. Pygeum fruit is a red berry, resembling a cherry when ripe. The bark (red, brown, or gray) is the part used for medicinal purposes. It has a "hydrocyanic acid"-like odor.[1-3]

HISTORY: The hard wood of pygeum is valued in Africa and is used to make wagons.[1] Powdered pygeum bark is used by African natives to treat urinary problems.[1,3]

PHARMACOLOGY: In France, *Pygeum africanum* extract (PAE) has become the primary course of treatment for enlarged prostate.[1] Drugs used to alleviate symptoms of benign prostatic hypertrophy (BPH) (or hyperplasia) include anticholinergics, muscle relaxants, calcium antagonists, prostaglandin inhibitors, beta-agonists, tricyclic antidepressants, and alpha blockers.[4] Pygeum clinical trials (mostly European) are encouraging, but more research is needed in the US. Usual dosage of PAE is 100 mg/day in 6- to 8-week cycles.[2]

Most trial results report improvement of BPH symptoms. Reduction in gland size and other parameters occur but are not as profound.[3] Pygeum is also therapeutic as an anti-inflammatory and increases prostatic secretions and decreases certain hormones in the glandular area, which reduces the hypertrophy. Other actions of pygeum include increase in bladder elasticity and histological modifications of glandular cells.[2]

Symptomatic relief from BPH using PAE has been documented.[5-12] The extract, in combination with mepartricin, was successful in treating urinary symptomatology in 22 subjects with varying stages of prostatic adenoma.[7] In a 74-patient study, extracts of pygeum and testosterone alleviated obstructive bladder symptoms caused by BPH.[8] Using PAE, nocturnal frequency, difficulty in initiation of urination, and bladder fullness were 3 parameters improved over placebo in 60 patients.[9] In a placebo-controlled, double-blind, multi-center evaluation, pygeum capsules (50 mg) were given twice daily for 60 days. Out of 263 patients in 8 locations, 66% (vs 31% placebo) showed marked clinical improvement in micturition disorders.[10] High-dose PAE (200 mg/day) administered to 18 patients for 60 days improved urinary symptoms and sexual behavior in another report.[11] PAE in combination with *Urtica dioica* in half doses was found to be as safe and effective as full doses (300 mg urtica and 25 mg PAE) in treating urine flow, residual urine, and nycturia.[12]

The extract displays anti-inflammatory activity, which may affect gland size. It has been demonstrated that macrophages (inflammatory cells) produce chemotactic mediators that worsen BPH development.[13]

Pygeum may help reverse sterility, which can be caused by insufficient prostatic secretions.[1] PAE has increased prostate secretions.[14] It has improved seminal fluid composition.[1] By improving an underlying problem, PAE may improve sexual function.[3,11]

When compared with saw palmetto in a double-blind trial, saw palmetto produced greater reduction of symptoms and was better tolerated; however, PAE may have greater effects on prostate secretion.[15]

The ferulic acid ester components are responsible for pygeum's endocrine system activity. N-docosanol reduces luteinizing hormone, testosterone, and prolactin levels. This is important because testosterone accumulation within the prostate (and subsequent conversion to the more potent form) is believed to be a major factor in prostatic hyperplasia. PAE's "phytoestrogenic" action markedly reduces volume of prostatic hypertrophy.[16] Fat-soluble components reduce cholesterol content within the prostate, decreasing accumulation of cholesterol metabolites.[3]

TOXICOLOGY: A low incidence of toxicity has been demonstrated. No side effects were reported in 18 patients taking 200 mg/day of pygeum for 60 days.[11] GI irritation ranging from nausea to severe stomach pain has been documented but with only a small percentage discontinuing therapy.[3] In 263 patients, GI adverse effects occurred in 5 patients with only 3 patients having to stop treatment.[10] It is recommended that pygeum be taken only under professional supervision.[1]

[1] Chevallier A. *Encyclopedia of Medicinal Plants*. New York, NY: DK Publishing, 1996;257.

[2] Bruneton J. *Pharmacognosy, Phytochemistry, Medicinal Plants* Paris, France: Lavoisier Publishing, 1995;142.

[3] Murray M. *The Healing Power of Herbs*. Rocklin, CA: Prima Publishing, 1995;286-93

[4] Dagues F, et al. *Rev Prat* 1995;45(3):337-41.

[5] Bassi P, et al. *Minerva Urol Nefrol* 1987;39(1):45-50.

[6] Menchini-Fabris G, et al. *Arch Ital Urol Nefrol Androl* 1988;60(3):313-22.

[7] Casella G, et al. *Arch Sci Med* 1978;135(1):95-98.

[8] Flamm J, et al. *Wien Klin Wochenschr* 1979;91(18):622-27.

[9] DuFour B, et al. *Ann Urol* 1984;18(3):193-95.

[10] Barlet A, et al. *Wien Klin Wochenschr* 1990;102(22):667-73.

[11] Carani C, et al. *Arch Ital Urol Nefrol Androl* 1991;63(3):341-45.

[12] Krzeski T, et al. *Clin Ther* 1993;15(6):1011-20.

[13] Paubert-Braquet M, et al. *J Lipid Mediat Cell Signal* 1994;9(3):285-90.

[14] Clavert A, et al. *Ann Urol* 1986;20(5):341-43.

[15] Mandressi A, et al *Urologia* 1983;50:752-57.

[16] Mathe G, et al. *Biomed Pharmacother* 1995;49(7-8):339-43.

SCIENTIFIC NAME(S): *Cinchona succirubra* Pav. ex Klotsch (red cinchona), *C. calisya* Wedd. and *C. ledgeriana* Moens ex Trim. (yellow cinchona). Family: Rubiaceae

COMMON NAME(S): Red bark, Peruvian bark, Jesuit's bark, China bark, cinchona bark, quina-quina, fever tree

---

♦♦♦♦ PATIENT INFORMATION ♦♦♦♦

Uses: Quinine has been used for the treatment of leg cramps caused by vascular spasm, internal hemorrhoids, varicose veins and pleural cavities after thoracoplasty, malaria, and associated febrile states.

Drug Interactions: Quinine may increase the pharmacologic and toxic effects of amantadine, astemizole, carbamazepine, digoxin, nondepolarizing muscle relaxants (eg, pancuronium, phenobarbital, warfarin).[1]

Side Effects: Quinine has been known to cause urticaria, contact dermatitis, and other hypersensitivity reactions.

BOTANY: Cinchonas are evergreen shrubs and trees that grow to heights of 15 to 30 m.[2] They are native to the mountainous areas of tropical Central and South America. The oblong seed capsule is ≈ 3 cm long and, when ripe, splits open at the base. Each capsule contains 40 to 50 seeds that are so light that ≈ 75,000 seeds equal 1 ounce.[3] At least 1 other genus (*Remijia*) of the same family has been reported to contain quinidine.[4]

HISTORY: The dried ground bark of the cinchona plant has been used for centuries to treat malaria, fever, indigestion, mouth and throat diseases, and cancer.[2,3,5] The name cinchona is said to be derived from the Countess of Chinchon, the wife of a viceroy of Peru, who it was long believed was cured in 1638 from a fever by the use of the bark;[4] however, the story has been widely disputed. Formal use of the bark to treat malaria was established in the mid-1800s when the British began worldwide cultivation of the plant[3] to ensure continuing availability.[4]

Bark extracts have been used to treat hemorrhoids, to stimulate hair growth, and to manage varicose veins. Quinine has been used as an abortifacient.[3] Extracts of cinchona have a bitter, astringent taste and have been used as flavoring for food and beverages. Although the use of quinine for malaria has been largely supplanted by treatment with semisynthetic anti-infectives, its use persists in some regions.

PHARMACOLOGY: Quinine is among the most potent of the cinchona alkaloids with respect to antimalarial activity,[2] although resistant strains of the pathogen have been identified. A second common use of quinine is for the treatment of leg cramps caused by vascular spasm.

Quinine is bacteriostatic, highly active in vitro against protozoa, and it inhibits yeast fermentation.[3] Quinine and the related quinidine have cardiodepressant activity, and quinidine is used for its antiarrhythmic activity. Quinine and quinidine are available as commercial products.[6] Quinine also has analgesic and antipyretic actions.[6]

A mixture of quinine and urea hydrochloride is injected as a sclerosing agent in the treatment of internal hemorrhoids, varicose veins, and pleural cavities after thoracoplasty.[3]

TOXICOLOGY: Ground cinchona bark and quinine have caused urticaria, contact dermatitis, and other hypersensitivity reactions. These reactions may occur in people using topical preparations containing cinchona extracts or quinine.[3] The ingestion of these alkaloids can result in the clinical syndrome "cinchonism." People who are hypersensitive to these alkaloids also may develop the syndrome, which is characterized by severe headache, abdominal pain, convulsions, visual disturbances and blindness, auditory disturbances such as ringing in the ears, paralysis, and collapse.[2]

Therapeutic doses of quinine have resulted in acute hemolytic anemia,[5] a limitation for its use in a small portion of the population who are glucose-6-phosphate dehydrogenase (G-6-PD) deficient.[6]

Quinidine and related alkaloids are rapidly absorbed from the GI tract, and a single 2 to 8 g oral dose of quinine may be fatal to an adult.[2,3,6]

Quinine use is discouraged during pregnancy because of fetal and abortifacient effects.[6] Treatment of overdose is generally supportive. Urinary acidification and renal dialysis can be employed if necessary.[6]

Quinine has been reported to interact with several drugs. Most studies and case reports of quinine interactions with drugs have involved prescription doses of quinine (ie, ≥ 200 mg).[1] The effects of the amounts of quinine in tonic beverages (≈ 80 mg/32 oz) needs to be assessed. Until this information is available, it would be prudent to limit the amount of quinine ingestion with drugs reported to interact.

Amantandine: Quinine may inhibit the renal clearance of amantadine, resulting in elevated serum concentrations of amantadine and an increased risk of toxicity (eg, ataxia, mental confusion).[1] When this interaction was studied in healthy male and female subjects, 200 mg of quinine inhibited renal clearance of amantadine only in male subjects. Additional controlled studies are needed to confirm the gender difference.

Astemizole: Quinine may inhibit the metabolism of astemizole, producing elevated serum concentrations of astemizole and increasing the risk of life-threatening cardiotoxicity.[1] A single 430 mg dose of quinine may result in elevated plasma concentrations of astemizole and its desmethyl metabolite. Consumption of 80 mg/day of quinine in beverages can elevate astemizole levels but the prolongation of the QT interval may not be clinically important.

Carbamazepine: Quinine may inhibit the metabolism of carbamazepine, producing elevated carbamazepine serum concentrations and increasing the pharmacologic and adverse effects.[1] Administration of 600 mg of quinine to healthy volunteers receiving carbamazepine increased phenobarbital levels by ≈ 37%.[1]

Digoxin: Quinine may decrease the biliary clearance of digoxin, resulting in elevated serum concentrations of digoxin and increasing the risk of toxicity.[1] In studies, administration of 250 to 1200 mg daily of quinine increased serum digoxin levels by as much as 75%. However, digoxin toxicity has not been reported.

Nondepolarizing muscle relaxants: Quinine may enhance the effects of nondepolarizing muscle relaxants (eg, pancuronium).[1] Recurarization was reported in a patient receiving 1800 mg daily of quinine for malaria after reversal from anesthesia and administration of 6 mg pancuronium.

Phenobarbital: Quinine may inhibit the metabolism of phenobarbital, producing elevated phenobarbital serum

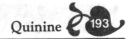
concentrations and increasing the pharmacologic and adverse effects.[1] Administration of 600 mg quinine to healthy volunteers receiving phenobarbital increased phenobarbital levels by $\approx$ 35%.

Warfarin: Quinine may inhibit the hepatic synthesis of clotting factors, resulting in a potentiation of the anticoagulant effects of warfarin and increasing the risk of hemorrhage.[1] While case reports have documented an increase in the anticoagulant effect of warfarin, retrospective and controlled studies have not confirmed this possible interaction.

[1] Tatro D,ed. *Drug Interaction Facts* St. Louis, MO: Facts and Comparisons, 1999 (updated quarterly).

[2] Leung AY. *Encyclopedia of Common Natural Ingredients Used in Food, Drugs, and Cosmetics.* New York, NY: John Wiley and Sons, 1980.

[3] Morton JF. *Major Medicinal Plants.* Springfield, IL: C.C. Thomas Publisher, 1977.

[4] Evans WC. *Trease and Evans' Pharmacognosy,* 13th ed. Philadelphia, PA: W.B. Saunders, 1989.

[5] Duke JA. *Handbook of Medicinal Herbs.* Boca Raton, FL: CRC Press, 1985.

[6] Hebel SK, Burnham TH, eds. *Drug Facts and Comparisons* St. Louis, MO: Facts and Comparisons, 1996.

Rose Hips

SCIENTIFIC NAME(S): Commonly derived from *Rosa canina* L., *R. rugosa* Thunb., *R. acicularis* Lindl. or *R. cinnamomea* L. Numerous other species of rose have been used for the preparation of rose hips. Family: Rosaceae

COMMON NAME(S): Rose hips, "heps"

꽃꽃꽃 PATIENT INFORMATION 꽃꽃꽃

Uses: Rose hips provide a source of vitamin C for natural vitamin supplements.

Side Effects: There have been no reported side effects except in those exposed to rose hips dust who have developed severe respiratory allergies.

BOTANY: Rose hips are the ripe ovaries or seeded fruit of roses forming on branches after the flower.[1]

HISTORY: Rose hips are a natural source of vitamin C, which has led to their widespread use in natural vitamin supplements, teas, and various other preparations including soups and marmalades.[2] Although these products have been used historically as nutritional supplements, they also have been used as mild laxatives and diuretics.

PHARMACOLOGY: Vitamin C is used as a nutritional supplement for its antiscorbutic properties. Because a significant amount of the natural vitamin C in rose hips may be destroyed during drying and processing, many "natural vitamin supplements" have some form of vitamin C added to them. One must read the label carefully to determine what proportion of the vitamin C is derived from rose hips vs other sources.

Unfortunately, this information is not always available on the package label.

The laxative activity of rose hips may be related to the presence of malic and citric acids or to purgative glycosides (multiflorin A and B).[3]

TOXICOLOGY: Rose hips ingestion generally is not associated with toxicity. More than 100 g of plant material would have to be ingested to obtain a 1200 mg dose of vitamin C, an impractical amount to ingest. Most people do not have any side effects from ingesting small gram quantities of the plant. Adverse effects associated with the long-term ingestion of multi-gram doses of vitamin C (ie, oxalate stone formation)[4] have not been reported with rose hips. Production workers exposed to rose hips dust have developed severe respiratory allergies, with mild-to-moderate anaphylaxis.[1]

[1] Kwaselow A, et al. *J Allergy Clin Immunol* 1990;85(4):704.

[2] Tyler VE. *The New Honest Herbal.* Philadelphia, PA: G.F. Stickley Co., 1987.

[3] Leung AY. *Encyclopedia of Common Natural Ingredients Used In Food, Drugs and Cosmetics.* New York, NY: John Wiley and Sons, 1980.

[4] Roth DA, et al. *JAMA* 1977;237(8):768.

Rosemary

SCIENTIFIC NAME(S): *Rosmarinus officinalis* L. Family: Labiatae or Lamiaceae. Bog rosemary (*Andromeda* species) and wild or marsh rosemary (*Ledum palustre* L.) are members of the family Ericaceae and are not related to rosemary.

COMMON NAME(S): Rosemary, Old Man

❧❧❧ PATIENT INFORMATION ❧❧❧

Uses: Rosemary has decreased capillary permeability and fragility, and extracts have been used in insect repellents. The plant may have anticancer properties.

Side Effects: Ingestion of large quantities of rosemary can result in stomach and intestinal irritation and kidney damage.

BOTANY: Rosemary grows as a small evergreen shrub with thick aromatic leaves.[1] The plant has small pale blue flowers that bloom in late winter and early spring.[2,3] Although rosemary is native to the Mediterranean, it is now cultivated worldwide.

HISTORY: Rosemary is a widely used culinary herb. Tradition holds that rosemary will grow only in gardens of households where the "mistress" is truly the "master."[4] The plant has been used in traditional medicine for its astringent, tonic, carminative, antispasmodic, and diaphoretic properties. Extracts and the volatile oil have been used to promote menstrual flow and as abortifacients.[4,5] Rosemary extracts are commonly cosmetic ingredients, and a rosemary lotion is said to stimulate hair growth and prevent baldness.[6]

PHARMACOLOGY: The clinical value of rosemary is difficult to establish because of the lack of studies. Diosmin has been reported to decrease capillary permeability and fragility.[4] A derivative of rosemaricine has been shown to induce significant smooth muscle and analgesic effects in vitro.[1] Rosemary extracts are reported to have antioxidant properties comparable to those of butylated hydroxytoluene and butylated hydroxy-anisole. Carnosic acid and labiatic acid are reported to be the active compounds.[1] The plant may have anticancer properties.[2] Extracts have been used as insect repellents.[2]

TOXICOLOGY: Although the oil is used safely as a flavoring and the whole leaves are used as a potherb, ingestion of large quantities of the oil can be associated with toxicity.[7] Toxicity is characterized by stomach and intestinal irritation and kidney damage.[3] There is no valid role for rosemary oil as an abortifacient. Bath preparations containing the oil may cause erythema, and toiletries can cause dermatitis in sensitive individuals.[6]

[1] Leung AY. *Encyclopedia of Common Natural Ingredients Used in Food, Drugs and Cosmetics.* New York, NY: John Wiley and Sons, 1980.

[2] Simon JE. *Herbs: An Indexed Bibliography, 1971-1980.* Hamden, CT: Shoe String Press, 1984.

[3] Osol A, et al, eds. *The Dispensatory of the United States of America,* 25th ed. Philadelphia, PA: JB Lippincott, 1955.

[4] Tyler VE. *The New Honest Herbal.* Philadelphia, PA: G.F. Stickley Co., 1987.

[5] Dobelis IN, ed. *Magic and Medicine of Plants.* Pleasantville, NY: Reader's Digest, 1986.

[6] Duke JA. *Handbook of Medicinal Herbs.* Boca Raton, FL: CRC Press, 1985.

[7] Spoerke DG. *Herbal Medications.* Santa Barbara, CA: Woodbridge Press, 1980.

Sage

SCIENTIFIC NAME(S): *Salvia officinalis* L. (Dalmatian sage), *S. lavandulaefolia* Vahl. (Spanish sage). Family: Labiatae or Lamiaceae

COMMON NAME(S): Garden sage, true sage, scarlet sage, meadow sage

---

❧❧❧ PATIENT INFORMATION ❧❧❧

Uses: Sage has no proven medical effects but may be antispasmodic and carminative.

Side Effects: The only side effects reported with the ingestion of sage include cheilitis, stomatitis, dry mouth, or local irritation.

BOTANY: Sage is a small, evergreen perennial plant with short woody stems that branch extensively and can attain heights of 0.6 to 0.9 m.[1] Its violet-blue flowers bloom from June to September. The plant is native to the Mediterranean region and grows throughout much of the world. This plant should not be confused with red sage or the brush sage of the desert.

HISTORY: Dried sage leaf is used as a culinary spice and as a source of sage oil, which is obtained by steam distillation. Traditionally, sage and its oil have been used for the treatment of a wide range of illnesses; the name *Salvia* derives from the Latin word meaning "healthy" or "to heal."[2,3] Extracts and teas have been used to treat digestive disorders, as a tonic, and as an antispasmodic. The plant has been used topically as an antiseptic and astringent and to manage excessive sweating.[4] Sage has been used internally as a tea for the treatment of dysmenorrhea, diarrhea, gastritis, and sore throat. The dried leaves have been smoked to treat asthma. Despite these varied uses, there is little evidence that the plant exerts any significant pharmacologic activity.

The plant's fragrance is said to suppress fish odor. Sage oil is used as a fragrance in soaps and perfumes. It is a widely used food flavoring, and sage oleoresin is also used in the culinary industry.

PHARMACOLOGY: Sage extracts have strong antioxidative activities, with labiatic acid and carnosic acid reported to be the active compounds.[1] The phenolic acid salvin and its monomethyl ether found in sage have antimicrobial activity, especially against *Staphylococcus aureus*.[1] There is some evidence that sage oil may exert a centrally mediated antisecretory action; the carminative effect likely is due to the irritating effects of the volatile oil.[5]

TOXICOLOGY: Although sage oil contains thujone, the oil does not have a reputation for toxicity. The oil is non-irritating and nonsensitizing when applied topically to human skin in diluted concentrations.[1] Cheilitis and stomatitis have been reported in some cases following sage tea ingestion.[4] Others have reported that ingestion of large amounts of the plant extract may cause dry mouth or local irritation.

[1] Leung AY. *Encyclopedia of Common Natural Ingredients Used in Food, Drugs, and Cosmetics.* New York, NY: John Wiley and Sons, 1980.

[2] Dobelis IN, ed. *Magic and Medicine of Plants.* Pleasantville, NY: Reader's Digest Association, Inc., 1986.

[3] Simon JE. *Herbs: an indexed bibliography, 1971-1980.* Hamden, CT: Shoe String Press, 1984.

[4] Duke, JA. *Handbook of Medicinal Herbs.* Boca Raton, FL: CRC Press, 1985.

[5] Spoerke DG, Jr. *Herbal Medications.* Santa Barbara, CA: Woodbridge Press, 1980.

SCIENTIFIC NAME(S): *Hypericum perforatum* L. Family: Hypericaceae

COMMON NAME(S): St. John's wort, klamath weed, John's wort, amber touch-and-heal, goatweed, rosin rose, millepertuis

---

❧❧❧ PATIENT INFORMATION ❧❧❧

Uses: St. John's wort has been used to treat depression.

Drug Interactions: None known, although concomitant use with prescription antidepressants is not recommended.[1] Excessive doses may potentiate existing[2] monoamine oxidase inhibitor therapy and serotonin reuptake inhibitor therapy.[3]

Side Effects: Side effects are rare but have included rash caused by photosensitivity.

BOTANY: St. John's wort is an aromatic perennial native to Europe but now found throughout the US and parts of Canada. The plant is an aggressive weed found in the dry ground of roadsides, meadows, woods, and hedges. It generally grows to a height of 30 to 60 cm, except on the Pacific coast where it has reached heights of 1.5 m.[4] The plant has oval leaves and yields golden-yellow flowers, which bloom from June to September. It is said that the blooms are at their brightest coincidental with the feast day of John the Baptist (June 24).[5] The petals contain black or yellow glandular dots and lines. Harvest of the plant for medicinal purposes must occur July to August, and it must be dried immediately to avoid loss of potency.[6]

HISTORY: This plant has been used as an herbal remedy for its anti-inflammatory and healing properties since the Middle Ages. Although it fell into disuse, interest in St. John's wort was revived during the past decade, and it is now a component of numerous herbal preparations for the treatment of anxiety and depression. The plant has been used in traditional medicine as an antidepressant, diuretic, and treatment for gastritis and insomnia. An olive oil extract of the fresh flowers acquires a reddish color after standing in the sunlight for several weeks. This "red oil" has been taken internally for the treatment of anxiety but has also been applied externally to relieve inflammation and promote healing. Its topical application is believed to be particularly useful in the management of hemorrhoids. Although it is often listed as a folk treatment for cancer, there is no scientific evidence to document an antineoplastic effect.[5,6]

PHARMACOLOGY: Most of the research associated with this plant has focused on the pharmacologic activity of hypericin, the best known component of St. John's wort. This compound was thought to exert its tranquilizing effect by increasing capillary blood flow.[7]

The observed MAO inhibition seen with hypericin could be caused by a photo-catalyzed reaction in vitro, which would probably not be operative in the CNS. A paper by Bladt and Wagner examined *Hypericum* fractions in vitro and ex vivo and reported no evidence of MAO inhibition except at 1 mm, probably an unrealistic concentration.[8]

An extract of St. John's wort *(Psychotonin M)* elicited responses in experimental animal studies that were characteristic for antidepressant activity.[9] The antidepressant activity of this particular commercial product was further evaluated in 6 women with clinically evident depressive symptoms. After 4 to 6 weeks of treatment with only *Psychotonin M*, all patients showed a quantitative improvement in anxiety, dysphoric mood, loss of interest, and more than half a dozen other psychometric measurements.[10]

Many reports (1994 to present), including a study using the Hamilton depression scale, evaluate St. John's wort to be clinically effective in the treatment of mild-to-moderate depression,[11-13] rating close to 70% treatment response.[14] A meta-analysis evaluating 23 randomized trials, including 1757 mild–to-moderate severely depressed patients, was conducted to investigate St. John's wort (vs placebo and other conventional antidepressants). St. John's wort was significantly superior to placebo and "similarly effective" as conventional antidepressants. Side effects occurred in close to 20% of patients on *Hypericum* and 53% of patients on standard antidepressants.[15] Other reviews yielded similar outcomes.[6,11,16]

Pharmacokinetics of hypericin and pseudohypericin have been performed in humans, and although similar in structure, they possess substantial pharmacokinetic differences.[17] Single-dose and steady-state pharmacokinetics have also been evaluated.[18] A daily dose of *Hypericum*, as determined by trials and studies, is 200 to 900 mg of alcohol extract.[6] Other unidentified components inhibit catechol-o-methyltransferase and suppress interleukin-6 release. The latter suppression probably affects mood through neurohormonal pathways. The benzodiazepine inhibition of benzodiazepine binding in vitro by amentoflavone, another constituent in *Hypericum* species has been reported.[19] St. John's wort has also been extensively studied for its antiviral activity.

Hypericin was investigated in hopes of finding an effective treatment against human immunodeficiency virus (HIV).[5,20]

Hypericin and pseudohypericin exert effects against a wide spectrum of other viruses as well, including influenza virus, herpes simplex virus types I and II, sindbis virus, poliovirus, retrovirus infection in vitro and in vivo, murine cytomegalovirus, and hepatitis C.[6,21,22] The mechanisms by which the 2 components exert their antiviral effects do not seem to be interruption of transcription, translation, or viral protein transport, but some unconventional mechanisms. Recent reports find that exposure of hypericin to fluorescent light markedly increases its antiviral activity.[5] *Hypericum* is discussed as a photodynamic agent and may be helpful in future therapeutics and diagnostics.[23]

Extracts of the plant have been active against gram-negative and gram-positive bacteria in vitro.[24] In one report, *Hypericum* extract showed bacteriostatic activity at a dilution of 1:200,000 and bactericidal action at 1:20,000.[6] St. John's wort has also been used to treat otitis infection in 20% tincture form. The tannin component of the plant probably exerts an astringent action that contributes to the plant's traditional use as a wound-healing agent.[21] A report on the polycyclic dione, hypericin, as a potential antiglioma therapy has been presented.[25]

Other uses include: Oral and topical administration of hypericin for treatment of vitiligo (failure of skin to form melanin),[26] anti-inflammatory, and antiulcerogenic properties from the component amentoflavone (a biapigenin derivative)[27] and folk uses such as hemorrhoid and burn treatment.[6]

TOXICOLOGY: In controlled human studies of a standardized extract, no adverse effects, including changes in

EEG, ECG, or laboratory test parameters, were observed following treatment for up to 6 weeks.[9]

A reaction resembling sedative-hypnotic intoxication occurred in a patient following ingestion of St. John's wort and paroxetine.[3] The reaction did not occur when the patient took the herbal product alone.

When ingested, hypericin can induce photosensitization, characterized by inflammation of the skin and mucous membranes following exposure to light. While this reaction is observed rarely in humans, it is of more significance in animals that graze on the plant.[21] A case report of photosensitivity occurring in a 61-year-old female discusses "recurring elevated itching erythematous lesions" from 3 years of taking St. John's wort for depression. The rash was reversible after discontinuation of the medication.[28]

Slight in vitro uterotonic activity from St. John's wort has been reported in animals, suggesting avoidance of use during pregnancy.[21]

The volatile oil of St. John's wort is an irritant.[21]

[1] Blumenthal M, et al. *Popular Herbs in the US Market: Therapeutic Monographs.* Austin, TX: American Botanical Council, 1997.

[2] Newall CA, et al. *Herbal Medicines: A Guide for Health-Care Professionals.* London, England: Pharmaceutical Press, 1996;250-52.

[3] Gordon J. *Am Fam Physician* 1998;57:950-53.

[4] Awang DVC. *CPJ-RPC* 1991 Jan:33.

[5] Tyler VE. *The New Honest Herbal.* Philadelphia, PA: G.F. Stickley Co., 1987.

[6] Bombardelli E, et al. *Fitoterapia* 1995;66(1):43-68.

[7] Suzuki O, et al. *Planta Med* 1984;2:272.

[8] *J Geriatr Psychiatry Neurol* 7 1994;(Suppl 1): S57-S59.

[9] Okpanyi VSN, et al. *Arzneimittelforschung* 1987;37:10.

[10] Muldner VH, et al. *Arzneimittelforschung* 1984;34:918.

[11] Ernst E. *Fortschr Med* 1995;113(25):354-55.

[12] Mueller W, et al. *Deutsche Apotheker Zeitung* 1996 Mar 28;136:17-22, 24.

[13] DeSmet P, et al. *BMJ* 1996 Aug 3;313:241-42.

[14] Harrer G, et al. *Phytomedicine* 1994;1:3-8.

[15] Linde K, et al. *BMJ* 1996;313(7052):253-58.

[16] Witte B, et al. *Fortschritte Der Medizin* 1995;113(28):404-8.

[17] Staffeldt B, et al. *J Geriatr Psychiatry Neurol* 1994 Oct 7;(Suppl 1):547-53.

[18] Kerb R, et al. *Antimicrob Agents Chemother* 1996;40(9):2087-93.

[19] Baureithel K, et al. *Pharm Acta Helv* 1997;72(3):153-57.

[20] Castleman M. *The Healing Herbs.* Emmaus, PA: Rodale Press, 1991.

[21] Newall C, et al. *Herbal Medicines.* London, England: Pharmaceutical Press, 1996;250-52.

[22] Taylor R, et al. *J Ethnopharmacol* 1996;52(3):157-63.

[23] Diwu Z. *Photochem Photobiol* 1995;61(6):529-39.

[24] Barbagallo C, et al. *Fitoterapia* 1987;58:175.

[25] Couldwell W, et al. *Neurosurgery* 1994;35(4):705-10.

[26] Duke JA. *Handbook of Medicinal Herbs.* Boca Raton, FL: CRC Press, 1985.

[27] Berghofer R, et al. *Planta Med* 1989;55:91.

[28] Golsch S, et al. *Hautarzt* 1997;48(4):249-52.

SCIENTIFIC NAME(S): *Sassafras albidum* (Nuttal) Nees, synonymous with *S. officinale* Nees et Erbem. and *S. variifolium* Kuntze. Family: Lauraceae

COMMON NAME(S): Sassafras, saxifras, ague tree, cinnamon wood, saloop

---

❧❧❧ PATIENT INFORMATION ❧❧❧

Uses: Sassafras has been used for eye inflammation, insect bites and stings, lice, rheumatism, gout, sprains, swelling, and cutaneous lesions but is now banned in the US, even for use as a flavoring or fragrance.

Side Effects: Besides containing a cancer-causing agent, sassafras can induce vomiting, stupor, and hallucinations. It can also cause abortion, diaphoresis, and dermatitis.

BOTANY: Sassafras is the name applied to three species of trees, two native to eastern Asia, and one native to eastern North America. Fossils show that sassafras was once widespread in Europe, North America, and Greenland. The trees grow up to $\approx$ 30 m in height and 1.8 m in diameter, though they are usually smaller. Sassafras bears leaves 10 to 15 cm long that are oval on older branches but mitten-shaped or three-lobed on younger shoots and twigs. All parts of the tree are strongly aromatic. The drug is obtained by peeling the root (root bark).[1]

HISTORY: American Indians have used sassafras for centuries and told early settlers that it would cure a variety of ills. The settlers exported it to Europe, where it was found to be ineffective.[2]

Over the years, the oil from the roots and wood has been used as a scent in perfumes and soaps. The leaves and pith, when dried and powdered, have been used as a thickener in soups. The roots are often dried and steeped for tea, and sassafras was formerly used as a flavoring in root beer. Its use as a drug or food product has been banned by the FDA as carcinogenic; however, its use and sale persist throughout the US. Medicinally, sassafras has been applied to insect bites and stings to relieve symptoms.[2]

PHARMACOLOGY: Sassafras has been used as a sudorific agent,[3] a flavoring agent for dentifrices, root beers, and tobaccos, and for treatment of eye inflammation.[4] Extracts of the roots and bark have been found to mimic insect juvenile hormone in *Oncopeltus fasciatus*.[5] The oil has been applied externally for relief of insect bites and stings and for lice. Other external uses include treatment of rheumatism, gout, sprains, swelling, and cutaneous eruptions.[4,6]

The plant has been reported to have antineoplastic activity[7] and to induce cytochrome P488 and P450 enzymes.[6] Sassafras is said to antagonize certain alcohol effects.[4] Alcohol extracts of the related *S. randaiense* Rehder exhibit antimicrobial and antifungal activity in vitro, and this activity appears to be due to the presence of magnolol and isomagnolol.[8]

TOXICOLOGY: Sassafras oil and safrole have been banned for use as flavors and food additives by the FDA because of their carcinogenic potential. Safrole and its metabolite, 1'-hydroxysafrole, act as nerve poisons and have caused malignant hepatic tumors in animals. Based on animal data and a margin-of-safety factor of 100, a dose of 0.66 mg safrole per kg body weight is considered hazardous for humans; the dose obtained from sassafras tea may be as high as 200 mg (3 mg/kg).[1,9] One study showed that even a safrole-free

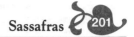

extract produced malignant mesenchymal tumors in > 50% of black rats treated. These tumors corresponded to malignant fibrous histiocytomas in humans.[10]

Oil of sassafras is toxic in doses as small as 5 ml in adults.[11] Ingestion of 5 ml produced shakes, vomiting, high blood pressure and high pulse rate in a 47-year-old female.[12] Another case of a 1 tsp dose of sassafras oil in a young man also caused vomiting, along with dilated pupils, stupor, and collapse.[4] There have been additional reports of the oil causing death,[6] abortion,[4] and liver cancer.[1,4,6] Safrole is a potent inhibitor of liver microsome hydroxylating enzymes; this effect may result in toxicity caused by altered drug metabolism.[9] Symptoms of sassafras oil poisoning in humans may include vomiting, stupor, lowering of body temperature, exhaustion, tachycardia, spasm, hallucinations, paralysis, and collapse.[1,6]

Additionally, sassafras can cause diaphoresis[13] and contact dermatitis in certain individuals.[4] A case study reported oil of sassafras in combination as a teething preparation, which resulted in false-positive blood tests for diphenylhydantoin in a 4-month-old child.[14]

[1] Bisset N. *Herbal Drugs and Phytopharmaceuticals* Stuttgart, Germany: CRC Press, 1994;455-56.

[2] Winter R. *The People's Handbook of Allergies and Allergens* Chicago, IL: Contemporary Books, 1984.

[3] *Merck Index*, 10th ed. Rahway, NJ: Merck and Co. 1983.

[4] Duke J. *CRC Handbook of Medicinal Herbs* CRC Press:Boca Raton, FL. 1989;430-31.

[5] Jacobson M, et al. *Lloydia* 1975;38:455.

[6] Newall C, et al. *Herbal Medicine* London, England: Pharmaceutical Press, 1996;235-36.

[7] Hartwell JL. *Lloydia* 1969;32:247.

[8] El-Feraly F, et al. *J Nat Prod* 1983 Jul-Aug;46:493-98.

[9] Segelman AB. *JAMA* 1976;236:477.

[10] Benedetti MS, et al. *Toxicology* 1977;7:69.

[11] Spoerke DG. *Herbal Medications* Santa Barbara, CA: Woodridge Press Publishing Co. 1980.

[12] Grande G, et al. *Vet Hum Toxicol* 1987 Dec;29:447.

[13] Haines J. *Postgrad Med* 1991;90(4):75-76.

[14] Jones M, et al. *Am J Dis Child* 1971 Sep;122:259-60.

SCIENTIFIC NAME(S): *Serenoa repens* (Bartr.) Small. This plant is sometimes referred to as *S. serrulata* (Michx.) Nichols or *Sabal serrulatum* Schult. Family: Palmae

COMMON NAME(S): Saw palmetto, sabal, American dwarf palm tree, cabbage palm

---

❧❧❧ PATIENT INFORMATION ❧❧❧

Uses: Recent studies suggest that extracts of saw palmetto may be beneficial in the management of prostate enlargement.

Side Effects: No significant adverse effects are reported with saw palmetto, but it may cause headaches and, if taken in large amounts, diarrhea. It should not be used by pregnant women or those of childbearing potential.

BOTANY: The saw palmetto is a member of the fan palms and grows to $\approx$ 3 m with leaf clusters that can each attain a length of $\geq$ 60 cm. The plant grows from the Carolinas to Texas. Saw palmetto produces a brownish black berry that is harvested commercially.

HISTORY: Saw palmetto berry tea has been used for years for the management of GU problems, to increase sperm production, to increase breast size, and to increase sexual vigor. Early in the century, it was used as a mild diuretic and as a treatment for prostatic enlargement. However, the therapeutic value of the tea came under question and saw palmetto was eventually dropped from the National Formulary.[1]

PHARMACOLOGY: Although assessments based on earlier research indicated that the plant was of no therapeutic value, a number of more recent studies suggest that extracts of the plant may be beneficial in the management of prostatic enlargement (benign prostatic hypertrophy [BPH]).

A hexane extract of the berries has been shown to have antiandrogenic properties through a direct action on the estrogen receptors and by inhibiting the enzyme testosterone-5-alpha-reductase.[2] Saw palmetto extract has been shown to inhibit DHT binding to cellular and nuclear receptor sites, thereby increasing the metabolism and excretion of DHT.[3] A double-blind placebo-controlled study evaluated the hormonal effects of saw palmetto extract given to men with BPH for 3 months prior to operation. The study found that saw palmetto had an estrogenic and antiprogesterone effect as determined by estrogen and progesterone receptor activity.[4]

The results from numerous double-blinded trials and open trials of the effects of saw palmetto extract in BPH have been reported. Typically, these studies have been small and of $\approx$ 3 months' duration.

In one of the larger trials,[2] 110 patients each received either a hexane extract of saw palmetto or placebo under double-blind conditions for 30 days. Active treatment consisted of 320 mg/day of a commercially available 80 mg tablet preparation. Treatment was assessed based on objective measures such as nocturia, intensity of dysuria, flow rate, postmicturition residue, and subjective patient and physician assessments. *S. repens* extracts were statistically superior to placebo for every parameter after 30 days of treatment. In a study of 45 patients with BPH, prazosin (eg, *Minipress*) was found to be only marginally more effective than saw palmetto extract when given for 12 weeks, as measured by flowmetry and subjective assessments of irritation.[5]

Extracts of *S. repens* have been shown to inhibit both cyclooxygenase and 5-lipoxygenase, thereby contributing to its anti-inflammatory effect.[6]

TOXICOLOGY: In most controlled trials, the incidence of side effects was low and consisted mainly of headache. No changes in blood chemistry parameters have been noted during therapy. Large amounts of the berry are reported to cause diarrhea.[7] Although the plant has been classified an "Herb of Undefined Safety," no important adverse events have been reported.[8] Because of its potential hormonal effects, the product should not be used by pregnant women or those of childbearing potential. Similarly, little experience exists with the extract when given to children or patients suffering from hormonal-dependent illnesses other than benign prostatic hypertrophy (ie, prostate or breast cancers).

[1] Elghamry MI, et al. *Experientia* 1969;25:828.
[2] Champault G, et al. *Br J Clin Pharmacol* 1984;18:461.
[3] Sultan C, et al. *J Steroid Biochem* 1984;20:515.
[4] DiSilverio F, et al. *Eur Urol* 1992;21:309.
[5] Semino M, et al. *Arch Esp Urol* 1992;45:211.
[6] Breu W, et al. *Arzneimittelforschung* 1992;42:547.
[7] Spoerke DG. *Herbal Medications*. Santa Barbara, CA: Woodbridge Press, 1980.
[8] Duke JA. *Handbook of Medicinal Herbs*. Boca Raton, FL: CRC Press, 1985.

Schisandra

SCIENTIFIC NAME(S): *Schisandra chinensis* Baillon, *S. arisanensis* Hayata, *S. sphenanthera* Rehd, *S. rubriflora* Franch. Family: Schizandraceae

COMMON NAME(S): Schisandra, schizandra; gomishi, hoku-gomishi, kita-gomishi (Japanese); wu-wei-zu (Chinese)

❧❧❧ PATIENT INFORMATION ❧❧❧

Uses: Schisandra has been used as a tonic and restorative, as well as for liver protection, nervous system effects, respiratory treatment, GI therapy and others.

Side Effects: Research indicates that side effects are infrequent, although schisandra has the ability to produce profound CNS depression and may interfere with the metabolism of other concurrently administered drugs.

BOTANY: The family Schizandraceae (Schisandraceae) comprises 2 genera (*Schisandra* and *Kadsura*). *Schisandra* spp are climbing, aromatic trees with white, pink, yellow, or reddish male or female flowers. The fruits are globular and red with several kidney-shaped seeds. The fruit is harvested in autumn when fully ripened.[1] *S. chinensis* is native to northeastern and north central China and is found in eastern Russia.

HISTORY: Schisandra is one of the many traditional Chinese medicines that are recommended for coughs and various nonspecific pulmonary diseases.[2] It has been studied extensively in Chinese and Japanese literature. Schisandra had been used for healing purposes for > 2000 years. It is often used as an ethanolic tincture. The Chinese name for the plant, "wu-wei-zu," means "five-flavored herb" because of the flavor of the five main "elemental energies" of the plant. The fruit has a salty, sour taste.[1]

PHARMACOLOGY: Besides serving as a tonic and restorative, schisandra has other reported uses, such as liver protection, nervous system effects, respiratory treatment, GI therapy, adaptogenic properties, and others.

Liver: The lignan components in schisandra possess definite liver protectant effects. The active principles appear to be lignans such as wu-wei-zu C, shisantherin D, deoxygomisin A, gomisin N, and gomisin C. Active hepatoprotective constituents all appear to share 1 or 2 methylene dioxy group.[2,3] Animal studies on gomisin A offer convincing evidence of liver protection, including protective actions against halothane-induced hepatitis,[4] carbon tetrachloride, d-galactosamine, and dl-ethionine toxicity,[5,6] hepatic failure induced by bacteria,[7] and preneoplastic hepatic lesions.[8-11] Gomisin A's mechanism for tumor inhibition may be a result of its ability to improve bile acid metabolism.[12] Gomisin A causes hepatic cell proliferation, improves liver regeneration, hepatic blood flow, and liver function recovery in rats.[13] These effects are caused by protection of the hepatocyte plasma membrane.[14]

Ethanol extracts of schisandra have been found to increase liver weight in rats and mice. This action has been attributed to schizandrin B and schizandrol B. In a mouse study, extract added to a semipurified basal diet over a 14-day period increased the enzymatic metabolism of the mutagens benzo[a]pyrene (BaP) and aflatoxin B (AFB) and increased cytochrome P450 activity. Despite this increased level of metabolism, schisandra extract increased the in vitro mutagenicity of AFB. However, chemicals inducing similar patterns of enzymes have been found to reduce the in vivo binding of AFB to DNA.[15] It is also recognized that the schizandrins and ≈ 6 related compounds may temporarily inhibit or lower the activity of hepatic ALT. This has been observed in animals pretreated with hepatotoxins.[16-18]

Nervous System: Schisandra is a nervous system stimulant, increasing reflex responses and improving mental alertness. In China, the berries are used to treat mental illnesses such as depression. It is also used for irritability and memory loss.[1] Schisandra in combination with other herbs has improved memory retention disorder and facilitated memory retention deficit in animal testing. This suggests a possible use in treating age-related memory deficits in humans.[19] Schisandra (also in combination with *Zizyphus spinosa* and *Angelica sinensis*) has accelerated neurocyte growth and may prevent atrophy of neurocyte process branches.[20] Schisandra has been evaluated for its inhibitory effects on the CNS as well. In Chinese medicine, it is used as a sedative for insomnia.[1] This inhibition mechanism has been evaluated and may be related to effects on dopaminergic receptors.[21] Gomisin A has also inhibited spontaneous and methamphetamine-induced motor activity in animals.[22]

Respiratory: Schisandra is used to treat respiratory ailments such as shortness of breath, wheezing, and cough.[1]

GI: In the rat intestine, schisandra extract reduces BaP metabolism, which is the opposite effect from that in the liver. Experiments show that it increases the activity of glutathione S-transferase. In the intestine, schisandra shifts BaP metabolism in favor of diols and 3-hydroxybenzo[a]pyrene and away from BaP- 4,5-epoxide and the mutagenic BaP quinones. Schisandra does not increase intestinal cytochrome P450 activity.[23] Schisandra has been used for treatment of diarrhea and dysentery.[1] One report found schisandra extract to have no significant effects on gastric secretory volume, gastric pH, and acid output,[24] while another study found schisandra to have inhibitory effects on gastric contraction and stress-induced gastric ulceration when administered IV and orally in rats.[22] Metabolism of schisandra has been reported.[25-27] It has been used to balance fluid levels, improve sexual stamina, treat rashes, stimulate uterine contractions, and improve failing senses.[1] One report found antibacterial effects in alcohol and acetone extracts of the fruit.[3]

TOXICOLOGY: Schisandra has the capability to produce profound CNS depression. Because of its documented effects on hepatic and gastric enzyme activity, it is possible that schisandra may interfere with the metabolism of other concurrently administered drugs. The full spectrum of the clinical effects of the plant on the liver are not well documented, and the safety of the plant has not been established scientifically. However, research does not report any incidence of toxic side effects.

[1] Chevallier A. *Encyclopedia of Medicinal Plants* New York, NY: DK Publishing, 1996.

[2] Hikino H, et al. *Planta Med* 1984;50:213.

[3] Maeda S, et al. *Yakugaku Zasshi* 1982;102(6):579–88.

[4] Jiaxiang N, et al. *J Appl Toxicol* 1993;13(6):385-88.

[5] Ko K, et al. *Planta Med* 1995;61(2):134-37.

[6] Takeda S, et al. *Nippon Yakurigaku Zasshi* 1986;87(2):169-87.

[7] Mizoguchi Y, et al. *Planta Med* 1991;57(4):320-24.

[8] Nomura M, et al. *Cancer Lett* 1994;76(1):11-18.

[9] Ohtaki Y, et al. *Biol Pharm Bull* 1994;17(6):808-14.

[10] Nomura M, et al. *Anticancer Res* 1994;14(5A):1967-71.

[11] Miyamoto K, et al. *Biol Pharm Bull* 1995;18(10):1443-45.

[12] Ohtaki Y, et al. *Anticancer Res* 1996;16(2):751-55.

[13] Takeda S, et al. *Nippon Yakurigaku Zasshi* 1986;88(4):321-30.

[14] Nagai H, et al. *Planta Med* 1989;55(1):13-17.

[15] Hendrich S, et al. *Food Chem Toxicol* 1986;24:903.

[16] Tiangtong B, et al. *Chin Med J* 1980;93:41.

[17] Maeda S, et al. *Jpn J Pharmacol* 1985;38:347.

[18] Pao T, et al. *Chung Hua I Hsueh Tsa Chih* 1974 May;54:275-77.

[19] Nishiyama N, et al. *Biol Pharm Bull* 1996;19(3):388-93.

[20] Hu G, etal. *Chin Pharm J* 1994 Jun;29:333-36.

[21] Zhang L, et al. *Chung Kuo I Hsueh Ko Hsueh Yuan Hsueh Pao* 1991;13(1):13-16.

[22] Maeda S, et al. *Yakugaku Zasshi* 1981 Nov;101:1030-41.

[23] Salbe AD, et al. *Food Chem Toxicol* 1985;23:57.

[24] Hernandez D, et al. *J Ethnopharmacol* 1988 May/Jun;23:109-14.

[25] Hendrich S, et al. *Food Chem Toxicol* 1936;24(9):903-12.

[26] Chi Y, et al. *Yao Hsueh Hsueh Pao* 1992;27(1):57-63.

[27] Chi Y, et al. *Eur J Drug Metab Pharmacokinet* 1993;18(2):155-60.

SCIENTIFIC NAME(S): *Scutellaria laterifolia* L. Family: Labiatae

COMMON NAME(S): Scullcap, skullcap, helmetflower, hoodwort, mad-dog weed

---

ഇ⭑ഇ⭑ PATIENT INFORMATION ഇ⭑ഇ⭑

Uses: Scullcap is not recognized as having therapeutic activity although recent studies suggest that it might have anti-inflammatory activity.

Side Effects: If taken in a normal dose, scullcap does not seem to exhibit any adverse effects.

BOTANY: Scullcap, a member of the mint family, is native to the US where it grows in moist woods. Scullcap is an erect perennial that grows to 0.6 to 0.9 m in height. Its bluish flowers bloom from July to September. Official compendia (eg, NF VI) recognized only the dried overground portion of the plant as useful; however, some herbal texts listed all parts as medicinal.[1] The aerial parts of the plant are collected during the flowering period, typically August and September. A number of species have been used medicinally, and the most common European species has been *S. baicalensis* Georgii, a native of East Asia.

HISTORY: Scullcap appears to have been introduced into traditional American medicine toward the end of the 1700s as a treatment for the management of hydrophobia. It was later used as a tonic, particularly in proprietary remedies for "female weakness."[2] The plant was reputed to be an herbal tranquilizer, particularly in combination with valerian but has since fallen into disuse.

PHARMACOLOGY: Over the past 15 years, Japanese researchers have investigated the activity of the related plant *S. baicalensis*. Animal studies indicate that extracts of the plant have a demonstrable anti-inflammatory effect. Although the mechanism of action is not well understood, it is believed that hot water extracts of *Scutellaria* and the active metabolites of the flavonoids baicalin and wogonin glucuronide (baicalein and wogonin, respectively) are potent inhibitors of the enzyme sialidase.[3] In another study, isoscutellarein-8-*O*-glucuronide from the leaf was found to be a potent inhibitor of the enzyme.[4] Serum sialic acid increases cancers, rheumatic diseases, infections, and inflammations, and a sialidase inhibitor, such as scullcap extract, may have a therapeutic application. Teas prepared from *Scutellaria* species have demonstrable in vitro antibacterial and antifungal activity.[5]

TOXICOLOGY: There is no evidence to indicate that *Scutellaria* is toxic when ingested at "normal" doses. According to the FDA, overdose of the tincture causes giddiness, stupor, confusion, twitching of the limbs, intermission of the pulse, and other symptoms similar to convulsions.[6]

---

[1] Meyer JE. *The Herbalist*. Hammond, IN: Hammond Book Co., 1934.

[2] Tyler VE. *The New Honest Herbal*. Philadelphia, PA: G.F. Stickley Co., 1987.

[3] Nagai T, et al. *Planta Med* 1989;55:27.

[4] Nagai T, et al. *Biochem Biophys Res Comm* 1989;163:25.

[5] Franzblau SG, et al. *J Ethnopharmacol* 1986;15:279.

[6] Duke JA. *Handbook of Medicinal Herbs*. Boca Raton, FL: CRC Press, 1985.

Senna

SCIENTIFIC NAME(S): *Cassia acutifolia* Delile, syn. with *Cassia senna* L. and *C. angustifolia* Vahl. Family: Fabaceae

---

❧❧❧ PATIENT INFORMATION ❧❧❧

Uses: Senna is most commonly used as a laxative.

Side Effects: The chronic use of senna has resulted in pigmentation of the colon, reversible finger clubbing, cachexia, and a dependency on the laxative.

BOTANY: *C. acutifolia* is native to Egypt and the Sudan while *C. angustifolia* is native to Somalia and Arabia. Plants known as "wild sennas" (*C. hebecarpa* Fern. and *C. marilandica* L.) grow on moist banks and woods in the eastern US. This plant should not be confused with "cassia," a common name for cinnamon. Senna is a low branching shrub, growing to ≈ 0.9 m in height. It has a straight woody stem and yellow flowers.[1] The top parts are harvested, dried, and graded. The hand-collected senna is known as Tinnevally senna. Leaves that have been harvested and graded mechanically are known as Alexandria senna. There are more than 400 known species of *Cassia*.[1]

HISTORY: Senna was first used medicinally by Arabian physicians in the ninth century A.D.[1] It was used in traditional Arabic and European medicine as a cathartic. The leaves have been brewed and the tea administered for its strong laxative effect. Because it is often difficult to control the concentration of the active ingredients in the tea, an unpredictable effect may be obtained. Therefore, standardized commercial dosage forms have been developed, and these concentrates are available as liquids, powders, and tablets in *otc* laxatives. The plant derives its name from the Arabic "sena" and from the Hebrew word "cassia," which means "peeled back," a reference to its peelable bark.

PHARMACOLOGY: Senna is a potent laxative. Its cathartic effects can be obtained from a tea prepared from 5 or 10 ml of dried leaves.

Senna's use in treating constipation is well documented. It is a popular laxative, especially in the elderly.[2] Many reports are available discussing senna's role in constipation,[3,4] its use in the elderly,[5-9] in psychiatric patients,[10] in spinal cord injury patients,[11] and in pregnancy, where it is the stimulant laxative of choice.[12] In cancer treatment protocols, senna also has reversed the constipating effects of narcotics and may prevent constipation if given with the narcotic.[13] However, it may cause more adverse effects than other laxatives, primarily abdominal pain.[14] Castor oil was superior to senna for chronic constipation sufferers in another report.[15]

Senna may affect intestinal transit time.[16-18] Its effectiveness as part of a cleansing regimen to evacuate the bowels in preparation for such tests as colonoscopies or barium enemas is documented.[19-29] Results from these studies include reduced ingestion of commercial *Golytely* solution and simethicone when given with senna[24] and more effective colon cleansing with senna in combination with polyethylene glycol electrolyte lavage solution, compared to the solution alone.[25] Senna has also been studied in chronic constipation,[30] and as long-term laxative treatment.[31] Several mechanisms are postu-

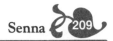

lated as to how senna acts as an effective laxative. Sennosides irritate the lining of the large intestine, causing contraction, which results in a bowel movement $\approx$ 10 hours after the dose is taken.[1] The anthraquinone glycosides are hydrolyzed by intestinal bacteria to yield the active, free anthraquinones. Alternately, it has been suggested that the glycosides are absorbed in small quantities from the small intestine, hydrolyzed in the liver, and the resultant anthraquinones are secreted into the colon.[32] One report using human intestinal flora showed sennoside A converts to rheinanthrone, the active principle causing peristalsis of the large intestines. Sennosides A and B also play a role in inducing fluid secretion in the colon.

Prostaglandins may also be involved in the laxative actions.[33] One report suggests prostaglandin-mediated action of sennosides.[34] Indomethacin can partly inhibit the actions of sennosides A and B.[33] However, conflicting reports argue that prostaglandins do not contribute to the laxative effect.[35,36]

Metabolism of anthranoid laxatives has been reported,[37,38] as has the metabolism of sennosides.[39-41] The kinetics of senna constituents rhein and aloe-emodin have been investigated.[42]

TOXICOLOGY: Chronic use of any laxative, in particular irritant laxatives such as senna, often results in a "laxative-dependency syndrome" characterized by poor gastric motility in the absence of repeated laxative administration. Other reports of laxative abuse include laxative-induced diarrhea,[43,44] osteomalacia, and arthropathy associated with prolonged use.[45]

The chronic use of anthroquinone glycosides has been associated with pigmentation of the colon (*melanosis coli*).

Several cases of reversible finger clubbing (enlargement of the ends of the fingers and toes) have been reported following long-term abuse of senna-containing laxatives.[46-48] One report described a woman who developed finger clubbing following ingestion of 4 to 40 *Senokot* tablets per day for $\approx$ 15 years.[49] Clubbing reversed when the laxative was stopped. The mechanism may be related to either increased vascularity of the nail beds or a systemic metabolic abnormality secondary to chronic laxative ingestion.

Senna abuse has been associated with the development of cachexia and reduced serum globulin levels after chronic ingestion.[50]

Risk assessment for senna's use during pregnancy has been addressed.[51] One review suggests senna to be the "stimulant laxative" of choice during pregnancy and lactation.[12] Uterine motility was not stimulated by sennosides in one report in pregnant ewes.[52] None of the breast-fed infants experienced abnormal stool consistency from their mothers' ingestion of senna laxatives. The constituent rhein, taken from milk samples varied in concentration from 0 to 27 ng/ml, with 89% to 94% of values < 10 ng/ml.[53,54] Nonstandardized laxatives are not recommended during pregnancy.[33]

Generally, senna may cause mild abdominal discomfort such as cramping. Prolonged use may alter electrolytes. Patients with intestinal obstruction should avoid senna.[33]

Various case reports of senna toxicity are available and include coma and neuropathy after ingestion of a senna-combination laxative,[55] hepatitis after chronic use of the plant,[56] occupational asthma and rhinoconjunctivitis from a factory worker exposed to senna-containing hair dyes,[57] and asthma and allergy symptoms from workers in a bulk laxative manufacturing facility.[58]

[1] Chevallier A. *Encyclopedia of Medicinal Plants* New York, NY: DK Publishing, 1996;72.

[2] Heaton K, et al. *Dig Dis Sci* 1993;38(6):1004-8.

[3] Marlett J, et al. *Am J Gastroenterol* 1987;82(4):333-37.

[4] Godding E. *Pharmacology* 1988;36(Suppl)1:230-36.

[5] Maddi V. *J Am Geriatr Soc* 1979 Oct;27:464-68.

[6] Passmore A, et al. *BMJ* 1993;307(6907):769-71.

[7] Kinnunen O, et al. *Pharmacology* 1993;47(Suppl)1:253-55.

[8] Passmore A, et al. *Pharmacology* 1993;47(Suppl)1:249-52.

[9] Pahor M, et al. *Aging* 1995;7(2):128-35.

[10] Georgia E. *Curr Ther Res* 1983 Jun;33(Sec 1);1018-22.

[11] Cornell S, et al. *Nurs Res* 1973 Jul-Aug;22:321-28.

[12] Gattuso J, et al. *Drug Saf* 1994;10(1):47-65.

[13] Cameron J. *Cancer Nurs* 1992;15(5):372-77.

[14] Sykes N. *J Pain Sympt Manage* 1996; 11(6):363-69.

[15] Pawlik A, et al. *Herba Polonica* 1994;40(1-2):64-67.

[16] Rogers H, et al. *Br J Clin Pharmacol* 1978 Dec;6:493-97.

[17] Sogni P, et al. *Gastroenterol Clin Biol* 1992;16(1):21-24.

[18] Ewe K, et al. *Pharmacology* 1993;47(Suppl)1:242-48.

[19] Staumont G, et al. *Pharmacology* 1988;36(Suppl)1:49-56.

[20] Han R. *Chung Hua Hu Li Tsa Chih* 1989;24(5):273-75.

[21] Hangartner P, et al. *Endoscopy* 1989;21(6):272-75.

[22] Labenz J, et al. *Med Klin* 1990;85(10):581-85.

[23] Borkje B, et al. *Scand J Gastroenterol* 1991;26(2):162-66.

[24] Wildgrube H, et al. *Bildgebung* 1991;58(2):63-66.

[25] Ziegenhagen D, et al. *Gastrointest Endosc* 1991;37(5):547-49.

[26] Bailey S, et al *Clin Radiol* 1991;44(5):335-37.

[27] Fernandez S, et al. *Rev Esp Enferm Dig* 1995;87(11):785-91.

[28] Tooson J, et al. *Postgrad Med* 1996;100(2):203-4, 207-12, 214.

[29] Ziegenhagen D, et al. *Z. Gastroenterol* 1992;30(1):17-19.

[30] Mishalany H. *J Pediatr Surg* 1989;24(4):360-62.

[31] Ralevic V, et al. *Gastroenterology* 1990;99(5):1352-57.

[32] Bowman WC, et al. *Textbook of Pharmacology*, 2nd ed., Blackwell Scientific Publications, 1980.

[33] Newall C, et al. *Herbal Medicines*, London, England: Pharmaceutical Press, 1996;243-44.

[34] Beubler E, et al. *Pharmacology* 1988;36(Suppl)1:85-91.

[35] Mascolo N, et al. *Pharmacology* 1988;36(Suppl)1:92-97.

[36] Mascolo N, et al. *J Pharm Pharmacol* 1988;40(12):882-84.

[37] deWitte P, et al. *Hepatogastroenterology* 1990;37(6):601-5.

[38] deWitte P. *Pharmacology* 1993;47(Suppl)1:86-97.

[39] Lemli J. *Pharmacology* 1988;36(Suppl)1:126-28.

[40] Hietala P, et al. *Pharmacology* 1988;36(Suppl)1:138-43.

[41] Lemli J. *Ann Gastroenterol Hepatol (Paris)* 1996;32(2):109-12.

[42] Krumbiegel G, et al. *Pharmacology* 47(Suppl)1:120-24.

[43] Cummings J, et al. *BMJ* 1974 Mar 23;1:537-41.

[44] Morris A, et al. *Gastroenterology* 1979 Oct;77:780-86.

[45] Frier B, et al. *Br J Clin Pract* 1977 Jan-Feb-Mar;31:17-19.

[46] Prior J, et al. *Lancet* 1978;ii:947.

[47] Malmquist J, et al. *Postgrad Med* 1980 Dec;56:862-64.

[48] Armstrong R, et al. *BMJ* 1981 Jun 6;282:1836.

[49] FitzGerald O, et al. *Ir J Med Sci* 1983:152:246.

[50] Levin D, et al. *Lancet* 1981;1:919.

[51] Anonymous. *Pharmacology* 1992;44(Suppl)1:20-22.

[52] Garcia-Villar R. *Pharmacology* 1988;36(Suppl)1:203-11.

[53] Faber P, et al. *Pharmacology* 1988;36(Suppl)1:212-20.

[54] Faber P, et al. *Geburtshilfe Frauenheilkd* 1989;49(11):958-62.

[55] Dobb G, et al. *Med J Aust* 1984 Apr 14;140:495-96.

[56] Beuers U, et al. *Lancet* 1991;337(8737):372-73.

[57] Helin T, et al. *Allergy* 1996;51(3):181-84.

[58] Marks G. *Am Rev Respir Dis* 1991;144(5):1065-69.

SCIENTIFIC NAME(S): *Squalus acanthias* (spiny dogfish shark), *Sphyrna lewini* (hammerhead shark) and other shark species

COMMON NAME(S): As above.

❧❧❧❧ PATIENT INFORMATION ❧❧❧❧

Uses: Shark cartilage has been touted as a cancer control agent, but no studies have proven this theory. Squalamine has been identified as a potent antibiotic with fungicidal and antiprotozoal activity.

Side Effects: No adverse effects have appeared on either substance.

HISTORY: Shark cartilage is prepared from the cartilage of freshly caught sharks in the Pacific Ocean. The cartilage is cut from the shark, cleaned, shredded, and dried. One of the main processing plants for dogfish shark is in Costa Rica.[1,2]

Squalamine was originally isolated from shark stomachs but has subsequently been synthesized.[1] This compound is still under experimental evaluation.

PHARMACOLOGY: Many claims have been made that shark cartilage can cure cancer. The rationale includes the fact that sharks rarely get cancer, that sharks are cartilaginous fish, and that cartilage is avascular and contains agents that inhibit vascularization (angiogenesis). The reasoning then follows that sharks do not get cancer because the inhibited vascularization prevents the formation of tumors; hence, giving it to humans may inhibit tumor angiogenesis and thus cure cancer.[1]

In late 1992, incomplete and unpublished clinical studies in Havana, Cuba, purported to show some progress in terminally ill cancer patients. The National Cancer Institute reviewed these studies and decided against researching shark cartilage.[1] Recently, however, the FDA granted an IND application for a shark cartilage product, *Benefin,* by Lane Labs-USA, Inc. to investigate benefits in prostate cancer and AIDS-related Kaposi's sarcoma.[3]

Future work should continue to focus on the isolation of the responsible proteins or small molecules. The tetranectin-like protein from the reef shark is important because, in humans, tetranectin enhances plasminogen activation catalyzed by the tissue plasminogen activator. It may also play a role in cancer metastasis. Research along these lines has demonstrated the presence of a broad-spectrum aminosterol antibiotic in the dogfish shark, which they named squalamine.[4] It shows significant bactericidal activity against gram-negative and gram-positive bacteria. It is also fungicidal and induces activity against protozoa.[4] This discovery implicates a unique steroid acting as a potential host-defense agent in vertebrates and provides unique concepts of chemical design for a new family of much needed broad-spectrum antibiotics.

TOXICOLOGY: No toxicity data have appeared in current literature on either shark cartilage or squalamine.

---

[1] Masslo Anderson J. *MD Magazine* 1993;37:43.
[2] Moss RW. *Cancer Therapy: The Independent Consumers Guide to Non-Toxic Treatment & Prevention.* New York, NY: Equinox Press, 1992.
[3] Hunt TJ, et al. *Am J Health-Syst Pharm* 1995;52:1756.
[4] Moore KS, et al. *Proc Nat Acad Sci USA* 1993;90(4):1354.

Slippery Elm

SCIENTIFIC NAME(S): *Ulmus rubra* Muhl. Also known as *U. fulva* Michx.
Family: Ulmaceae

COMMON NAME(S): Slippery elm, red elm

❧❧❧❧ PATIENT INFORMATION ❧❧❧❧

Uses: Parts of slippery elm have been used externally as emollients, while
powdered bark has been included in throat lozenges.

Side Effects: Extracts from slippery elm have caused contact dermatitis and the
pollen has been reported as allergenic.

BOTANY: The slippery elm tree is native to eastern Canada and eastern and central US, where it grows in moist woods to heights of 20 m.

HISTORY: The dried inner bark has been used in traditional medicine for more than a century in the US. Collected in the spring, the inner bark yields a thick mucilage or demulcent that was used in North American medicine to treat urinary tract inflammations and applied topically for cold sores and boils. A decoction of the leaves was used as a poultice to remove discoloration around blackened or bruised eyes.[1] A preparation of elm mucilage was official in the United States until late in the 19th century.

PHARMACOLOGY: Because of the mucilage content of slippery elm, preparations of the plant have been used externally as emollients. Powdered bark is incorporated into lozenges to provide demulcent action in the treatment of throat irritation.[2] Preparations of the plant are reported to have antiherpetic and antisyphilitic activity.[3]

TOXICOLOGY: An oleoresin from several *Ulmus* species has been reported to cause contact dermatitis,[1] and the pollen is allergenic.[3] Preparations of slippery elm were used as abortifacients, a practice which has not remained popular.

---

[1] Lewis WH, et al. *Medical Botany*. New York, NY: John Wiley and Sons, 1977.
[2] Morton JF. *Major Medicinal Plants*. Springfield, IL: C.C. Thomas, 1977.
[3] Duke JA. *Handbook of Medicinal Herbs*. Boca Raton, FL: CRC Press, 1985.

SCIENTIFIC NAME(S): *Glycine max* L. Leguminosae/Fabaceae

COMMON NAME(S): Soy, soybean, soya

❧❧❧ PATIENT INFORMATION ❧❧❧

Uses: Soy is commonly used as a source of fiber, protein, and minerals. The isoflavone compounds in soybeans may have anticancer effects, alleviate menopausal symptoms, prevent osteoporosis, and combat cardiovascular and GI problems.

Side Effects: Overall tolerance to soybeans is good to excellent for most patients. Although there are no strong studies, the effects on infant development by phytoestrogens in soy-based formulas is of concern. Soy dust has caused an asthma epidemic.

BOTANY: The soybean is an annual plant that grows ~ 0.3 to 1.5 m tall. Bean pods, stems, and leaves are covered with short, fine hairs. The pods contain up to 4 yellow-to-brownish oval seeds. The cotyledons account for most of the seed's weight and contain most of the oil and protein.[1]

HISTORY: Soybeans were cultivated in China as far back as the 11th century B.C. Described by Chinese Emperor Shung Nang in 2838 B.C., they were said to have been China's most important crop. Cultivation of the plant went to Japan, then Europe, and eventually to the US in the early 1800s. The US now produces half of the world's soybeans. Soybeans possess several benefits, including anticarcinogenic effects, improvement in cardiovascular and intestinal problems, and relief of menopausal symptoms. Soybeans are also an important source of nutrition.[1-3]

Soy is an important food source and has been used in Asian cultures for thousands of years. These cultures consume 2 to 3 ounces of soy per day, as compared with Western diets that contain ~ 1/10 of that amount.[3] Soybean products include soybean milk, soybean flour, soybean curd, sufu, tofu (cheese-like cake high in protein and calcium), tempeh (Indonesian main dish), fermented soybean paste (miso), soybeans sprouts, soy sauce, soybean oil, textured soy proteins (in meat extenders), soy protein drinks, and livestock feeds. Because of its low cost, good nutritional value, and versatility, soy protein is also used as part of food programs in less-developed countries. It is also used in infant formulas (most often if milk protein allergy exists).[1]

PHARMACOLOGY: Isoflavones from the soybean have hormonal and nonhormonal actions. Hydrolysis of isoflavone glycosides by intestinal glucosidases yields genistein, daidzein, and glycitein. These may also become further metabolized to additional metabolites including equol and p-ethyl phenol. This metabolism is highly individualistic and can vary, for example, with carbohydrate intake altering intestinal fermentation. Isoflavones undergo enterohepatic circulation and are secreted into bile. Plasma half-life of genistein and daidzein is ≈ 8 hours, with peak concentration being achieved in 6 to 8 hours in adults. Elimination is via urine, primarily as glucuronide conjugates.[4] Phytoestrogens may play important roles in cancer prevention, menopausal symptoms, osteoporosis, cardiovascular disease, and GI disorders. Proposed mechanisms of the phytoestrogens include estrogenic and antiestrogenic effects, induction of cancer cell differentiation, inhibition of tyrosine kinase and DNA topoisomerase activity, angiogenesis suppression, and antioxidant effects.[5]

Anticancer: Soybeans are one of the foods highest in anticancer activity.[6] Inhibition of early cancer markers in epithelial cells has been demonstrated by genistein.[7] Genistein's anticancer effects may be related to its ability to reduce expression of stress response related genes. Induction of stress proteins in tumor cells protects them against death, so inhibition of this stress response by the isoflavone is beneficial.[8] When foods with weak estrogen-like compounds such as soy are consumed by women, their blood estrogen levels drop, decreasing a breast cancer risk.[2] Soy has lengthened the menstrual cycle, decreasing the number of cycles in a lifetime. This reduces the incidence of each estrogen surge, which occurs early in each cycle, and may play another important role in fighting breast cancer. Menstrual cycles in Asian women are 2 to 3 days longer than those of western women.[2] Soy protein delayed menstruation by 1 to 5 days in one report. The mitotic rate for breast tissue is 4 times as great in the luteal phase as during the follicular phase. With longer cycles, longer follicular phases are present, which in addition, protects against breast cancer. Breast cancer rates are 0.2% in England but only 0.05% in Japan.[9] Genistein exhibited antiproliferative effects against breast cancer cell growth.[10] Asian women experience lower breast cancer incidence, which may be related to the high content of soy products in their diet. Soy supplementation as adjuvant treatment in early breast cancer patients may decrease risk of cancer recurrence.[11] A diet rich in legumes, especially soybeans, has been associated with a reduction of risk in endometrial cancer in a Hawaiian, case-controlled study in 332 diagnosed endometrial cancer patients.[12] Male cancer preven-

tative effects have also been documented from soy. Genistein decreased benign prostatic hypertrophy and prostate cancer growth in vitro, suggesting the isoflavones to be of potential therapeutic benefit.[13] Asian men consuming low-fat, high-fiber, soy-based diets have a lower incidence of prostate cancer than European or North American men. Isoflavonoids are present in prostatic fluid, and the metabolism of them in males has been reported.[14]

Menopausal symptoms/osteoporosis: Women of menopausal age suffering from decreased estrogen production may need to replace this important hormone. In standard hormone replacement therapy (HRT), a combination of estrogen and progesterone is commonly prescribed. This combination not only helps to alleviate menopausal symptoms, but the progesterone component prevents osteoporosis and reduces uterine cancer risk compared with using estrogens alone. HRT has also been shown to reduce risk of coronary heart disease.[15] However, HRT is less effective than estrogens alone in protection against heart disease and may increase the risk of breast cancer.[4] In addition, HRT regimens have low acceptance rates among postmenopausal women.[15] Soy products may offer a favorable but not necessarily safer alternative to conventional HRT. Hot flashes and postmenopausal symptoms, including bone mineral loss, can be reduced by 45 g of soyflour.[2] Hot flashes were decreased by 45% in one report in postmenopausal women given soy powder, as compared with a 30% reduction with placebo powder.[4] Soy phytochemical consumption may even prevent osteoporosis.[16] A mechanism that may help explain isoflavones' role in bone loss prevention is as follows: Estrogens attach to estrogen receptor (ER) sites in certain areas of the body,

"ER alpha," and the more recently found "ER beta." ER alpha is mostly present in the female reproductive system, where ER beta predominates in other estrogen-responsive tissue such as bladder and bone. This may help explain why estrogen has beneficial actions in bone and elsewhere. Genistein binds to ER alpha (weakly) but complexes ER beta as well as estrogen does. This bound portion then exerts its beneficial actions.[4]

Cardiovascular disease/lipid alterations: Increased consumption of soy in Asian populations is associated with decreased rates in cardiovascular disease.[16] A vegetarian diet, consisting of soy-based products was given to 32 coronary heart disease patients who discontinued their conventional hyperlipidemic medications. The diet resulted in normalization of serum lipids, with the best results associated with the group who maintained this diet for the longest period of time.[17] In another report, although arterial elasticity was improved 26% with soy isoflavone intake (80 mg/day) in 21 women, plasma lipids in this trial were unaffected.[18] Another study also concluded no differences in serum lipids from soy isoflavone supplementation. However, these effects were evaluated in patients with average serum cholesterol levels.[19]

GI benefits: Soybean fiber can prevent constipation, reducing the incidence of bowel disease.[2] Fiber-supplemented soy formula in one report reduced the duration of diarrhea in 44 infants.[20]

TOXICOLOGY: Tolerance to soy preparations in a 164-patient study was good to excellent for most patients.[17] The effects of phytoestrogens in soy-based infant formulas is of concern and may have some biological impact.[21,22] Daily exposure of infants to the isoflavones in soy-based formula, in one report, was found to be 13,000 to 22,000 times higher than estradiol concentrations in early life.[23] Effects of these soy isoflavones on steroid-dependent developmental processes in babies should be studied. Carefully controlled, large-scale clinical trials in this infant population should be a priority.[24,25] Inhalation of soy dust caused an asthma epidemic in 26 patients exposed to an unloading of the product in Barcelona. Skin prick tests confirmed exposure to soy in all cases.[26] Specific immunoglobulins such as IgE, are associated with this type of "soy bean asthma."[27] Soybeans can be treated with proteases to reduce allergenicity.[28]

[1] Ensminger A, et al. *Foods and Nutrition Encyclopedia*, 2nd ed. Boca Raton, FL: CRC Press, 1994;2017-35.

[2] Polunin M. *Healing Foods*. New York, NY: DK Publishing, 1997;70.

[3] Craig S, et al. *The Complete Book of Alternative Nutrition*. Emmaus, PA: Rodale Press, 278-79.

[4] Anonymous. *The Soy Connection*, Chesterfield, MO: United Soybean Board, 1998 Spring;6:#2.

[5] Kurzer M, et al. *Annu Rev Nutr* 1997;17:353-81.

[6] Craig W. *J Am Diet Assoc* 1997;97(10 Suppl 2):S199-S204.

[7] Katdare M, et al. *Oncol Rep* 1998;5(2):311-15.

[8] Zhou Y, et al. *J Natl Cancer Inst* 1998;90(5):381-88.

[9] Cassidy A, et al. *Am J Clin Nutr* 1994;60:333-40.

[10] Barnes S. *Breast Cancer Res Treat* 1997;46(2-3):169-79.

[11] Stoll B. *Ann Oncol* 1997;8(3)223-25.

[12] Goodman M, et al. *Am J Epidemiol* 1997;146(4):294-306.

[13] Geller J, et al. *Prostrate* 1998;34(2):75-79.

[14] Morton M, et al. *Cancer Lett* 1997;114(1-2):145-51.

[15] Clarkson T, et al. *Proc Soc Exp Biol Med* 1998;217(3):365-68.

[16] Barnes S. *Proc Soc Exp Biol Med* 1998;217(3):386-92.

[17] Medkova I, et al. *Ter Arkh* 1997;69(9):52-55.

[18] Nestel P, et al. *Arterioscler Thromb Vasc Biol* 1997;17(12):3392-98.

[19] Hodgson J, et al. *J Nutr* 1998;128(4):728-32.

[20] Vanderhoof J, et al. *Clin Pediatr* 1997;36(3):135-39.

[21] Bluck L, et al. *Clin Chem* 1997;43(5):851-52.

[22] Huggett A, et al. *Lancet* 1997;350(9080):815-16.

[23] Setchell K, et al. *Lancet* 1997;350(9070):23-27.

[24] Sheehan D. *Proc Soc Exp Biol Med* 1998;217(3):379-85.

[25] Irvine C, et al. *Proc Soc Exp Biol Med* 1998;217(3):247-53.

[26] Pont F, et al. *Arch Bronconeumol* 1997;33(9):453-56.

[27] Codina R, et al. *Chest* 1997;111(1):75-80.

[28] Yamanishi R, et al. *J Nutr Sci Vitaminol* 1996;42(6):581-87.

SCIENTIFIC NAME(S): *Spirulina* spp. Family: Oscillatoriaceae

COMMON NAME(S): Spirulina, dihe, tecuitlatl, blue-green algae

---

⋙⋘ PATIENT INFORMATION ⋙⋘

Uses: Spirulina has been reported to enhance antibody production, improve dietary hyperlipidemia, reduce gastric secretory activity, exert a preventative effect on liver triglycerides, and cause tumor regression.

Side Effects: Spirulina is nontoxic in humans.

BIOLOGY: The term spirulina encompasses several thousand species of cyanophyta (blue-green algae). These organisms are microscopic, corkscrew-shaped filaments, and can be found around the world. In some locations they impart a dark green color to bodies of water. They are noted for their characteristic behavior in carbonated water and their energetic growth in laboratory cultures.[1]

HISTORY: Spirulina has been known at least since the 16th century. Spanish explorers found the Aztecs harvesting a "blue mud" that probably consisted of spirulina. The mud, which was dried to form chips or formed into cheese-like loaves, was obtained from Lake Texcoco, in what is now Mexico. Spirulina was similarly harvested by natives of the Sahara Desert, where it was known by the name *dihe*. Spirulina has been sold in the US as a health food or food supplement since about 1979. It is available as a fine powder or tablet. Some authors have suggested using spirulina as a source of protein.[2]

PHARMACOLOGY: Promoters of spirulina have claimed that it can be used as a diet pill. The theory is that high levels of phenylalanine act to inhibit the appetite. However, an FDA review found no evidence to support this claim.[3,4]

The nutritional value of spirulina depends on the method of processing: Protein in concentrates prepared from disintegrated cellular material has greater bioavailability than preparations of whole cells.[5,6] An examination of 3 commercial preparations of spirulina indicated that > 80% of what is thought to be vitamin B_{12} may actually be analogs that have little or no nutritional value for humans.[7] *S. fusiformis* is a valuable source of vitamin A in rats.[8] Spirulina as a beta-carotene source is questionable compared with standard sources, but the spirulina-fed rats exhibited better growth patterns than standard.[9] *S. maxima's* effects to alter vitamins A and E storage and use have been reported in rats.[10] Availability of iron from spirulina fed to rats is comparable to rats being fed standard ferrous sulfate.[11] Spirulina alone or in combination is a good dietary supplement during pregnancy in animals as well.[12]

Extract of spirulina and dunaliella algae injected into induced oral carcinoma in animals resulted in 70% partial tumor regression.[13] A similar study reported the absence of gross tumors in experimental oral cancer in hamsters.[14] Tumor regression is accompanied by significant induction of tumor necrosis factor, suggesting a possible mechanism of tumor destruction.[15] A later evaluation confirms spirulina's chemopreventative effects in human oral leukoplakia in tobacco chewers in India (45% lesion regression vs 7% placebo).[16]

S. platensis and its constituent polysaccharide "calcium spirulan" were found to inhibit replication of several enveloped viruses. These include herpes simplex I, cytomegalovirus, mumps, and measles viruses, influenza A virus, and HIV-1. Inhibition of virus entry into host cells appears to be the mechanism.[17]

Spirulina has been reported to enhance antibody production,[18] improve dietary hyperlipidemia,[19] reduce gastric secretory activity,[20] exert a preventative effect on liver triglycerides,[21,22] and provide radioprotection (against gamma radiation) in mouse bone marrow cells.[23]

TOXICOLOGY: Nutritional tests have established spirulina as nontoxic to humans.[2] However, spirulina can contain amounts of mercury as high as 10 ppm. Consumption of 20 g of spirulina per day could produce a mercury consumption above the maximum 180 mcg considered prudent for safety.[24] Reported mean heavy metal levels include arsenic 0.42 ppm, cadmium 0.1 ppm, lead 0.4 ppm, and mercury 0.24 ppm. Microbial contamination may occur if spirulina is grown on the effluent of fermented animal wastes.[25] Spirulina can concentrate radioactive di- and trivalent metallic ions.[26] Some spirulina manufacturers report that microbiological data for standard plate counts, fungi, yeasts, and coliforms conform to US standards for spray-dried powdered milk.

[1] Guerin-Dumartrait E, et al. *Ann Nutr Aliment* 1975;29:489.
[2] Clement G. In Tannenbaum SR & Wang DI, eds. *Single-Cell Proteins II*. Cambridge, MA: MIT Press, 1975.
[3] *FDA Consumer* 1981 Sep:3.
[4] *ACSH News & Views* 1982 Apr,3
[5] Omstedt P, et al. In Tannenbaum SR & Wang DI, eds. *Single-Cell Proteins II* Cambridge, MA: MIT Press, 1975.
[6] Ciferri O. *Microbiol Rev* 1983;47:551.
[7] Herbert V, et al. *JAMA* 1982;248:3096.
[8] Annapurna V, et al. *Plant Foods Hum Nutr* 1991;41(2):125-34.
[9] Kapoor R, et al. *Plant Foods Hum Nutr* 1993;43(1):1-7.
[10] Mitchell G, et al. *J Nutr* 1990;120(10):1235-40.
[11] Kapoor R, et al. *Plant Foods Hum Nutr* 1993;44(1):29-34.
[12] Kapoor R, et al. *Plant Foods Hum Nutr* 1993;43(1):29-35.
[13] Schwartz J, et al. *J Oral Maxillofac Surg* 1987;45(6):510-15.
[14] Schwartz J, et al. *Nutr Cancer* 1988;11(2):127-34.
[15] Shklar G, et al. *Eur J Cancer Clin Oncol* 1988;24(5):839-50.
[16] Mathew B, et al. *Nutr Cancer* 1995;24(2):197-202.
[17] Hayashi T, et al. *J Nat Prod* 1996;59(1):83-87.
[18] Hayashi O, et al. *J Nutr Sci Vitaminol* 1994;40(5):431-41.
[19] Iwata K, et al. *J Nutr Sci Vitaminol* 1990;36(2):165-71.
[20] Cristea E, et al. *Farmacia* 1992 Jan-Dec;40:73-82.
[21] Michele D, et al. *Farmacia* 1992 Jan-Dec;40:119-26.
[22] Gonzalez de Rivera C, et al. *Life Sci* 1993;53(1):57-61.
[23] Qishen P, et al. *Toxicol Lett* 1989;48(2):165-69.
[24] Johnson PE, et al. *Nutr Res* 1986;6:85.
[25] Wu JF, et al. *Bull Environ Contam Toxicol* 1981;27:151.
[26] Tseng CL, et al. *Radioisotopes (Japan)* 1986;35:540.

SCIENTIFIC NAME(S): *Melaleuca alternifolia* (Cheel) Family: Myrtaceae

COMMON NAME(S): Tea tree oil

❧❧❧ PATIENT INFORMATION ❧❧❧

Uses: Tea tree oil has been used mainly for its antimicrobial effects. Tea tree oil should be applied topically. Do not ingest orally.

Side Effects: Use of tea tree oil has resulted in allergic contact eczema and dermatitis.

BOTANY: There are many plants known as "tea trees," but *Melaleuca alternifolia* is responsible for the "tea tree oil," which has recently gained popularity. Native to Australia, the tea tree is found in coastal areas. It is an evergreen shrub that can grow to 6 m tall. Its narrow, 4 cm, needle-like leaves release a distinctive aroma when crushed. The fruits grow in clusters, and its white flowers bloom in the summer.[1]

HISTORY: Tea tree oil (TTO) was first used in surgery and dentistry in the mid-1920s. Its healing properties were also used during World War II for skin injuries to those working in munition factories. Tea tree oil's popularity has resurfaced within the last few years with help from promotional campaigns, and the oil may be present in soaps, shampoos, and lotions.[1]

PHARMACOLOGY: Tea tree oil has been used mainly for its antimicrobial effects without irritating sensitive tissues. It has been applied to cuts, stings, acne, and burns. In hospitals, TTO has been used in soap and soaked in blankets to make an antibacterial covering for burn victims. When run through air-conditioning ducts, TTO has been shown to exert bactericidal effects.[1] A considerable amount of literature has become available on this topic.

Disc diffusion and broth microdilution methods have been used to determine antimicrobial effects against 8 TTO constituents. Terpin-4-ol was active against all test organisms including *Candida albicans, Escherichia coli, Staphylococcus aureus*, and *Pseudomonas aeruginosa*. Other constituents of the oil (such as linalool and α-terpineol) had some antimicrobial activity as well.[2,3] In addition, constituents terpin-4-ol, α-terpineol, and α-pinene were found to possess antimicrobial effects against *Staphylococcus epidermidis* and *Propionibacterium acnes*.[4]

TTO may be useful in removing "transient skin flora while suppressing but maintaining resident flora."[5] TTO was also shown to be an effective topical treatment of monilial and fungal dermatoses and superficial skin infections in 50 subjects for 6 months with minimal or no side effects reported.[6] A report suggests TTO to be useful in treatment of "methicillin-resistant *S. aureus* (MRSA) carriage." In this evaluation, all 66 isolates of *S. aureus* were susceptible to the essential oil (64 isolates being MRSA, 33 being mupirocin-resistant).[7]

TTO's activity against anaerobic oral bacteria has been surveyed.[8] A case report exists, discussing antibacterial efficacy of TTO in a 40-year-old woman with anaerobic vaginosis.[9]

In a randomized, double-blind study comparing the efficacy of 10% (w/w) tea tree oil cream with 1% tolnaftate (and placebo creams) against tinea pedis (athlete's foot), TTO was found to be as effective as tolnaftate in reducing symptoms but no more effective than placebo in achieving mycological cure.[10] In a report on onychomycosis (nail fungus), TTO (100%) vs clotrimazole solution (1%) application yielded similar results in treatment. Both therapies had high recurrence rates.[11]

TTO can be added to baths or vaporizers to help treat respiratory disorders. Related oils have been used for nasal antiseptic purposes, pulmonary anti-inflammatory use, and coughs.[1,12,13] TTO is also used in perfumery and aromatherapy.[2]

TOXICOLOGY: Allergic contact eczema was found to be caused primarily by the α-limonene constituent (in TTO) in 7 patients tested. In this same report, alpha-terpinene and aromadendrene additionally caused dermatitis in 5 of the patients.[14] Eucalyptol was found to be the contact allergan in a Dutch report.[15]

Contact allergy due to TTO may be related to cross-sensitization to colophony.[16] A case report describes a petechial body rash and marked neutrophil leukocytosis in a 60-year-old man who ingested ≈ ½ teaspoonful of the oil (for common cold symptoms). He recovered 1 week later.[17]

TTO in comparison to conifer resin acids was found to exhibit no cytotoxic activity in vitro using human epithelial and fibroblast cells.[18]

Another case report describes ataxia and drowsiness as a result of oral TTO ingestion (< 10 ml) by a 17-month-old male. He was treated with activated charcoal, which was only partially successful, but after a short time appeared normal and was discharged 7 hours after ingestion.[19]

[1] Low T, et al. (contributing editors). *Reader's Digest (Aust) Magic and Medicines of Plants.* Surry Hills, NSW, 2010 Australia: PTY Limited 1994;349.
[2] Bruneton J. *Medicinal Plants.* Seacus, NY: Lavoisier Publ. Inc., 1995;461.
[3] Osol, et al, eds. *The Dispensatory of the United States of America.* Philadelphia, PA: JB Lippincott, 1960;1750.
[4] Carson C, et al. *J Appl Bacteriol* 1995;78(3):264-69.
[5] Carson C, et al. *Microbios* 1995;82(332):181-85.
[6] Raman A, et al. *Letters in Applied Microbiology* 1995;21(4):242-45.
[7] Hammer K, et al. *Am J Infect Control* 1996;24(3):186-89.
[8] Shemesh A, et al. *Aust J Pharm* 1991 Sep;72:802-3.
[9] Carson C, et al. *J Antimicrob Chemother* 1995;35(3):421-24.
[10] Shapiro S, et al. *Oral Microbiology and Immunology* 1994;9(4):202-8.
[11] Blackwell A. *Lancet* 1991 Feb 2;337:300.
[12] Tong M, et al. *Australas J Dermatol* 1992;33(3):145-49.
[13] Buck D, et al. *J F Pract* 1994;38(6):601-5.
[14] Knight T, et al. *J Am Acad Dermatol* 1994;30(3):423-27.
[15] Van der Valk P, et al. *Ned Tijdschr Geneeskd* 1994;138(16):823-25.
[16] Selvaag E, et al. *Contact Dermatitis* 1994;31(2):124-25.
[17] Elliott C. *Med J Aust* 1993 Dec 6;159:830-31.
[18] Soderberg T, et al. *Toxicology* 1996;107(2):99-109.
[19] Del Beccaro M. *Vet Hum Toxicol* 1995;37(6):557-58.

SCIENTIFIC NAME(S): *Dipteryx odorata* (Aubl.) Willd. Also *D. oppositifolia* may be used. Family: Fabaceae (Leguminosae)

COMMON NAME(S): Tonka bean, tonga bean, tongo bean, tonco seed, tonquin bean, torquin bean, cumaru, tonco bean

---

◆◆◆ PATIENT INFORMATION ◆◆◆

Uses: Tonka bean contains coumarin, which is used as a flavoring in foods and tobacco and as a fragrance in cosmetics. Otherwise, tonka beans have no proven pharmacological effects.

Side Effects: If ingested in safe amounts, tonka beans do not have any potent side effects. When fed to animals in higher doses, ingredients in the tonka bean have caused severe hepatic damage, growth retardation, and testicular atrophy. Large doses of the fluid extract can result in cardiac paralysis.

BOTANY: Members of the genus *Dipteryx* are native to South America (Venezuela, Guyana, and Brazil), and are typically large trees bearing single-seeded fruits ≈ 3 to 5 cm in length. The fruit is dried with the seed removed. If not processed further, the fruit is known as "black beans." The beans are macerated in rum and then air-dried. This forms a crystalline deposit of coumarin, and the seeds appear to be frosted. Tonka beans are rounded at one end and bluntly pointed at the other. The bean is black and deeply wrinkled longitudinally. The bean has a fragrant odor and a bitter taste.[1]

HISTORY: Tonka beans contain coumarin, which imparts a pleasant fragrance to cakes, preserves, tobacco, soaps, and liqueurs.[2,3] The seeds are sometimes cured in rum.[4] According to the FDA Code of Federal Regulations Section 189.130, food containing any coumarin as a constituent of tonka beans or tonka extracts is deemed im-

pure.[5] Synthetic coumarin has, to some extent, replaced the natural product. South American natives mix the seed paste with milk to make a thick nutty flavored beverage. Extracts have been used in traditional medicine to treat cramps and nausea. Seed extracts are administered rectally for schistosomiasis in China. The fruit has been said to have aphrodisiac properties.

PHARMACOLOGY: There are no well-controlled studies describing the pharmacologic effects of tonka beans or their components. Synthetic coumarin has been developed to replace the natural product in some cases. A related compound, warfarin (eg, *Coumadin*) is a potent anticoagulant.[6,7]

TOXICOLOGY: Dietary feeding of coumarin to rats and dogs has been associated with extensive hepatic damage, growth retardation, and testicular atrophy.[2] Large oral doses of the fluid extract can result in cardiac paralysis.[2]

---

[1] Evans WC. *Pharmacognosy.* London, England: Bailliere Tindall, 1989.

[2] Duke JA. *Handbook of Medicinal Herbs.* Boca Raton, FL: CRC Press, 1985.

[3] Lewis WH, et al. *Medical Botany. Plants affecting man's health.* New York: John Wiley and Sons, 1977.

[4] Mabberley DJ. *The Plant-Book.* Cambridge, England: Cambridge University Press, 1987.

[5] Food and Drug Administration: Coumarin. 21 CFR 4-1-94 Edition. Ch. 1, Section 189.130.

[6] Olin BR, Hebel SK, eds. *Drug Facts and Comparisons.* St. Louis, MO: Facts and Comparisons, July 1992.

[7] Claus EP, et al. *Pharmacognosy,* 6th ed. Philadelphia, PA: Lea & Fegiber, 1970.

Turmeric

SCIENTIFIC NAME(S): *Curcuma longa* L. Synonymous with *C. domestica* Vahl. Family: Zingiberaceae

COMMON NAME(S): Turmeric, curcuma, Indian saffron

≈≈≈ PATIENT INFORMATION ≈≈≈

Uses: Turmeric is used as a spice. Recent investigations indicate that the strong antioxidant effects of several components of turmeric result in an inhibiton of carcinogenesis and may play a role in limiting the development of cancers.

Side Effects: There are no known side effects.

BOTANY: Turmeric is a perennial member of the ginger family characterized by a thick rhizome. The plant grows to a height of ≈ 0.9 to 1.5 m and has large oblong leaves. It bears funnel-shaped yellow flowers.[1] The plant is cultivated widely throughout Asia, India, China, and tropical countries. The primary (bulb) and secondary (lateral) rhizomes are collected, cleaned, boiled, and dried; and lateral rhizomes contain more yellow coloring material than the bulb.[2] The dried rhizome forms the basis for the culinary spice.

HISTORY: Turmeric has a warm, bitter taste and is a primary component of curry powders and some mustards. The powder and its oleoresins are used extensively as food flavorings in the culinary industry. The spice has a long history of use in Asian medicine. In Chinese medicine, it has been used to treat problems as diverse as flatulence and hemorrhage. It also has been used topically as a poultice, as an analgesic, and to treat ringworms.[3] The spice has been used for the management of jaundice and hepatitis.[2] The oil is sometimes used as a perfume component.

PHARMACOLOGY: Several soluble fractions of turmeric, including curcumin, have been reported to have antioxidant properties. Turmeric inhibits the degradation of polyunsaturated fatty acids.[4] The curcumins inhibit cancer at initiation, promotion, and progression stages of development.[5]

In smokers, turmeric given at a daily dose of 1.5 g for 30 days significantly reduced the urinary excretion of mutagens compared with controls; turmeric had no effect on hepatic enzyme levels or lipid profiles suggesting that the spice may be an effective antimutagen useful in chemoprevention.[6]

Ukonan-A, a polysaccharide with phagocytosis-activating activity has been isolated from *C. longa*,[7] and Ukonan-D has demonstrated strong reticuloendothelial system-potentiating activity.[8] Aqueous extract of *C. longa* has been shown to have cytoprotective effects that inhibit chemically induced carcinogenesis, forming a basis for the traditional use of turmeric as an anticancer treatment.[9]

A combination of turmeric and neem (*Azadirachta indica*) applied topically has been shown to effectively eradicate scabies in 97% of 814 people treated within 3 to 15 days.[10] Other pharmacologic properties of turmeric include choleretic, hypotensive, antibacterial, and insecticidal activity.

The choleretic (bile-stimulating) activity of curcumin has been recognized for almost 40 years, and these compounds have been shown to possess strong antihepatotoxic properties.[11]

TOXICOLOGY: No reports of toxicity have been reported following the ingestion of turmeric. No change in weight was observed following chronic treat-

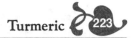

ment, although changes in heart and lung weights were observed; a decrease in white and red blood cell levels were observed. Although a gain in weight of sexual organs and an increase in sperm motility was observed, no spermatotoxic effects were found.[12]

[1] Dobelis IN, ed. *Magic and Medicine of Plants*. Pleasantville, NY: Reader's Digest Association, Inc., 1986.

[2] Evans WC. *Trease and Evans' Pharmacognosy*, 13th ed. London, England: Balliere Tindall, 1989.

[3] Leung AY. *Encyclopedia of Common Natural Ingredients Used in Food, Drugs and Cosmetics*. New York, NY: John Wiley and Sons, 1980.

[4] Reddy AC, et al. *Mol Cell Biochem* 1992;111:117.

[5] Nagabhushan M, et al. *J Am Coll Nutr* 1992;11:192.

[6] Polasa K, et al. *Mutagenesis* 1992;7:107.

[7] Gonda R, et al. *Chem Pharm Bull* 1992;40:990.

[8] Ibid. 1992;40:185.

[9] Azuine MA, et al. *J Cancer Res Clin Oncol* 1992;118:447.

[10] Charles V, et al. *Trop Geogr Med* 1992;44:178.

[11] Kiso Y, et al. *Phytochemistry* 1983;49:185.

[12] Qureshi S, et al. *Planta Med* 1992;58:124.

SCIENTIFIC NAME(S): *Arctostaphylos uva ursi* L. Sprengel. (Also referred to as *Arbutus uva ursi* L.). The related plants *A. adenotricha* and *A. coactylis* Fern et Macbr. have also been termed uva ursi by some authors. Family: Ericaceae

COMMON NAME(S): Uva ursi, bearberry, kinnikinnik, hogberry, rockberry, beargrape, manzanita

---

❧❧❧ PATIENT INFORMATION ❧❧❧

Uses: Uva ursi is useful in treating urinary tract infections; as a diuretic; to treat induced contact dermatitis, allergic reaction-type hypersensitivity, and arthritis in conjunction with prednisolone and dexamethasone.

Side effects: Ingestion of uva ursi in large doses has resulted rarely in ringing of the ears, nausea, vomiting, cyanosis, convulsions, collapse, and death. The product may also impart a green color to the urine and cause gastric discomfort.

BOTANY: Uva ursi is a low-growing evergreen shrub with creeping stems that form a dark green carpet of leaves. It can grow to ≈ 51 cm in height. The plant has small, dark, fleshy, leathery leaves and clusters of small white or pink bell-shaped flowers. It blooms from April to May and produces a dull orange berry. The plant grows abundantly throughout the northern hemisphere from Asia to the US.[1,2]

HISTORY: "Uva ursi" means "bear's grape" in Latin, probably because bears are fond of the fruit. Uva ursi was first documented in a 13th century Welsh herbal.[2] Teas and extracts of the leaves have been used as urinary tract antiseptics and diuretics for centuries. The plant has been used as a laxative, and the leaves have been smoked.[3] Bearberry teas and extracts have been used as vehicles for pharmaceutical preparations. In homeopathy, a tincture of the leaves is believed to be effective in the treatment of cystitis, urethritis, and urinary tract inflammations. The berries are not used medicinally. They are juicy but have an insipid flavor that improves upon cooking.[4]

PHARMACOLOGY: The constituent arbutin is hydrolyzed in gastric fluid to hydroquinone. In alkaline urine, hydroquinone is mildly astringent and is an effective antimicrobial agent. Despite this activity, large amounts of uva ursi must be consumed for any significant effect to occur and the urine must be alkalinized.[5] Evidence suggests that arbutin itself may contribute to the antiseptic activity of the plant because arbutin and crude leaf extracts have been shown to possess mild antimicrobial activity in vitro.[6] A report discusses liquid concentration of uva ursi possessing antiseptic and diuretic properties.[7] Uva ursi aerial part extracts were found to be most active against *Escherichia coli* and *Proteus vulgaris*.[8]

Antibacterial activity of arbutin-causing urinary tract infection is caused by β-glucosidase activity of the infective organism.[6] Uva ursi is one of the best natural urinary antiseptics and has been extensively used in herbal medicine.[2] The German Commission E monograph lists its use as "for inflammatory disorders of the lower urinary tract." An herbal remedy including uva ursi is used to treat "compulsive strangury, enuresis, and painful micturition."[1] One report discusses metabolite production of uva ursi;[9] other reports discuss bile expelling/lowering effects of the plant[10] and its beneficial effects in treating kidney stones.[11]

Several plant compounds (ursolic acid and isoquercetin) are mild diuretics and contribute to the plant's diuretic effect.

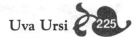

Uva ursi is a constituent in many *otc* herbal diuretic preparations. A report on bearberry reviews diuretic effects and other plant properties.[12]

Arbutin may increase inhibitory action of prednisolone and dexamethasone on induced contact dermatitis, allergic re-action-type hypersensitivity, and arthritis, suggesting uva ursi's therapeutic effects against immuno-inflammation.[13-16]

TOXICOLOGY: Hydroquinone is toxic in large doses.[17] Ingestion of 1 g of the compound resulted in ringing of the ears, nausea, vomiting, cyanosis, convulsions, and collapse. Death followed the ingestion of 5 g of hydroquinone.[18] These symptoms are rare; most commercial products have < 1 g of crude uva ursi per dose. Doses up to

20 g of uva ursi have not caused pharmacologic responses in healthy individuals.[19] Products containing uva ursi may turn urine green. The plant's astringent tannin content may cause gastric discomfort and usually limits the dose ingested.

The published report of the Expert Advisory Committee in Herbs and Botanical Preparations to the Canadian Health Protection Branch (January 1986) recommended that food preparations containing uva ursi provide labeling contraindicating their use during pregnancy and lactation because large doses of uva ursi are oxytocic.[18]

Individuals suffering from kidney disease should not use uva ursi. Do not take the plant for > 7 to 10 days at a time.[2]

[1] Bisset N. *Herbal Drugs and Phytopharmaceuticals.* Stuttgart, Germany: CRC Press, 1994.

[2] Chevallier A. *Encyclopedia of Medicinal Plants.* New York, NY: DK Publishing Inc., 1996.

[3] Spoerke DG. *Herbal Medications.* Santa Barbara, CA: Woodbridge Press Publishing Co., 1980.

[4] *Wild Edible and Poisonous Plants of Alaska.* Univ. of Alaska Cooperative Extension Service; 1985.

[5] Frohne D. *Planta Med* 1970;18:1.

[6] Jahodar L, et al. *Cesk Farm* 1985;34:174.

[7] Zaits K, et al. *Farmatsiia* 1975;24(1):40-42.

[8] Holopainen M, et al. *Acta Pharm Fenn* 1988 Apr;97: 197-202.

[9] Duskova J, et al. *Cesk Farm* 1991;40:83-85.

[10] Azhunova T, et al. *Farmatsiia* 1988 Feb;37(2):41-43.

[11] Grases F, et al. *Int Urol Nephrol* 1994;26(5):507-11.

[12] Houghton P, et al. *Pharm J* 1995 Aug;255:272-73.

[13] Kubo M, et al. *Yakugaku Zasshi* 1990;110(1):59-67.

[14] Matsuda H, et al. *Yakugaku Zasshi* 1990;110(1):68-76.

[15] Matsuda H, et al. *Yakugaku Zasshi* 1991;111(4-5):253-58.

[16] Matsuda H, et al. *Yakugaku Zasshi* 1992;112(9):673-77.

[17] Woodard T, et al. *Fed Proc* 1949;8:348.

[18] Newall C, et al. *Herbal Medicine.* London, England: Pharmaceutical Press, 1996.

[19] Tyler VE. *The Honest Herbal.* Philadelphia, PA: G.F. Stickley Co., 1981.

Valerian

SCIENTIFIC NAME(S): *Valeriana officinalis* L. A number of other members of the genus *Valeriana* have been used medicinally including *V. wallichii* DC. (*Centranthus ruber* (L.) DC) Family: Valerianaceae

COMMON NAME(S): Valerian, radix valerianae, Indian valerian (*V. wallichii*), red valerian

---

PATIENT INFORMATION

Uses: Valerian has been used for its sedative and hypnotic properties.

Side Effects: Valerian is generally recognized as safe, but some patients have experienced headaches, excitability, uneasiness, and cardiac disturbances.

BOTANY: Members of the genus *Valeriana* are herbaceous perennials widely distributed in the temperate regions of North America, Europe, and Asia. Of the ≈ 200 known species, *V. officinalis* is most often cultivated for medicinal uses. The dried rhizome contains a volatile oil with a distinctive offensive odor.[1] The fresh drug has no appreciable smell; it develops over time because of hydrolysis of compounds to isovaleric acid.[2]

HISTORY: Although the odor of the rhizome is disagreeable to many, in the 16th century the plant was considered a fragrant perfume. Preparations have been used as sedatives for centuries; their use persists especially in France, Germany, and Switzerland.

PHARMACOLOGY: Before the discovery of the valepotriates, bornyl acetate and isovalerate were thought to be responsible for valerian's mild sedative properties. However, because the volatile oil only accounted for about one-third of the sedative effect of the total extract, other compounds appear to contribute to the effect of valerian.[2]

Because no single component of valerian can account for the sedative activity of the extracts, it is being recognized that this activity is most likely an additive effect of several valerian components.

Valerenic acid and valeranone have antispasmodic properties[3] mediated by the influx of intracellular calcium; these compounds also have anticonvulsive, hypotensive, and sedative properties, perhaps by influencing serotonin, GABA, and norepinephrine levels.[4,5]

Controlled studies have confirmed a sedative-hypnotic effect. When 128 people were given 400 mg valerian extract, a commercial valerian preparation, or placebo (double-blind crossover design), valerian root produced an improvement in sleep quality. Night awakenings and somnolence the next morning were relatively unaffected by the valerian extract. The commercial preparation caused an increase in morning drowsiness. There were no changes in EEG in any group.[1] Similar results were found in a comparative study of 450 mg valerian aqueous extract, 900 mg extract, and placebo. The smaller dose produced a decrease in sleep latency; doubling the dose led to no further improvement but caused morning drowsiness.[6] There was no evidence of a "carry-over" sedative effect to the next night in either study. The effects appear to be similar to those of short-acting benzodiazepines.

TOXICOLOGY: The toxicity of valerian compounds appears to be low. Signs of toxicity included ataxia, hypothermia, and increased muscle relaxation. No toxicities have been reported in humans. In controlled clinical trials, headaches, excitability, uneasiness, and

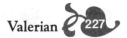

cardiac disturbances have been noted.[7] It is not clear how this plant interacts with barbiturates, benzodiazepines, and opiates in humans.

The valepotriates exhibit cytotoxic and antitumor activities[8] with alkylating activity comparable to mustard-like agents.[9] Although there is little evidence that the valepotriates are effec-

tive cytotoxic agents in vivo, there is some slight concern about the safety of valerian preparations, particularly following long-term use.[7]

V. officinalis has been classified as GRAS (generally recognized as safe) for food use; extracts and the root oil are used as flavorings for foods and beverages.

[1] Leathwood PD, et al. *Pharmacal Biochem Behav* 1982;17:65.

[2] Houghton PJ. *J Ethnopharmacol* 1988;22:121.

[3] Hazelhoff B, et al. *Arch Int Pharmacodyn* 1982;257:274.

[4] Hendriks H, et al. *Planta Med* 1985 Feb:28.

[5] Riedel E, et al. *Planta Med* 1982;46:219.

[6] Leathwood PD, et al. *Planta Med* 1985;51:144.

[7] Hobbs C. *HerbalGram* 1989;21:19.

[8] Bounthanh C, et al. *Planta Med* 1981;41:21.

[9] Braun R, et al. *Dtsch Apoth-Ztg* 1982;122:1109.

SCIENTIFIC NAME(S): *Hamamelis virginiana* L. Family: Hamamelidaceae

COMMON NAME(S): Witch hazel, hamamelis, snapping hazel, winter bloom, spotted alder, tobacco wood, hamamelis water

---

ᨠᨠᨠ PATIENT INFORMATION ᨠᨠᨠ

Uses: Witch hazel has astringent and hemostatic properties, making it useful as a skin astringent to promote healing in hemorrhoid treatment, diarrhea, dysentery, and colitis, as well as other skin inflammations such as eczema. It can also be gargled to treat mucous membrane inflammations of the mouth, throat, and gums. Witch hazel has been used to treat damaged veins, bruises, and sprains; it rapidly stops bleeding, making it useful as an enema.

Side Effects: Internal use is not recommended. Doses of 1 g of witch hazel will cause nausea, vomiting, or constipation, possibly leading to impactions. Hepatic damage may occur if the tannins are absorbed to an appreciable extent.

BOTANY: Witch hazel grows as a deciduous bush, often reaching ≈ 6 m in height. The plant is found throughout most of North America. Its broad, toothed leaves are ovate, and the golden yellow flowers bloom in the fall. Brown fruit capsules appear after the flowers, then when ripe, eject their two seeds away from the tree. The dried leaves, bark, and twigs are used medicinally.[1,2]

HISTORY: Witch hazel is a widely known plant with a long history of use in the Americas. One source lists > 30 traditional uses for witch hazel including the treatment of hemorrhoids, burns, cancers, tuberculosis, colds, and fever. Preparations have been used topically for symptomatic treatment of itching and other skin inflammations and in ophthalmic preparations for ocular irritations.[3]

The plant is used in a variety of forms including the crude leaf and bark, fluid extracts, a poultice, and most commonly as witch hazel water. The latter, also known as hamamelis water or distilled witch hazel extract, is obtained from the recently cut and partially dormant twigs of the plant. This plant material is soaked in warm water followed by distillation and the addition of alcohol to the distillate. Witch hazel water is the most commonly found commercial preparation, usually kept in most homes as a topical cooling agent or astringent.[2,3]

Traditionally, witch hazel was known to native North American people as a treatment for tumors and eye inflammations. Its internal use was for hemorrhaging. Eighteenth century European settlers came to value the plant for its astringency, and it is still used today for this and other purposes.[2]

PHARMACOLOGY: Witch hazel leaves, bark, and its extracts have been reported to have astringent and hemostatic properties. These effects have been ascribed to the presence of a relatively high concentration of tannins in the leaf, bark, and extract. Tannins are protein precipitants in appropriate concentrations.[4]

Witch hazel water is devoid of tannins but still retains its astringency, suggesting that other constituents may possess astringent qualities.[2]

The mechanism of witch hazel astringency involves the tightening of skin proteins, which come together to form a protective covering that promotes skin healing.[2] This quality is desirable in treatment of hemorrhoids (including preventive measures for recurring

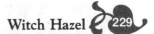

hemorroids).[5] A preparation of tea has been used in cases of diarrhea, dysentery, and colitis.[1,2,3,6]

Skin problems are also treated with witch hazel. Its drying and astringent effects help treat skin inflammations such as eczema. Witch hazel's action on skin lesions also protects against infection.[2] Skin lotions may also contain witch hazel for these purposes.[1] Inflammation of mucous membranes including mouth, throat, and gums may also be treated with witch hazel in the form of a gargle.[1]

Witch hazel is also used to treat damaged veins. Its ability to tighten distended veins and restore vessel tone is employed in varicose vein treatment and is also valuable for bruises and sprains.[1,2] This hemostatic property of witch hazel is said to stop bleeding instantly and, if used as an enema, offers a rapid cure for inwardly bleeding piles.[3]

TOXICOLOGY: Although the volatile oil contains the carcinogen safrole, this is found in much smaller quantities than in plants such as sassafras.[3] Although extracts of witch hazel are available commercially, it is not recommended that these extracts be taken internally because the toxicity of the tannins has not been well defined.[6] Although tannins are not usually absorbed following oral administration, doses of 1 g of witch hazel will cause nausea, vomiting, or constipation, possibly leading to impactions; hepatic damage may occur if the tannins are absorbed to an appreciable extent.[1,7] Witch hazel water is not intended for internal use. Teas can be brewed from leaves and twigs available commercially in some health-food stores, but their safety is undefined.

At least one report is available discussing contact allergy to witch hazel.[8]

[1] Bisset N. *Herbal Drugs and Phytopharmaceuticals.* Stuttgart, Germany: CRC Press, 1994.

[2] Chevallier A. *Encyclopedia of Medicinal Plants.* New York, NY: DK Publishing Inc., 1996.

[3] Duke JA. *Handbook of Medicinal Herbs*, Boca Raton, FL: CRC Press, 1985.

[4] Bate-Smith EC. *Phytochemistry* 1973;12:907.

[5] Weiner B, et al. *Nat Assoc Retail Drug J* 1983 Apr;105:45-49.

[6] Newall C, et al. *Herbal Medicine*. London, England: Pharmaceutical Press, 1996.

[7] Spoerke DG. *Herbal Medications*. Santa Barbara, CA: Woodbridge Press, 1980.

[8] Granlund H. *Contact Dermatitis* 1994;31(3):195.

Withania

SCIENTIFIC NAME(S): *Withania somnifera* Dunal; *W. coagulans* Dunal Family: Solanaceae

COMMON NAME(S): Withania, aswagandha, ashwagandha

꣼꣼ PATIENT INFORMATION ꣼꣼

Uses: Withania is a respiratory stimulant and smooth muscle relaxant. It has antihypertensive, anti-inflammatory, and immunosuppressant activity.

Side Effects: Studies show a potential for additive CNS depression to occur with the use of withania.

BOTANY: Withania is related to the tomato and potato plants. It is an erect evergreen shrub that grows to ≈ 1.5 meters. It is found throughout the drier regions of India, Afghanistan, and as far west as Israel.

HISTORY: Withania has always had a prominent place in Ayurvedic, Unani, and ancient Indian systems of medicine. Its use has been focused primarily on restoring the "balance of life forces" much in the same way as ginseng and eleutherococcus are used. It is often referred to as "Indian ginseng." The fresh berries have been used as an emetic. The dried fruits and roots are said to be sedative, diuretic, and anti-inflammatory, and they have been used for "chronic liver complications."[1] Withania has also been used to treat tumors and tuberculosis[2] and is used topically for the management of swelling and ulcerations.

PHARMACOLOGY: A total extract of the fruit has been reported to have CNS-depressant effects in mice, rabbits, and dogs. Antihypertensive activity has been demonstrated in animal studies, and it is a respiratory stimulant and a smooth muscle relaxant. Studies with albino rats showed alcoholic dried, total alkaloid, and aqueous extracts to cause CNS depression within 30 to 40 minutes of oral administration, as indicated by sedation, reduced exploratory and spontaneous activities, and hypothermia. The extracts stimulated respiration slightly and potentiated the sleep-ing time induced by pentobarbitone. There were no analgesic effects. Extracts increased the lethal effects of amphetamine. Studies of *W. ashwagandha* Kaul showed that an acetone extract of alkaloids caused mild CNS depression in dogs and mice and protected against supra-maximal electroshock seizures in rats. The extract caused hypothermia in mice and potentiated hypnosis induced by barbiturates, ethanol, and urethane. Its effects were not antagonized by LSD or dibenzyline. Alcoholic and aqueous extracts had no significant neurologic effects. Similarly, in another study, aqueous, aqueous-methanol, and methanol extracts failed to produce CNS depression in mice, leading to the conclusion that therapeutic sedation should not be expected from these extracts.[3]

Withania extracts have anti-inflammatory activity in rats with acute inflammation induced by egg albumin and against subacute inflammation induced by formalin. The dried alcoholic extract reduced granulation tissue formed in response to subcutaneous implantation of cotton wool pellets. In rats, alcoholic extracts of *W. somnifera* leaves showed slight activity against acute inflammation but were strongly anti-inflammatory against subacute inflammation. The activity of extract administered in a dose of 1g/kg was equivalent to that of 10 mg/kg of hydrocortisone and 50 mg/kg phenylbutazone.

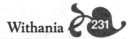

The extract has been reported to protect against carbon tetrachloride-induced hepatotoxicity.[4] A methanol extract of withania contains a compound different from withaferin-A that has antitumor activity in mice. The alkaloids in withania were not irritating to mucous membranes.[5] The leaves of *W. somnifera* contain components with antibacterial actions.[6]

Withaferin-A and withanolide-D induce immunosuppressant activity.[7,8] One study in rats and mice found that methanol-water extracts of the root ex-erted antistress activity as measured by a battery of tests including forced swimming, stress-induced gastric ulceration, and several forms of restraint stress.[9]

TOXICOLOGY: The LD-50 of methanolic extracts of withania root IP in mice is 1076 mg/kg; the LD-50 of withaferin-A is 1564 mg/kg by the same route. These data suggest that acute toxicity is not usually encountered with this plant.[7] The potential for additive CNS depression should be kept in mind.

[1] Budhiraja RD, et al. *Planta Med* 1977;32.154.
[2] Chakraborti SK, et al. *Experientia* 1974;30:852.
[3] Fontaine R, et al. *Planta Med* 1976;30:242.
[4] Sudhir S, et al. *Planta Med* 1986;36:61.
[5] Prasad S, et al. *Ind J Physiol Pharmacol* 1968;12:175.
[6] Das JM, et al. *Indian J Biochem Biophys* 1964;1:157.
[7] Bahr V, et al. *Planta Med* 1982;44:32.
[8] Shobat B, et al. *Biomedicine* 1978;28:18.
[9] Battacharya SK, et al. *Phytother Res* 1987;1:32.

Yarrow

SCIENTIFIC NAME(S): *Achillea millefolium* L.; Family: Compositae

COMMON NAME(S): Yarrow, thousand-leaf, mil foil, green arrow, wound wort, nosebleed plant

---

ತ⊱ೆ⊱ PATIENT INFORMATION ⊱ೆ⊱ೆ

Uses: Yarrow has been used to induce sweating and to stop wound bleeding. It can also reduce heavy menstrual bleeding and pain. It has been used to relieve GI ailments, for cerebral and coronary thromboses, to lower high blood pressure, to improve circulation, and to tone varicose veins. It has antimicrobial actions, is a natural source for food flavoring, and is used in alcoholic beverages and bitters.

Side Effects: Contact dermatitis is the most commonly reported side effect. It is generally not considered toxic.

BOTANY: The name yarrow applies to any of roughly 80 species of daisy plants native to the north temperate zone. *A. millefolium* L. has finely divided leaves and whitish, pink, or reddish flowers. It can grow up to 0.9 m in height. This hardy perennial weed blooms from June to November. Golden yarrow is *Eriophyllum confertiflorum*.[1,2]

HISTORY: Yarrow is native to Europe and Asia and has been naturalized in North America. Its use in food and medicine dates back to the Trojan War, around 1200 B.C.[3] In classical times, yarrow was referred to as "herba militaris" because it stopped wound bleeding caused by war.[2] Yarrow leaves have been used for tea, and young leaves and flowers have been used in salads. Infusions of yarrow have served as cosmetic cleansers and medicines. Sneezewort leaves (*A. ptarmica*) have been used in sneezing powder, while those of *A. millefolium* have been used for snuff.[1] Yarrow has been used therapeutically as a strengthening bitter tonic and astringent. Chewing fresh leaves has been suggested to relieve toothaches.[3,4] Yarrow oil has been used in shampoos for a topical healing effect.

PHARMACOLOGY: Yarrow is used as a sudorific to induce sweating. It is also classified as a wound-healing herb

because it stops wound bleeding.[4] It has been used for this purpose for centuries and is a component in some healing ointments, lotions, and percolates or extracts.[2,5] Its healing and regenerating effects have been reported when used as a constituent in medicated baths to remove perspiration and remedy inflammation of skin and mucous membranes.[5,6,7] One study reports wound-healing properties of yarrow oil in napalm burns.[8]

Chamazulene, a constituent in yarrow essential oil, has anti-inflammatory and antiallergenic properties.[9]

The yarrow component achilleine arrests internal and external bleeding.[2]

Yarrow helps regulate the menstrual cycle and reduces heavy bleeding and pain.[2,9] It has been used as an herbal remedy for cerebral and coronary thromboses.[9] Yarrow has also been used to lower high blood pressure, improve circulation, and tone varicose veins.[2,3]

Antispasmodic activity of yarrow has also been documented, probably caused by the plant's flavonoid fractions[2,9] or azulene.[9] Yarrow has relieved GI ailments such as diarrhea, flatulence, and cramping.[5] Yarrow's antimicrobial actions have also been documented. In

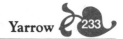

vitro fungistatic effect from the oil has been proven.[10] The oil has also exhibited marked activity against *S. aureus* and *C. albicans*.[11] Another report discusses antistaphylococcal activity from yarrow grass extract.[12] Antibacterial actions have also been demonstrated against *B. subtillus, E. coli, Shigella sonnei,* and *flexneri*.[9] Other actions of yarrow include growth inhibiting effects on seed germination caused by constituents phenylcarbonic acids, coumarins, herniarin, and umbelliferone,[13] marked hypoglycemic and glycogen-sparing properties.[14] Yarrow is a natural source for food flavoring and is used in alcoholic beverages and bitters.[9]

Thujone-free yarrow extract is generally recognized as safe (GRAS) for use in beverages.

TOXICOLOGY: Contact dermatitis is the most commonly reported adverse reaction from yarrow. Guaianolide peroxides from yarrow have caused this reaction,[15] as have α-peroxyachifolid,[16] 10 sesquiterpene lactones, and 3 polyines.[17] Terpinen-4-ol, a yarrow oil component, has irritant properties and may contribute to its diuretic actions.[9] Thujone, a known toxin and minor component in the oil, is in too low a concentration to cause any health risk.[9] Yarrow is not generally considered toxic.[3,9]

[1] Seymour ELD. *The Garden Encyclopedia.* Wise, 1936.

[2] Chevallier A. *Encyclopedia of Medicinal Plants.* New York, NY: DK Publishing, 1996;54.

[3] Duke J. *CRC Handbook of Medicinal Herbs.* Boca Raton, FL: CRC Press Inc., 1989;9-10.

[4] Loewenfeld C, et al. *The Complete Book of Herbs and Spices.* London, England: David E Charles, 1979.

[5] Bisset N. *Herbal Drugs and Phytopharmaceuticals.* Stuttgart, Germany: CRC Press Inc., 1994;342-44.

[6] Gafitanu E, et al. *Revista Medico-Chirurgicala A Societatii de Medici Si Naturalisti Din Iasi* 1988;92(1):121-22.

[7] Taran D, et al. *Voenno-Meditsinskii Zhurnal* 1989;(8):50-52.

[8] Popovici A, et al. *Rev Med* 1970;16(3-4):384-89.

[9] Newall C, et al. *Herbal Medicines.* London, England: Pharmaceutical Press, 1996;271-73.

[10] Kedzia B, et al. *Herba Polonica* 1990;36(3):117-25.

[11] Molochko V, et al. *Vestnik Dermatologii I Venerologii* 1990;(8):54-56.

[12] Detter A. *Pharmazeutische Zeitung* 1981 Jun 4;126:1140-42.

[13] Molokovskii D, et al. *Problemy Endokrinologii* 1989;35(6):82-87.

[14] Paulsen E, et al. *Contact Dermatitis* 1993;29(1):6-10.

[15] Chandler R, et al. *J Pharm Sci* 1982 Jun 71:690-93.

[16] Tozyo T, et al. *Chem Pharm Bull* 1994;42(5):1096-1100.

[17] Rucker G, et al. *Pharmazie* 1994;49(2-3):167-69.

SCIENTIFIC NAME(S): *Rumex crispus* L. Family: Polygonaceae

COMMON NAME(S): Yellow dock, curly dock, curled dock, narrow dock, sour dock, rumex

---

꙰꙰꙰ PATIENT INFORMATION ꙰꙰꙰

Uses: The roots of yellow dock exert a laxative effect.

Side Effects: The oxalate content of the leaves may result in GI symptoms or kidney damage. The stewed leaf stalks can be eaten as a potherb, but mature and uncooked leaves should be avoided. Overdose of the root may cause diarrhea, nausea, and polyuria.

BOTANY: A perennial herb that grows to ≈ 0.9 to 1.2 feet, yellow dock has narrow, slender light green leaves with undulated margins. It flowers in June and July.[1] Although native to Europe, it grows throughout the United States. The yellow, deep, spindle-shaped roots and rhizomes are used medicinally.

HISTORY: The spring leaf stalks of this plant have been used as a potherb in salads but are disagreeable to some because of their tart sour-sweet taste. The plant must be boiled and rinsed thoroughly before being eaten. Because of its astringent properties, the plant has been used (generally unsuccessfully) in the treatment of venereal diseases and skin conditions. The powdered root has been used as a natural dentifrice. Larger amounts have been given as a laxative and tonic.

PHARMACOLOGY: Little is known about the pharmacology of yellow dock. The anthroquinone content most likely contributes to the laxative effect of the plant. The tannin component, however, may cause constipation. The related plant *R. hymenosepalus* (dock) contains a tannin that, upon hydrolysis, yields leucodelphinidin and leucopelargonidin, 2 compounds with potential antineoplastic activity.[2]

TOXICOLOGY: The oxalate crystals damage mucosal tissue resulting in severe irritation and possible tissue damage. The ingestion of large amounts of oxalates may result in GI symptoms; systemic absorption of oxalates may result in kidney damage. The stewed leaf stalks can be eaten as a potherb, but mature and uncooked leaves should be avoided. Overdoses of the root extract may cause diarrhea, nausea, and polyuria.

One traditional remedy for dermatitis and rashes suggest applying the juice of *Rumex* spp. However, sensitive people may develop dermatitis after contact with yellow dock.

---

[1] Meyer JE. *The Herbalist.* Hammond, IN: Hammond Book Co., 1934.

[2] Lewis WH, et al. *Medical Botany.* New York, NY: John Wiley & Sons, 1977.

SCIENTIFIC NAME(S): *Pausinystalia yohimbe* (K. Schum.) Pierre. Synonymous with *Corynanthe johimbe*. Family: Rubiaceae.

COMMON NAME(S): Yohimbe, yohimbehe, yohimbine

༈༈༈ PATIENT INFORMATION ༈༈༈

Uses: Yohimbe has been investigated for the treatment of organic impotence, in particular with diabetes, and for use as an aphrodisiac.

Side Effects: Yohimbe may be toxic if ingested in high amounts. It causes severe hypotension, abdominal distress, and weakness and may cause CNS stimulation and paralysis.

BOTANY: This tree grows throughout the African nations of Cameroon, Gabon, and Zaire

HISTORY: The bark of the West African yohimbe tree is rich in the alkaloid yohimbine, and the crude bark and purified compound have long been hailed as aphrodisiacs. The bark has been smoked as a hallucinogen and has been used in traditional medicine to treat angina and hypertension. Today the drug is being investigated for the treatment of organic impotence.

PHARMACOLOGY: Yohimbine is generally classified as an α_2-adrenergic blocking agent. Small doses have a stimulant action in humans resulting in autonomic and psychic changes commonly associated with the subjective experience of anxiety.[1] Yohimbine has been reported to be an inhibitor of monoamine oxidase[2] but more likely has a weak calcium channel blocking effect.[3]

Yohimbine dilates blood vessels, thereby lowering blood pressure; however, its use as an antihypertensive agent has long been abandoned. The drug causes a significant increase in blood pressure after an oral dose of 5 mg in patients with orthostatic hypotension secondary to pure autonomic failure or multisystem atrophy. This response is associated with an increased heart rate and increased plasma noradrenaline levels.

Because yohimbine can cause dilation of peripheral and mucous membrane blood vessels along with CNS stimulation, the drug has been investigated for the treatment of organic impotence. It should be noted that the crude drug and yohimbine have a long history of use as aphrodisiacs.

Sexual-stimulant products available over-the-counter often contain yohimbine, sometimes combined with hormones such as methyltestosterone.

One older prescription product (*Afrodex*, Bentex Pharmaceuticals), which is no longer manufactured, combined 5 mg each of yohimbine HCl, methyltestosterone, and nux vomica in a capsule for the treatment of male climacteric and impotence. Although a number of clinical trials were conducted with this product,[4] the results were generally unimpressive, leading the *Medical Letter* to conclude that "there is still no good evidence that *Afrodex* and similar drugs have more than placebo effects."[5]

More recent investigations strongly suggest that higher doses of the drug (6 mg 3 times a day) may be effective in the treatment of organically impotent men.[6] One study found that 10 of 23 men treated with the drug derived a benefit from treatment. Eleven of the 23 men were diabetic patients.[7] One prescription product containing 5.4 mg yohimbine HCl (*Yocon*, Palisades Pharmaceuticals) is indicated as a sympathicolytic and mydriatic that also may have activity as an aphrodisiac. Yohimbine appears to be effective and may exert its activity by increasing the norepinephrine content of the corpus cavernosum.[8]

TOXICOLOGY: Yohimbine may be toxic if ingested in high doses. The drug causes severe hypotension, abdominal distress, and weakness. Larger doses may cause CNS stimulation and paralysis. This drug should not be used in the presence of renal or hepatic disease. It has been suggested that because of its monoamine oxidase inhibiting activity the usual precautions for concomitant drug use with this class of agents be followed.[2] Yohimbine may precipitate psychoses in predisposed individuals. The drug or crude product should never be self-administered but should only be taken under supervision of a physician.

[1] Ingram CG. *Clin Pharm Ther* 1962;3:345.
[2] Tyler VE. *The New Honest Herbal*. Philadelphia, PA: G.F. Stickley Co., 1987.
[3] Watanabe K, et al. *J Pharm Pharmacol* 1987;39:439.
[4] Miller WW. *Curr Ther Res* 1968;10:354.
[5] Anon. *Med Lett Drugs Ther* 1968;10:97.
[6] Anon. *Medical World News* 1982;23:115.
[7] Morales A, et al. *J Urol* 1982;128:45.
[8] Morales A, et al. *N Engl J Med* 1981;305:1221.

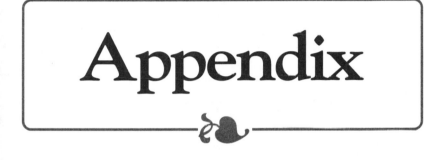

Appendix

There have been relatively few reports of interactions with the coadministration of herbs and conventional drug therapies. The table below profiles potential drug-herb interactions based on reported herbal constituents and known pharmacological actions. Many of the interactions are inconsequential. However, some could be serious depending on the herb quality, concentration, and sensitivity of the patient.

Monitoring is imperative. Always ask patients if unusual herbs or foods are being taken concomitantly with standard medications.

Report findings of interactions through FDA Medical Products Reporting Program (MedWatch) by phone at (301) 443-1240, or fax at 1-800-FDA-0178. Review MedWatch reports at www-.fda.gov/medwatch.

Herb/Conventional Drug Interactions[1]		
Medications/ Therapeutic Class	Potential Herbal Interactions	Possible Adverse Effects
Central Nervous System		
Analgesics	Herbal-containing principles with diuretic activity (eg, corn silk, dandelion, juniper, uva ursi)	These may pose an increased risk of toxicity with the anti-inflammatory analgesic drugs.
	Herbs containing agents with corticosteroid activity (eg, licorice, bayberry)	These may induce reduction in plasma-salicylate concentration.
	Herbs containing agents with sedative properties (eg, calamus, nettle)	Possible enhancement of sedative side effects.
Anticonvulsants	Herbs with active principles which have sedative effects (eg, calamus, nettle, ground ivy, sage, borage)	Possible increase in sedative side effects. May increase risk of seizure.
	Herbs with salicylates (eg, poplar, willow)	May cause transient potentiation of phenytoin therapy.
	Ayurvedic Shankapushpi[2]	May shorten phenytoin's half-life and diminish its effectiveness.
Antidepressants	Herbs containing sympathomimetic amines (eg, agnus castus alkaloids, calamus amines, cola alkaloids, broom alkaloids, licorice)[2]	Increased risk of hypertensive crisis with MAO inhibitors. May potentiate sedative side effects.
	Ginkgo biloba	Use with tricyclic antidepressants or other medications known to decrease the seizure threshold is not advised.
Antiemetic and antivertigo drugs	Herbs containing sedative principles (eg, calamus, nettle, ground ivy, sage, borage)	May increase activity of sedative side effects.
	Herbs containing anticholinergic principles	May be antagonistic.
Antiparkin-sonism agents	Herbs containing anticholinergic principles	Possible potentiation and increased risk of side effects.
	Herbs containing principles with cholinergic activity	Possible antagonism.
Antipsychotics	Herbs containing diuretic principles (eg, corn silk, dandelion, juniper)	Possible potentation of lithium action; increased risk of toxicity.
	Herbs with anticholinergic principles (eg, corkwood tree)	May reduce plasma levels of phenothiazines; possible increased risk of seizures.
	Ginseng, yohimbine, and ephedra[2]	Concomitant use with phenelzine and other MAO inhibitors may result in insomnia, headache, and tremulousness.

Herb/Conventional Drug Interactions[1]		
Medications/ Therapeutic Class	Potential Herbal Interactions	Possible Adverse Effects
Anxiolytics/ hypnotics (eg, alprazolam)	Several herbs with claimed sedative properties (eg, calamus, kava, nettle, ground ivy, sage, borage)	Potentiation.
Phenobarbital[2]	Thujone-containing herbs (eg, wormwood, sage) and gamolenic acid-containing herbs (eg, evening primrose oil, borage)	May lower seizure threshold.
Nonsteroidal anti-inflammatory drugs (NSAIDs)[2]	Feverfew	NSAIDs may reduce the effectiveness of feverfew perhaps mediated by its prostaglandin inhibition effects.
	Herbs with antiplatelet activity (eg, ginkgo biloba, ginger, ginseng, garlic)	May increase the risk of bleeding due to gastric irritation.
Stimulants	Ginseng (*Panax* spp.)	Increased risk of side effects.
Cardiovascular System		
Antiarrhythmic	Herbs with cardioactive principles	Antagonize or affect efficiency of therapy.
	Herbs with diuretic properties (eg, corn silk, dandelion, juniper, uva ursi)	If hypokalemia occurs, may be antagonistic.
Anticoagulants	Herbs containing coagulant or anticoagulant principles (coumarins; eg, alfalfa, red clover, chamomile, ginkgo biloba)	Possible risk of antagonism or potentiation.
	Garlic[2]	May decrease platelet aggregation.
	Ginger[2]	Inhibits thromboxane synthetase, prolonging bleeding time.
	Herbs with high salicylate content (eg, meadowsweet, poplar)	Possible risk of potentiation.
Antihyperlipidemic drugs	Herbs containing hypolipidemic principles (eg, black cohosh, fenugreek, garlic, plantain)	Possible additive effects.
Antihypertensives	Herbs containing hypertensive ingredients (eg, blue cohosh, cola, ginger)	May be antagonistic.
	Herbs containing principles with mineralocorticoid action (eg, licorice, bayberry)	
	Herbs containing hypotensive principles (eg, black cohosh, devil's claw, hawthorn)	Possible potentiation.
	Herbs containing high levels of amine compounds or sympathomimetic action (eg, Agnus castus, black cohosh, cola, maté, St. John's wort)	May be antagonistic.
	Herbs containing diuretic ingredients (eg, corn silk, dandelion, juniper, uva ursi)	Possible risk of potentiation.
Beta-adrenergic blocking agents	Herbs containing cardioactive principles (cardiac glycosides)	Possible antagonism.
	Herbs with high levels of amines or sympathomimetic action (eg, Agnus castus, black cohosh, cola, maté, St. John's wort)	Possible risk of severe hypertension.
Cardenolides (cardiac glycosides)	Herbs with cardioactive constituents (eg, mistletoe [viscotoxin, negative inotropic properties], cola nut [caffeine], figwort [cardioactive glycosides])	Decreased effectiveness or potentiation; increased potential for side effects.
	Hawthorn, Siberian ginseng, Kyushin, and uzara root[2]	May increase the risk of bleeding.

Herb/Conventional Drug Interactions[1]		
Medications/ Therapeutic Class	Potential Herbal Interactions	Possible Adverse Effects
Diuretics	Herbs containing diuretic properties (eg, corn silk, dandelion, gossypol, juniper, uva ursi)	Increased risk of hypokalemia.
	Herbals having hypotensive properties (eg, agrimony, black cohosh, devil's claw, mistletoe)	May cause difficulty in controlling diuresis.
Nitrates and calcium-channel blocking agents	Herbs with cardioactive constituents (eg, broom, squill)	Interferes with therapy (eg, broom may slow heart rate, cause arrhythmias).
	Herbs containing hypertensive principles (eg, bayberry, blue cohosh, cola)	Antagonistic effects.
	Herbs containing anticholinergic principles	Possible reduced buccal absorption of nitroglycerin.
Sympatho-mimetics	Herbs containing sympathomimetic amines (eg, aniseed, capsicum, parsley, vervain)	Possible increased risk of hypertension.
	Herb principles having hypertensive action (eg, bayberry, broom, blue cohosh, licorice)	
	Herb principles with hypotensive action (eg, agrimony, celery, ginger, hawthorn)	Antagonistic effects.
Anti-infective agents		
Antifungals	Herbs containing anticholinergic agents (eg, corkwood tree)	Possible decreased absorption of ketoconazole.
Endocrine System		
Antidiabetic drugs	Herbs containing hypo- or hyperglycemic principles (eg, alfalfa, fenugreek, ginseng)	Possible antagonism or potentiation of action.
	Herbs containing diuretic principles (eg, broom, buchu, corn silk, juniper)	Antagonistic effects.
	Chromium, karela[2]	May affect blood glucose levels, complicating insulin and chlorpropamide requirements, respectively.
Corticosteroids	Herbs containing diuretic principles (eg, broom, buchu, corn silk, juniper)	Possible risk of increased potassium loss.
	Herbs containing corticosteroid principles or action (eg, bayberry)	Increased risk of side effects (eg, sodium retention).
	Herbs, vitamins, and minerals with immunostimulating effects (eg, echinacea, astragalus, licorice, alfalfa sprouts, vitamin E, zinc)	May offset the immunosuppressive effects of corticosteroids.
Sex hormones	Herbs containing hormonal principles (eg, alfalfa, bayberry, black cohosh, licorice)	Potential interactions with existing therapy (eg, black cohosh may decrease the response to estrogens).
Drugs used to treat hyper- and hypothroidism	Herbs containing high levels of iodine	Interferes with therapy.
	Horseradish (eg, goiterogenic myrrh) and kelp[2]	
Drugs Used in Obstetrics and Gynecology		
Estrogens[2]	Herbs containing phytoestrogens (eg, dong quai, red clover, alfalfa, licorice, black cohosh, soybeans)	Concomitant use may result in symptoms of estrogen excess such as nausea, bloating, hypotension, breast fullness or tenderness, migraine, or edema.

Herb/Conventional Drug Interactions[1]		
Medications/ Therapeutic Class	Potential Herbal Interactions	Possible Adverse Effects
Oral contraceptives	Herbs containing principles with hormonal action (eg, black cohosh, licorice)	Possible interactions with exisitng drugs; may also reduce effectiveness of oral contraception.
Antineoplastics Drugs/Drugs with Immunosuppressive Activity		
Methotrexate	Herbs containing sufficient levels of salicylates (eg, willow, poplar, meadowsweet)	Possible increased risk of toxicity.
Immune-system affecting drugs	Herbs containing immunostimulant principles (eg, boneset, echinacea, mistletoe)	Possible antagonism or potentiation.
Drugs for Joint and Musculoskeletal Disorders		
Probenecid	Herbs containing sufficient levels of salicylates (eg, meadowsweet, poplar, willow)	Possible inhibition of uricosuric effect of probenecid.
Diuretics		
Acetazolamide	Herbs containing sufficient levels of salicylates (eg, meadowsweet, poplar, willow)	Increased potential for toxicity.
Anesthetics		
General anesthetics	Herbs containing hypotensive principles (eg, black cohosh, goldenseal, hawthorn)	Potentiation of hypotensive action.
Muscle relaxants	Herbs containing diuretic principles (eg, broom, buchu, corn silk)	Possible potentiation if hypokalemia occurs.
Depolarizing muscle relaxants	Herbs containing cardioactive principles (eg, cola, figwort, hawthorn)	Possible risk of arrhythmias.

[1] Adapted from "Herbal Medicines" by C. Newall, et al. The Pharmaceutical Press, London, 1996.

[2] Arch Intern Med 1998;158:2200-211.

Clinical Considerations for Specific Herb-Drug Interactions & Potential Adverse Effects of Herbs		
	Adverse Effects	Interactions and Clinical Concerns
Aloe (Cape aloe, Barbados aloe, Curaçao aloe; *Aloe vera* L., *A. perryi* Baker)	*External*: May cause allergic contact dermatitis.	*External*: Do not use in deep vertical (surgical) wounds; may delay healing.
	Internal: Excessive consumption of juice may cause painful intestinal contractions.	*Internal*: Juice and exudate. Possible loss of intestinal K^+ leading to a decrease in serum K^+. This may potentiate effects of **cardiac glycosides** and **antiarrhythmics**. Concurrent use of **thiazides, licorice, steroids,** and other **K^+-wasting drugs** may be potentiated by aloe juice. Avoid juice if pregnant. The dried leaf exudate (not gel or juice) contains anthraquinone glycosides which are irritating laxatives. Avoid in children under 12 years of age and during menstruation, nursing, stomach or intestinal inflammation, ulcerative colitis, Crohn's disease, inflamed hemorrhoids, intestinal obstruction, and kidney disorders.
Bilberry fruit (*Vaccinium myrtillus*)	Excessive consumption of dried fruits (high in tannins) may lead to constipation.	Because of reported antiaggregation effect on platelets (anthocyanosides), monitor patients on **antiplatelet drugs** and **anticoagulants**. Myrtillin has hypoglycemic effects; monitor patients with diabetes.
Cayenne (hot pepper; *Capsicum frutescens* L., *C. annuum* L.)	*External*: Strong initial burning sensation, particularly in sensitive areas (eg, eyes, face).	Use oily (olive oil) or acidic (vinegar) solutions to wash away irritating capsaicin. Eat bananas or yogurt, or drink milk to diminish GI irritation. Because it stimulates GI secretions, it may help protect against **NSAID** damage (30 minutes before giving NSAIDs). Cayenne reduces platelet aggregation and increases fibrinolytic activity; therefore, monitor patients taking **antiplatelet drugs** or **anticoagulants**.
	Internal: Stomach upset and discomfort. Diarrhea with burning sensations. Contraindicated in asthmatics because of bronchoconstrictive effects of capsaicin. Avoid use on damaged skin and in the presence of gastric ulcers.	
Chamomile (*Matricaria chamomilla* L. = German Chamomile)	Pollen in flowers may cause hypersensitivity leading to sneezing, runny nose, anaphylaxis, dermatitis, and GI upset. The dried flowering heads can be emetogenic if ingested in large amounts.	Should be consumed regularly for desired effect. This may delay concomitant drug absorption from the gut. Avoid during pregnancy because of emmenagogue effect.
English Chamomile (*Anthemis nobilis*) Compositae family (Asteraceae)	Avoid chamomile in individuals with known sensitivity to any members of the Compositae family (Asteraceae).	Excessive doses may interfere with **anticoagulant** therapy because of the coumarin constituents. English chamomile is reported to be an abortifacient and to affect the menstrual cycle.
Dong quai (*Angelica*) *polymorpha* Maxim. var. *sinensis*	Some species of *Angelica* are phototoxic or photosensitizing because of furanocoumarins. Lowers blood pressure. Possible CNS stimulation.	Contains vasodilatory and antispasmodic coumarin derivatives. Monitor warfarin patients. Possible synergism with calcium channel blockers. *Angelica Archangelica* L. is reported to be an abortifacient and to affect the menstrual cycle. *A. sinensis* has uterine-stimulant activity.

Clinical Considerations for Specific Herb-Drug Interactions & Potential Adverse Effects of Herbs		
	Adverse Effects	Interactions and Clinical Concerns
Echinacea spp. (*Echinacea angustifolia* DC., *E. purpurea* L. Moench and *E. pallida* Nutt. Britton) Compositae family	Cross-sensitivity in persons allergic to Compositae family pollen. Reported tingling and numbing sensation on tasting. Fever from freshly prepared juice.	Long-term use not recommended, particularly in people with autoimmune disorders (eg, lupus, rheumatoid arthritis). Also contraindicated in progressive disorders like multiple sclerosis, collagenosis, AIDS or HIV infection, and tuberculosis. Lack of toxicity data necessitates caution of excessive use, particularly during pregnancy.
Ephedra; Ma Huang (*Ephedra sinica*)	In large doses, ephedrine causes nervousness, headache, insomnia, dizziness, palpitations, skin flushing, tingling, vomiting, anxiety, and restlessness. Toxic psychosis could be induced by ephedrine. Skin reactions also have been observed in sensitive patients.	Contains the alkaloid ephedrine which is a CNS stimulant. Ephedrine stimulates the heart and increases heart rate. Dysrhythmias may occur when used in combination with **cardiac glycosides** or **anesthetics** (eg, halothane). Ephedrine constricts peripheral blood vessels and increases blood pressure; it has enhanced sympathomimetic effects when used with **guanethidine** and hypertensive crises are possible if used concomitantly with **MAOI antidepressants**. Avoid simultaneous use of **vasoconstrictor sympathomimetics**. Hypertension may occur when used with **oxytocin**, possibly severe with concomitant **beta blockers**. Bronchodilation, uterine contraction, and diuresis are other activities reported with ephedrine. Crude aerial parts have caused hyperglycemia as well as hypoglycemia. Patients with high blood pressure and diabetes should exercise caution when using these plants.
Feverfew (*Tanacetum parthenium*) Compositae family	Contact or chewing leaves may lead to aphthous ulcers. Dermatitis reported. Some abdominal pain, indigestion, diarrhea, flatulence, nausea, and vomiting reported.	May take several months (4 to 6) to see effects. Hence, it should not be discontinued abruptly. Can reduce platelet aggregation and increase fibrinolytic activity. Monitor patients on **anticoagulants** or **antiplatelet agents**. Has uterine-stimulant effects and should be avoided in pregnant women. Can modify menstrual flow. Avoid in children less than 2 years of age. Tachycardia has been reported. May prevent 5-HT (serotonin) release from platelets; possible potentiation of methysergide reported. A "post-feverfew" syndrome has been described with symptoms including nervousness, tension headaches, insomnia, stiffness/pain in joints, and tiredness. Some feel that feverfew should only be used for migraines when conventional drugs have failed. In ragweed family, cross-sensitivity possible.
Garlic	Considered non-toxic, but can cause oral and GI irritation.	Because of inhibition of platelet aggregation and increased fibrinolytic properties, monitor patients on **antiplatelet drugs** or **anticoagulants**. Therapeutic doses of garlic are not recommended for those with blood that clots slowly. Use caution in patients on anticoagulant therapy. May increase serum **insulin** levels, decreasing blood glucose. Garlic may also lower cholesterol and lipid levels. High doses are reported to induce anemia because of both decreased hemoglobin synthesis and hemolysis. May potentiate the antithrombotic effects of **aspirin**. Also is likely to be synergistic with **eicosapentenoic acid** (EPA) in fish oils. Doses of garlic greatly exceeding amounts used in food should not be taken during pregnancy and lactation.

Clinical Considerations for Specific Herb-Drug Interactions & Potential Adverse Effects of Herbs		
	Adverse Effects	Interactions and Clinical Concerns
Ginger (*Zingiber officinale* Roscoe)	High doses may cause GI irritation and discomfort when taken on an empty stomach. Fresh ginger is considered more effective. A 1/4 inch slice of fresh ginger equals ≈ 1 to 2 grams of powder.	Because ginger inhibits platelet aggregation, patients on **antiplatelet drugs** or **anticoagulants** should be monitored. Increased calcium uptake by heart muscle may alter **calcium channel blocker** effect. Contraindications include pregnancy (large amounts) and gallstones because of its cholagogue effect. Low doses are commonly used in the management of nausea of pregnancy (hyperemesis gravidarum). The German Commission E Monographs state that ginger should not be used for treatment of vomiting in pregnancy.
Ginkgo (*Ginkgo biloba* L.)	The extract may rarely cause GI discomfort and headache.	Therapeutic response may occur in 2 to 3 weeks and must be taken continuously. Inhibits platelet-activating factor (PAF); bleeding episodes reported. Use caution with patients on **antiplatelet drugs** and **warfarin**. No studies have been done on leaf extracts in pregnant and lactating women; it should be avoided in this population. Avoid the small oval fruits of the female tree because contact or ingestion of the fruit pulp has caused severe allergic reactions (eg, edema, erythema, blisters, itching). The bad smell is caused by butyric acid, but the toxin in the seed is 4-0-methylpyridoxine. Curiously, the boiled or cooked seeds are eaten and available canned in Asian food shops.
Ginseng (*Panax quinquefolium* L. = American ginseng; *P. ginseng* L. = Asian ginseng)	Generally low toxicity with high-quality standardized products. Breast tenderness in women, nervousness, and excitation have been reported, which diminish with lower doses or longer use. Women may experience estrogenic side effects.	Use in cyclic fashion (2 weeks on and 2 weeks off). Can cause diminished platelet adhesiveness, so monitor patients on **anticoagulants**. High doses may inhibit early stage of infection immune function. Ginseng may potentiate the action of MAOIs (inhibits uptake of various neurotransmitter substances), and at least 2 cases of suspected interaction with phenelzine have been reported. Generally ginseng is contraindicated in acute illness, any form of hemorrhage and during the acute phase of coronary thrombosis. Also avoidance is recommended in nervous, tense, hysteric, manic, and schizophrenic individuals. Do not use with **stimulants** (even **caffeine**), **antipsychotic drugs**, or while being treated with **hormones**. Use with caution in patients with diabetes, cardiac problems, hypo- and hypertensive disorders, and in patients receiving **steroid therapy**. If possible, avoid during pregnancy and lactation.
Eleutherococcus or Siberian Ginseng (not the same as Panax ginseng but in the same family) (Araliaceae); *Eleutherococcus senticosus* (Rupr. & Maxim.) Maxim; synonymous with *Acanthopanax senticosus*	High doses associated with irritability, insomnia, and anxiety. Other adverse effects include skin eruptions, headache, diarrhea, hypertension, and pericardial pain in rheumatic heart patients.	Possible estrogenic effect in females. Side effects, toxicity, contraindications, and warnings similar to those for *Panax* species (see ginseng). Russian experience suggests this product not be used for people under the age of 40 and that only low doses be taken on a daily basis. Patients are advised to abstain from alcohol, sexual activity, bitter substances, and spicy foods. Avoid during pregnancy and lactation. Possible assay interference with **digoxin**; concomitant therapy increased digoxin level to greater than 5 mg/ml without symptoms of toxicity (case report).

Clinical Considerations for Specific Herb-Drug Interactions & Potential Adverse Effects of Herbs		
	Adverse Effects	Interactions and Clinical Concerns
Goldenseal (*Hydrastis canadensis* L.)	Has CNS-stimulant properties. May interfere with the ability of the colon to manufacture the B vitamins or decrease their absorption.	Has been used in conjunction with standard antimicrobial therapy. Because of hypoglycemic properties, monitor diabetics. Has been used prophylactically for traveler's diarrhea (eg, 1 week before, during, and 1 week after travel). Do not use for greater than 2 months at a time. Contraindicated in patients with hypertension. Berberine has coagulant activity and can antagonize the action of **heparin**. It also has cardiac-stimulant properties. Do not use goldenseal as a douche because of its potential local ulcerative effects. Do not use locally for purulent ear discharge because of possibility of rupturing ear drum. Hydrostine, beberine, etc., alkaloids are potentially toxic, and thus excessive use should be avoided. Symptoms of alkaloid toxicity include stomach upset, nervous symptoms, depression, exaggerated reflexes, convulsions, paralysis, and death from respiratory failure. Alkaloids are also uterine stimulants and should be avoided during pregnancy. Avoid use during lactation.
Hawthorn (*Crataegus oxyacanthoides* Therill.; *C. monogyna* Jacq. Rosaceae family	High doses may lead to hypotension and sedation. Nausea, fatigue, sweating, and rash on the hands have been reported.	May take up to 2 weeks to see effects. Hawthorn's polymeric procyanidins may increase the activity of **cardiotonic drugs** like digitalis or they may reduce the toxicity of the cardiac glycosides via coronary vasodilating and antiarrhythmic effects. Because of cardioactive, hypotensive, and coronary vasodilatory properties of hawthorn, monitor other drugs with these actions (eg, **antihypertensives**) or avoid use. Hawthorn extracts have uteroactivity (reduction in tone and motility); avoid in pregnancy and lactation.
Kava-Kava (*Piper methysticum* Frost)	Masticated kava causes numbness of mouth (local anesthetic action). Monitor for excessive CNS depression.	Contraindicated in pregnancy because of loss of uterine tone. Avoid in lactation because of possible passage of pyrone compounds into milk. Also avoid in endogenous depression because of the sedative properties of the pyrones (kwain, methysticin, yangonin). Chronic ingestion of kava drink has led to "kawaism," characterized by dry, flaking, discolored skin, and reddened eyes. Because of euphoric effects, avoid other **CNS stimulants** or **depressants**. Heavy kava users are more likely to complain of poor health including low weight, reduced protein levels, "puffy faces," scaly rashes, increases in HDL and cholesterol counts, hematuria, blood cell abnormalities (eg, decreased platelets, lymphocytes), and pulmonary hypertension. Using kava along with **benzodiazepine** drugs (eg, alprazolam [*Xanax*]) may cause "semicomatose state" because of interaction. Avoid concomitant use.
LaPacho (Pau d'arco, Tahubo, *Tabeluia ipe, T. avellanedae*)	Chronic administration may lead to moderate-to-severe anemia. Wholebark decoction has no reports of human toxicity.	Purchase standardized products containing at least 2% to 4% lapachol. The various quinone derivatives (lapachol, 2-methylanthra-quinone, etc.) have proven antibacterial, antiviral, antiparasitic, anti-inflammatory, and anticancer activity. Concomitant use of similar-acting agents may have synergistic effects. Anti-vitamin K activity has been reported for lapachol, but the presence of several vitamin K-like substances in the whole bark suggests that this may not be a problem.

	Clinical Considerations for Specific Herb-Drug Interactions & Potential Adverse Effects of Herbs	
	Adverse Effects	Interactions and Clinical Concerns
Licorice (*Glycyrrhiza glabra* L.)	Low doses are safe and widely used in true licorice candy products. Excessive or prolonged ingestion (over several ounces per day of candy) can result in symptoms known as pseudoaldosteronism (hypertension; sodium, chloride, and water retention; hypokalemia; weight gain). Low levels of plasma renin activity, aldosterone, and antidiuretic hormone also may be seen. Most "licorice" candy in the US is flavored with anise oil. Read the label carefully to determine if it has licorice mass. If so, this is real licorice. European licorice is real licorice, containing large amounts of the root extract. Deglycyrrhizenated licorice is available to avoid steroidal effects.	Aldosterone-like effects may be reversed using a high-potassium and low-sodium diet. Avoid licorice in hypertensive patients, in those with renal or liver failure, or cardiovascular disease. Also, avoid with **cardiac glycoside** therapy since licorice may potentiate its action. It may also increase levels of endogenous **corticosteroids** as well as those of systemically or topically administered steroids. Hypokalemia can aggravate glucose intolerance, and licorice may interfere with existing hypoglycemic therapy. Excessive consumption during pregnancy and lactation should be avoided. Licorice has uterine-stimulant action and may affect the menstrual cycle. Licorice is contraindicated in gall bladder disease, kidney disease, pheochromocytoma and other adrenal tumors, diseases which cause low serum potassium levels (eg, 1° and 2° aldosteronism and severe chronic alcoholism), diseases that may result from low potassium levels (eg, certain kinds of flaccid paralysis of limb disorders), fasting, anorexia, bulimia, and untreated hypothyroidism.
Milk thistle (*Silibum marianum* L. Gaertn.) Compositae family	Generally non-toxic. Possible loose stools related to increased bile flow. Some individuals may show mild allergic response.	Loose stools can be controlled with oat bran or psyllium. Phosphatidylcholine-bound silymarin is claimed to be more effective. Helps prevent liver damage from various hepatotoxins and drugs (eg, **butyrophenones, phenothiazines, acetaminophen, halothane, phenytoin,** and **ethanol,** due to liver membrane-stabilizing and antioxidant effects of the flavolignans [silybin, silydianin, silychristin]). Silybin reduces biliary cholesterol and increases bile secretion, cholate excretion, and bilirubin excretion. Be aware of related drugs and avoid milk thistle. Also keep in mind potential effects of milk stimulation and steroid secretory modulation. Widely used in Europe for Amanita mushroom poisoning.
Peppermint (*Mentha* X *piperita* L.)	*External*: Possible contact dermatitis.	Use with caution in patients with hiatal hernia because peppermint relaxes the esophageal sphincter, thus potentiating esophageal reflux. Has wide range of effects causing concern about related drugs with similar or antagonistic action. Peppermint has carminative, antispasmodic, choleretic, and external analgesic action. Widely used as a tea (infusion) and as enteric-coated capsule for treating irritable bowel syndrome (1 to 2 capsules with 0.2 ml per capsule) 3 times daily with meals. Topical preparations of peppermint and menthol increase dermatitis potential when used in conjunction with heating pads. Contraindicated in pregnancy because of its emmenogogue effect and in gallstones because of its choleretic activity.
	Internal: Local mouth irritation and burning, skin rash, heartburn, and muscle tremor. Hypersensitivity reactions (skin rash) have been reported as well as heartburn, bradycardia, and muscle tremor.	
Herbs with phototoxic principles (eg, St. John's wort, celery, angelica)	Phototoxicity	Avoid UV or solarium light therapy or sun tanning because of potential photosensitizing effects.

Clinical Considerations for Specific Herb-Drug Interactions & Potential Adverse Effects of Herbs		
	Adverse Effects	Interactions and Clinical Concerns
St. John's wort (*Hypericum perforatum* L.) Hypericaceae family	Photosensitivity well documented with high doses because of hypericin. Pollen in flowers may cause severe allergic reaction and anaphylaxis.	Usually taken with food to prevent GI irritation or upset. The predominant mechanism of action is unclear but has been shown to be similar to **SSRIs** and **MAOIs**; therefore, concomitant use with these agents is not recommended. Also use caution with foods and drugs that interact with SSRIs and MAOIs. Contraindicated in pregnancy because of its emmenagogue and abortifacient effects and its uterine stimulant action. Avoid UV or solarium light therapy or sun tanning because of its potential photosensitizing effects. Also avoid in severe endogenous depression since it only has been shown to be effective in mild-to-moderate depression. St. John's wort enhances the sleeping time of **narcotics** and antagonizes the effects of **reserpine**. Avoid use in pregnancy and lactation.
Saw palmetto (*Serenoa repens* [Bartr.]) Small, Palmae family	Possible gastric side effects.	Because of well documented antiandrogen and antiestrogenic activity, avoid taking with any **hormone** therapy including oral contraceptive and hormone replacement therapy. Also has shown immunostimulant and anti-inflammatory activity; hence, watch for patients taking drugs that may increase or decrease these effects. For reproducible effects, it is recommended that the fat-soluble saw palmetto extracts standardized to contain 85% to 95% fatty acids and sterols be taken at the recommended dosage of 160 mg twice daily. Effects occur in 4 to 6 weeks. No demonstrated effect on serum prostate-specific antigen levels. Because of antiestrogenic effect, avoid during pregnancy and in patients with breast cancer.
Systemic lupus erythematosus	Alfalfa	Contraindicated.
Valerian (*Valeriana officinalis* L.) Valerianacea family	Strong disagreeable odor, rare morning drowsiness, headache, excitability, uneasiness, and cardiac disturbances.	Can reduce morning sleepiness. Can potentiate effects of other **CNS depressants**. Reduction of caffeine consumption combined with exercise can increase effectiveness of this mild sedative. The volatile components of valerian can increase the sleeping time induced by **pentobarbital**. Acts on GABA receptor and is potentially additive to **benzodiazapines**. The depressant action of valerian is reported not to be synergistic with alcohol. Avoid in pregnancy and lactation. Related species (*V. wallichi*) have shown abortifacient properties and can affect the menstrual cycle. The valepotriate compounds are unstable and this may affect shelf life and efficacy of product.

[1] The Review of Natural Products. St. Louis, MO: Facts and Comparisons.

[2] Newell C, et al. Herbal Medicines. London: The Pharmaceutical Press, 1996.

[3] DeSmet P, et al. Adverse Effects of Herbal Drugs. NY: Springer-Verlag, 1992-1995:1-3.

[4] Murray, M. The Healing Power of Herbs. CA: Prima Publishing, 2nd ed., 1995.

[5] Brinker, F. Herb Contraindications and Drug Interactions. Oregon: Eclectic Institute, Inc., 1997.

[6] McDermott, J. Herbal Chart for Health Care Professionals. *Pharmacy Today*, 1997 Feb.

[7] Bergner, P. Herb-Drug Interactions in Medical Herbalism. *J for Herbal Practitioners*.

PHARMACOLOGY: Diuretics remain among the most frequently prescribed drugs in the United States. In addition to the widespread use of prescription diuretics, over-the-counter (OTC) and natural diuretics continue to play an important role in the self-treatment of menstrual distress, edema, and hypertension.

Numerous OTC menstrual distress preparations contain xanthine alkaloids such as caffeine and theobromine, which are most often derived from inexpensive natural sources. Of these compounds, only caffeine has been found to be both safe and effective for use as an OTC diuretic. In its review of these products, the FDA Advisory Review Panel on Menstrual Drug Products concluded that the frequently used dandelion root (*Taraxacum officinale* Wiggers), a preparation once thought to have strong diuretic properties, is safe but ineffective in the treatment of dysmenorrhca. Nor is there evidence that dandelion is an effective diuretic.

Teas and extracts of buchu (*Barosma betulina*) and quack grass (*Agropyron* spp.) are popular, but their diuretic activity is probably no greater than that of the xanthine alkaloids in coffee or ordinary tea. Significant toxicity from buchu and quack grass have not been reported.[1]

Diuretic teas that should be avoided include juniper berries (*Juniperus communis*), which contain a locally irritating volatile oil capable of causing renal damage, and shave grass or horsetail (*Equisetum* spp.) a weakly diuretic plant that contains several toxic compounds including aconitic acid, equisitine (a neurotoxin), and nicotine.[2] In grazing animals, the ingestion of horsetail has caused excitement, convulsions, and death. Thiamine deficiency has been reported in sheep after the experimental administration of shave grass.

Other teas, such as ephedra (ma huang), contain the mildly diuretic stimulant ephedrine. These teas should be used with caution by hypertensive patients.

All plants and herbal extracts included in OTC products for use as diuretics are not toxic; however, the majority are either clinically ineffective or no more effective than caffeine. The following table lists plants that have been reported to possess diuretic activity. This list has been compiled from old materia medica, herbals, and when documentation is available, the scientific literature. There is generally little scientific evidence to justify the use of most of these plants as diuretics. Some are toxic even in very low doses. The fact that some have been used for centuries in herbal medicine does not necessarily attest to their effectiveness; rather it suggests that such plants have a relatively broad margin of safety and their use does not usually result in toxicity.

HERBAL DIURETICS		
Scientific Name	*Common Name*	*Part Used*
Abutilon indicum	—	Bark
Acalypha evrardii	—	Flower, leaf
Acanthus spinosus	—	Entire plant
Acorus calamus*	**Calamus**	**Rhizome**
Adonis vernalis	Pheasant's eye herb	Above ground
Agave americana	Agave	Roots
Agrimonia eupatoria	**Agrimony**	**Entire plant**
Agropyron	**Couch grass**	**Rhizomes, roots, stems**

HERBAL DIURETICS

Scientific Name	Common Name	Part Used
Alchemilla arvensis	**Lady's mantle**	**Entire plant**
Alisma plantago	—	Entire plant
Allium cepa	Onion	Bulb
Ammi visnaga	—	**Fruit**
Anemone spp.*	Windflower	Entire plant
Apium graveolens*	**Celery**	**Stalk, oil**
Apocynum cannabinum*	—	Entire plant
Arctostaphylos uva-ursi*	**Uva ursi**	**Leaves**
Arctium lappa	**Burdock**	**Root**
Asparagus officinale	**Asparagus**	**Roots**
Bacopa monnieri	—	Entire plant
Barosma spp.	**Buchu**	**Leaves**
Begonia cucullata	Begonia	Entire plant
Betula alba*	Betula	Leaves, twigs
Blumea lacera	—	Entire plant
Boerhaavia diffusa	—	Entire plant
Borago officinalis	**Borage**	**Leaves, tops**
Buddleja americana	—	Bark, leaf, root
Callistris arborea	—	Gum
Calystegia soldanella	—	Entire plant
Camellia sinensis	Common tea	Leaves
Capsella bursa-pastoris	Shepherd's purse	Above ground
Carex arenaria	—	Entire plant
Chamaelirium luteum	—	Root
Chelidomium majus	Celandine	Root, leaves, latex
Chicorium intybus	**Chicory**	**Root**
Chimaphilia umbellata	Pipsissewa	Above ground
Claytonia sibirica	—	Entire plant
Clematis spp*	—	**Entire plant**
Coffea arabica	Coffee	Fruit
Collinsonia canadensis	Stoneroot	Root
Convallaria majalis*	Lily of the valley	Flowering tops
Costus spicatus	—	Sap
Curanga fel-terrae	—	Leaf
Cynanchium vincetoxicum	—	Entire plant
Cytisus scoparius*	**Broom**	**Flowering tops**
Daucus carota	**Carrot**	**Root**
Digitalis purpurea*	**Foxglove**	**Leaves**
Drosera rotundifolia	Drosera	Entire plant

HERBAL DIURETICS		
Scientific Name	*Common Name*	*Part Used*
Ephedra spp.	**Ephedra**	**Stems**
Equisetum spp.	**Horsetail**	**Above ground**
Eryngium yuccifolium	—	Entire plant
Fumaria officinalis	**Fumitory**	**Flowering tops**
Gaillardia pinnatifida	—	Entire plant
Galega officinalis	Goat's rue	All but root
Galium aparine	Cleavers	Above ground
Glycyrrhiza glabra	**Licorice**	**Rhizome, root**
Helianthus annus	Sunflower	Seeds
Hemidesmus indicus	—	Entire plant
Herniaria glabra	Rupturewort	Above ground
Hibiscus spp.	**Hibiscus**	**Flowers**
Hydrangea arborescens*	Hydrangea	Roots
Hypericum perforatum	**St. John's Wort**	**Entire plant**
Hypochoeris scarzonerae	—	Entire plant
Ilex paraguayensis*	**Maté**	**Leaves**
Iris florentina	Orris	Peeled rhizome
Juniperus communis*	**Juniper**	**Berries**
Laportea meyeniana	—	Leaf, root
Levisticum officinale	**Lovage**	**Roots**
Paullinia cupana	**Guarana**	**Seeds**
Petroselinum crispum*	**Parsley**	**Leaves, seeds**
Peumus boldus	**Boldo**	**Leaves**
Pinus silvestris	Pine	Cones
Psoralae corylifolia	—	Seeds
Rafnia perfoliata	—	Leaf
Rehmannia lutea	—	Entire plant
Sambucus nigra	**Elderberry**	**Flowers**
Santalum album	**Sandalwood**	**Oil**
Sassafras albidum	**Sassafras**	**Root**
Senecionis herba	Senecio herb	Above ground
Serenoa repens	**Saw palmetto**	**Ripe fruits**
Smilax spp.	Sarsaparilla	Roots
Solanum dulcamara*	**Bittersweet**	**Twigs, branches**
Spiranthes diuretica	—	Entire plant
Tagetes multifida	—	Entire plant
Taraxacum officinale	**Dandelion**	**Leaves**
Theobroma cacao	**Cocoa**	**Seeds**

HERBAL DIURETICS		
Scientific Name	Common Name	Part Used
Trianthema portula-castrum	—	Leaves
Tribulus terrestris	—	Fruit
Urginea maritima*	**Squill**	**Bulb**
Urtica dioica*	**Nettle**	**Leaves**
Viola odorata	Violet	Leaves, flowers
Withania som-nifera*	**Withania**	**Root**

* Noted as toxic in reference; all others should not be considered safe for general use in the absence of valid safety. Plants in **bold** are described in their own monograph in this system.

[1] *Med Let* 1979;21:29.

[2] DerMarderosian AH. *Am Druggist* 1980 Aug:35.

Alabama

Alabama Poison Center, Tuscaloosa
2503 Phoenix Dr.
Tuscaloosa, AL 35405
800/462-0800 (AL only)
205/345-0600

Regional Poison Control Center
The Children's Hospital of Alabama
1600 7th Ave. S.
Birmingham, AL 35233-1711
205/939-9201
205/933-4050
800/292-6678 (AL only)

Alaska

Anchorage Poison Control Center
Providence Hospital Pharmacy
P.O. Box 196604
Anchorage, AK 99519-6604
907/261-3193
800/478-3193 (AK only)

Arizona

Samaritan Regional Poison Center
Good Samaritan Regional Medical Center
Ancillary-1
1111 E. McDowell Rd.
Phoenix, AZ 85006
602/253-3334
800/362-0101 (AZ only)

Arizona Poison and Drug Information Center

Arizona Health Sciences Center
1501 N. Campbell Ave., Rm. 1156
Tucson, AZ 85724
800/362-0101 (AZ only)
520/626-6016

Arkansas

Arkansas Poison and Drug Information Center
University of Arkansas for Medical Sciences
4301 W. Markham St. – 552
Little Rock, AR 72205
800/376-4766

Southern Poison Center, Inc.
875 Monroe Ave., Ste. 104
Memphis, TN 38163
901/528-6048
800/288-9999 (TN only)

California

California Poison Control System – Fresno
Valley Children's Hospital
3151 N. Millbrook, IN31
Fresno, CA 93703
800/876-4766 (CA only)

California Poison Control System – San Diego Division
UCSD Medical Center
200 W. Arbor Dr.
San Diego, CA 92103-8925
800/876-4766 (CA only)

California Poison Control System – Sacramento Division

UCDMC – HSF
Rm. 1024
2315 Stockton Blvd.
Sacramento, CA 95817
800/876-4766 (CA only)

Colorado

Rocky Mountain Poison and Drug Center
8802 E. 9th Ave.
Denver, CO 80220-6800
800/332-3073 (outside metro-CO only)
800/446-6179 (Las Vegas, NV only)
303/739-1123 (Denver metro)

Connecticut

Connecticut Regional Poison Center
University of Connecticut Health Center
263 Farmington Ave.
Farmington, CT 06030
800/343-2722 (CT only)

Delaware

The Poison Control Center
3600 Sciences Center, Ste. 220
Philadelphia, PA 19104-2641
800/722-7112 (PA only)
215/386-2100

District of Columbia

National Capital Poison Center
3201 New Mexico Ave., NW, Ste. 310
Washington, DC 20016
202/625-3333
202/362-8563 (TTY)

Florida

Florida Poison Information Center – Jacksonville
University of Florida Health Science Center – Jacksonville
655 W. 8th St.
Jacksonville, FL 32209
904/549-4480
800/282-3171 (FL only)

Florida Poison Information Center – Miami
University of Miami, School of Medicine
Department of Pediatrics
P.O. Box 016960 (r-131)
Miami, FL 33101
305/585-5253
800/282-3171 (FL only)

Florida Poison Information Center – Tampa
Tampa General Hospital
P.O. Box 1289
Tampa, FL 33601
813/253-4444 (Tampa)
800/282-3171 (FL only)

Georgia

Georgia Poison Center
Hughes Spalding Children's Hospital
Grady Health System
80 Butler St. SE, P.O. Box 26066
Atlanta, GA 30335-3801
800/282-5846 (GA only)
404/616-9000

Hawaii

Hawaii Poison Center
Kapiolani Medical Center for Women and Children
Honolulu, HI 96826
800/362-3585 (outer islands of HI only)
800/362-3586
808/941-4411

Idaho

Rocky Mountain Poison and Drug Center
8802 E. 9th Ave.
Denver, CO 80220-6800
800/860-0620 (ID only)
303/739-1123

Illinois

BroMenn Poison Control Center
BroMenn Regional Medical Center
Franklin at Virginia
Normal, IL 61761
309/454-6666

Interstate Center – Cardinal Glennon Children's Hospital
Regional Poison Center
1465 S. Grand Blvd.
St. Louis, MO 63104
800/366-8888 (Western IL only)

Indiana

Indiana Poison Center
Methodist Hospital of Indiana
1-65 at 21st St.,
P. O. Box 1367
Indianapolis, IN 46206-1367
800/382-9097 (IN only)
317/929-2323

Interstate Center – Kentucky Regional Poison Center of Kosair Children's Hospital
P.O. Box 35070
Louisville, KY 40232-5070
502/589-8222 (southern IN only)

Iowa

Iowa Poison Center
St. Luke's Regional Medical Center
2720 Stone Park Blvd.
Sioux City, IA 51104
712/277-2222
800/352-2222

Interstate Center – The Poison Center
Children's Memorial Hospital
8301 Dodge St.
Omaha, NE 68114
800/955-9119

Kansas

Mid-America Poison Control Center
University of Kansas Medical Center
3901 Rainbow Blvd., Room B-400
Kansas City, KS 66160-7231
913/588-6633
800/332-6633 (KS only and Kansas City metro area)

Interstate Center – Cardinal Glennon Children's Hospital
Regional Poison Center
1465 S. Grand Blvd.
St. Louis, MO 63104
800/366-8888 (Topeka, KS only)

Kentucky

**Kentucky Regional
Poison Center of
Kosair Children's
Hospital**
P.O. Box 35070
Louisville, KY
40232-5070
502/629-7275
800/722-5725 (KY only)

**Kentucky Regional
Poison Center**
Medical Towers S.,
Ste. 572
234 E. Gray St.
Louisville, KY 40202
502/589-8222

Louisiana

**Louisiana Drug and
Poison Information
Center**
School of Pharmacy
Northeast Louisiana
University
Monroe, LA 71209-6430
800/256-9822 (LA only)
318/362-5393

Maine

**Maine Poison Control
Center**
Maine Medical Center
Department of
Emergency Medicine
22 Bramhall St.
Portland, ME 04102
207/871-2950
800/442-6305 (ME only)

Maryland

**Maryland Poison
Center**
20 N. Pine St.
Baltimore, MD 21201
410/528-7701
800/492-2414 (MD only)

**National Capital Poison
Center (D.C. suburbs
only)**
3201 New Mexico
Avenue, NW, Ste. 310
Washington, DC 20016
202/625-3333
202/362-8563 (TTY)

Massachusetts

**Massachusetts Poison
Control System**
300 Longwood Ave.
Boston, MA 02115
617/232-2120
800/682-9211 (MA only)

Michigan

**Blodgett Regional
Poison Center**
1840 Wealthy, SE
Grand Rapids, MI 49506
800/POISON-1
(800/746-7661)
800/356-3232 (TTY
only)

**Children's Hospital of
Michigan Poison
Control Center**
4160 John R. Harper
Office Bldg., Ste. 616
Detroit, MI 48201
800/764-7661 (MI only)
313/745-5711

**Marquette General
Hospital Poison
Center**
420 W. Magnetic St.
Marquette, MI 49855
906/225-3497
800/562-9781

Minnesota

**Hennepin Regional
Poison Center**
Hennepin County
Medical Center
701 Park Ave.
Minneapolis, MN 55415
612/347-3141
800/764-7661 (MN only)
612/337-7387 (petline)

**Minnesota Regional
Poison Center**
8100 34th Ave. S.
P.O. Box 1309
Minneapolis, MN
55440-1309
800/222-1222 (MN only)
612/221-2113
800/764-7661

**North Dakota Poison
Information Center**
MeritCare Medical
Center
720 4th St. N.
Fargo, ND 58122
701/234-5575
800/732-2200 (ND, MN,
SD only)

Mississippi

**Mississippi Regional
Poison Control Center**
University of Mississippi
Medical Center
2500 N. State St.
Jackson, MS 39216
601/354-7660

**Southern Poison
Center, Inc.**
875 Monroe Ave.,
Ste. 104
Memphis, TN 38163
901/528-6048
800/288-9999 (TN only)

Missouri

**Cardinal Glennon
  Children's Hospital
  Regional Poison
  Center**
1465 S. Grand Blvd.
St. Louis, MO 63104
314/772-5200
800/366-8888 (MO,
  Western IL, and
  Topeka, KS only)
800/392-9111 (MO only)

**Children's Mercy
  Hospital Poison
  Control Center**
2401 Gillham Rd.
Kansas City, MO 64108
816/234-3430

**Interstate Center – The
  Poison Center**
8301 Dodge St.
Omaha, NE 68114
800/955-9119

Montana

**Rocky Mountain Poison
  and Drug Center**
8802 E. 9th Ave.
Denver, CO 80220-6800
800/525-5042 (MT only)
303/739-1123

Nebraska

The Poison Center
8301 Dodge St.
Omaha, NE 68114
402/354-5555 (Omaha
  only)
800/955-9119 (NE and
  WY only)

Nevada

**Rocky Mountain Poison
  and Drug Center**
8802 E. 9th Ave.
Denver, CO 80220-6800
800/446-6179 (Las
  Vegas, NV only)
303/739-1123

Washoe Poison Center
Washoe Medical Center
77 Pringle Way
Reno, NV 89520-0109
702/328-4129

New Hampshire

**New Hampshire Poison
  Information Center**
Dartmouth-Hitchcock
  Medical Center
1 Medical Center Dr.
Lebanon, NH 03756
603/650-8000
603/650-5000 (between
  11 p.m. and 8 a.m.)
800/562-8236 (NH only)

New Jersey

**New Jersey Poison
  Information and
  Education System**
201 Lyons Ave.
Newark, NJ 07112
800/764-7661 (NJ only)

New Mexico

**New Mexico Poison and
  Drug Information
  Center**
University of New
  Mexico
Health Sciences Library,
  Room 125
Albuquerque, NM
  87131-1076
505/272-2222
505/843-2551
800/432-6866 (NM only)

New York

**Central New York
  Poison Control Center**
SUNY Health Science
  Center
750 E. Adams St.
Syracuse, NY 13210
315/476-4766
800/252-5655 (NY only)

**Finger Lakes Regional
  Poison Center**
University of Rochester
  Medical Center
601 Elmwood Ave.,
  Box 321
Rochester, NY 14642
800/333-0542 (NY only)
716/275-3232
716/273-4155

**Hudson Valley Regional
  Poison Center**
Phelps Memorial
  Hospital Center
701 N. Broadway
Sleepy Hollow, NY
  10591
800/336-6997 (NY only)
914/366-3030

**Long Island Regional
  Poison Control Center**
Winthrop University
  Hospital
259 First St.
Mineola, NY 11501
516/542-2323

**New York City Poison
  Control Center**
NYC Department of
  Health
455 First Ave., Rm. 123
New York, NY 10016
212/340-4494
212/POISONS
212/447-2205
212/689-9014

**Western New York
  Regional Poison
  Control Center**
Children's Hospital of
  Buffalo
219 Bryant St.
Buffalo, NY 14222
800/888-7655 (NY
  Western regions only)
716/878-7654

North Carolina

Carolinas Poison Center
Carolinas Medical Center
5000 Airport Center
  Parkway, Ste. B
P.O. Box 32861
Charlotte, NC
  28232-2861
704/355-4000
800/848-6946 (NC only)

North Dakota

**North Dakota Poison
  Information Center**
MeritCare Medical
  Center
720 4th St. N.
Fargo, ND 58122
701/234-5575
800/732-2200 (ND, MN,
  SD only)

Ohio

**Central Ohio Poison
  Center**
700 Children's Dr.
Columbus, OH
  43205-2696
614/228-1323
800/682-7625 (OH only)
614/228-2272 (TTY)

**Cincinnati Drug and
  Poison Information
  Center**
Regional Poison Control
  Center
2368 Victory Parkway,
  Ste. 300
Cincinnati, OH 45206
513/558-5111
800/872-5111 (OH only)
330/379-8562

**Greater Cleveland
  Poison Control Center**
11100 Euclid Ave.
Cleveland, OH 44106
216/231-4455

Oklahoma

**Oklahoma Poison
  Control Center**
Children's Hospital
940 NE 13th St.
Oklahoma City, OK
  73104
405/271-5454
800/POISON-1

Oregon

Oregon Poison Center
Oregon Health Sciences
  University
3181 SW Sam Jackson
  Park Rd., CB 550
Portland, OR 97201
503/494-8968
800/452-7165 (OR only)

Pennsylvania

**Central Pennsylvania
  Poison Center**
Penn State University
  Hospital
Milton S. Hershey
  Medical Center
Hershey, PA 17033
800/521-6110
717/531-6111

**The Poison Control
  Center**
3600 Sciences Center,
  Ste. 220
Philadelphia, PA 19104
800/722-7112 (PA only)
215/386-2100

**Pittsburgh Poison
  Center**
3705 Fifth Ave.
Pittsburgh, PA 15213
412/681-6669

Rhode Island

Lifespan Poison Center
593 Eddy St.
Providence, RI 02903
401/444-5727

South Dakota

Iowa Poison Center
St. Luke's Regional
  Medical Center
2720 Stone Park Blvd.
Sioux City, IA 51104
712/277-2222
800/352-2222

Tennessee

**Middle Tennessee
  Poison Center**
The Center for Clinical
  Toxicology
Vanderbilt University
  Medical Center
1161 21st Ave. S.
501 Oxford House
Nashville, TN
  37232-4632
615/322-6435 (local)
800/288-9999 (TN only)
800/936-2034

**Southern Poison
  Center, Inc.**
875 Monroe Ave.,
  Ste. 104
Memphis, TN 38163
901/528-6048
800/288-9999 (TN only)

Texas

**Central Texas Poison
  Center**
Scott and White
  Memorial Hospital
2401 S. 31st St.
Temple, TX 76508
800/764-7661 (TX only)
254/724-7401

**North Texas Poison
  Center**
5201 Harry Hines Blvd.
P.O. Box 35926
Dallas, TX 75235
800/764-7661 (TX only)

South Texas Poison Center
University of Texas Health Science Center
Forensic Science Bldg., Rm. 146
7703 Floyd Curl Dr.
San Antonio, TX 78284-7849
800/764-7661 (TX only)

Southeast Texas Poison Center
The University of Texas Medical Branch
301 University Ave.
Galveston, TX 77555-1175
409/765-1420
800/764-7661 (TX only)

Texas Poison Center Network at Amarillo
P.O. Box 1110
1501 S. Coulter
Amarillo, TX 79175
800/764-7661

West Texas Regional Poison Center
4815 Alameda Ave.
El Paso, TX 79905
800/764-7661

Utah

Utah Poison Control Center
410 Chipeta Way, Ste. 230
Salt Lake City, UT 84108
801/581-2151
800/456-7707 (UT only)

Vermont

Vermont Poison Center
Fletcher Allen Health Care
111 Colchester Ave.
Burlington, VT 05401
802/658-3456

Virginia

Blue Ridge Poison Center
University of Virginia Health System
P.O. Box 437
Charlottesville, VA 22908
804/924-5543
800/451-1428 (VA only)

National Capital Poison Center (Northern VA only)
3201 New Mexico Ave., NW, Ste. 310
Washington, DC 20016
202/625-3333
202/362-8563 (TTY)

Virginia Poison Center
Virginia Commonwealth University
P.O. Box 980522
Richmond, VA 23298-0522
800/552-6337 (VA only)
804/828-9123

Washington

Washington Poison Center
155 NE 100th St., Ste. 400
Seattle, WA 98125
206/526-2121
800/732-6985 (WA only)
206/517-2394 (TDD)
800/572-0638 (TDD)

West Virginia

West Virginia Poison Center
3110 MacCorkle Ave. SE
Charleston, WV 25304
800/642-3625 (WV only)
304/348-4211

Wisconsin

Poison Center of Eastern Wisconsin
P.O. Box 1997
Milwaukee, WI 53201
414/266-2222
800/815-8855 (WI only)

Wyoming

The Poison Center
8301 Dodge St.
Omaha, NE 68114
402/354-5555 (Omaha)
800/955-9119 (WY and NE only)

The burgeoning field of biomedical science has created an information glut that often makes finding useful facts a problem. There are more than 900 biomedical journals and newsletters published in the United States alone (Kruzas AT, Medical Health Information Directory, Gale Research Co, Detroit, 1980). Of these, only a few address the study of natural products.

A full appreciation of natural products requires an understanding of their origin, history, nomenclature, chemistry, pharmacology, toxicology, availability, and therapeutic uses. Little more than a dozen journals deal specifically with these topics. Many of the remaining scientific and medical journals represent excellent secondary sources of information about natural products.

Table 1 presents a selected list of American and foreign periodicals devoted to the study of natural products. Books continue to be valuable sources of data about natural products. Many original works, no longer in publication, continue to set the standards in their fields (eg, Ernest Guenther's, The Essential Oils, Vols. 1–5 D, Van Nostrand Co, NY, 1948–1952). Table 2 is not an all-inclusive book list; rather, it offers suggestions for a well-rounded library on natural products.

With the increasing use of computer-accessible data bases, on-line indexing systems have become critical in the retrieval of references describing natural products. The biomedical field has at its disposal a variety of computer-based abstracting/indexing services. Of these, few specialty indexing services are available for the field of natural products (Table 3). Several excellent broad-based services do, however, provide quite adequate access to information about natural products.

It is hoped that this review of information sources will make the task of data retrieval and evaluation somewhat less overwhelming.

TABLE 1: Periodicals

Acta Botanica Indica, Society for Advancement of Botany, Meerut, India

American Journal of Natural Medicine – Impakt Communications, Green Bay, WI

Botanical Review – The New York Botanical Gardens, Bronx, NY

Bulletin on Narcotics– United Nations, New York, NY

Canadian Journal of Botany, NRC Research Press, Ottawa, Canada

Canadian Journal of Herbalism, Ontario Herbalists' Association, Ontario, Canada

Economic Botany, The Society for Economic Botany, The New York Botanical Garden, Bronx, NY

European Journal of Herbal Medicine: Phytotherapy, The National Institute of Medical Herbalists, Exeter, Devon, UK

Herb Companion, Interweave Press, Loveland, CO

Herb Quarterly, San Anselmo, CA

HerbalGram, The Journal of the American Botanical Council and the Herb Research Foundation, Austin, TX

International Herb Association Newsletter, International Herb Association, Mundelein, IL

International Journal of Aromatherapy, The American Alliance of Aromatherapy, Depoe Bay, OR

Journal of Economic and Taxonomic Botany, The Society for Economic and Taxonomic Botany, Scientific Publishers, India

Journal of Ethnopharmacology, The Journal of The International Society of Ethnopharmacology, Elsevier Science, Philadelphia, PA

Journal of Natural Products, The American Chemical Society and the American Society of Pharmacognosy, Columbus, OH

Medical Anthropology: Cross-Cultural Studies in Health and Illness, Gordon and Breach Science Publishers, International Publishers Distributor, Newark, NJ

TABLE 1: Periodicals

Medical Herbalism: A Journal for the Clinical Practitioner, Bergner Communications, Boulder, CO

Natural Health, Natural Health Limited Partnership, Brookline Village, MA

Natural Product Letters, Harwood Academic Publishers, International Publishers Distributor, Newark, NJ

Natural Product Reports, The Royal Society of Chemistry, Cambridge, UK

NCAHF Newsletters, The National Council Against Health Fraud, Inc., Loma Linda, CA

Pharmaceutical Biology (formerly *International Journal of Pharmacognosy*), Swets & Zeitlinger Publishers, Royersford, PA

Phytochemistry: The International Journal of Plant Biochemistry and Molecular Biology, The Journal of the Phytochemical Society of Europe and the Phytochemical Society of North America, Pergamon Press, Elsevier Science, New York, NY

Phytomedicine: International Journal of Phytotherapy and Phytopharmacology, Gustav Fischer Verlag, Jena, Germany

Phytotherapy Research, John Wiley & Sons, Inc., New York, NY

Plant Foods for Human Nutrition (formerly *Qualitas Plantarum*), Kluwer Academic Publishers, Hingham, MA

Planta Medica: Natural Products and Medicinal Plant Research, Thieme, New York, NY

Toxicon: An Interdisciplinary Journal on the Toxins Derived from Animals, Plants and Microorganisms, Elsevier Science, New York, NY

Veterinary and Human Toxicology, American College of Veterinary Toxicologists, Manhattan, KS

Z. Naturforsch. Verlag der Zeitschrift fur Naturforschung, Tubingen, Germany

TABLE 2: Books

Aikman L. *Nature's Healing Arts: From Folk Medicine to Modern Drugs.* Washington, DC: National Geographic Society; 1977.

TABLE 2: Books

Baslow H. *Marine Pharmacology: A Study of Toxins and Other Biologically Active Substances of Marine Origin.* Baltimore: Williams & Wilkins Co; 1969.

Beal JL, Reinhard E, eds. *Natural Products as Medicinal Agents: Plenary Lectures of the International Research Congress on Medicinal Plant Research, Strasbourg, July 1980.* Stuttgart: Hippokrates Verlag; c1981.

Blackwell WH. *Poisonous and Medicinal Plants.* Englewood Cliffs, NJ: Prentice Hall; 1990.

Bricklin M. *The Practical Encyclopedia of Natural Healing.* New rev ed. Emmaus, PA: Rodale Press; 1983.

British Herbal Pharmacopoeia. Great Britain: British Herbal Medicine Association; 1996.

Bucherl W, Buckley EE, Deulofeu V, eds. *Venomous Animals and Their Venoms.* 3 vols. New York: Academic Press; 1968-71.

Castleman M. *The Healing Herbs: The Ultimate Guide to the Curative Power of Nature's Medicines.* Emmaus, PA: Rodale Press; 1991.

Densmore F. *How Indians Use Wild Plants for Food, Medicine, and Crafts.* Washington, DC: Government Printing Office; 1928. Reprint, New York: Dover; 1974.

Der Marderosian AH, Liberti LE. *Natural Product Medicine: A Scientific Guide to Foods, Drugs, Cosmetics.* Philadelphia: G.F. Stickley; 1988.

Duke JA. *CRC Handbook of Medicinal Herbs.* Boca Raton, FL: CRC Press; 1985.

Evans WC. *Trease and Evans' Pharmacognosy.* 14th ed. London: WB Saunders; 1996.

Facciola S. *Cornucopia: A Source Book of Edible Plants.* Vista, CA: Kampong Publications; 1990.

Foster S. *Tyler's Honest Herbal: A Sensible Guide to the Use of Herbs and Related Remedies.* 4th ed. New York: Haworth Herbal Press; 1998.

Halstead BW. *Poisonous and Venomous Marine Animals of the World.* 2d rev. ed. Princeton, NJ: Darwin Press; 1988.

Henslow G. *The Plants of the Bible: Their Ancient and Mediaeval History Popularly Described.* London: Masters; 1906.

TABLE 2: Books

Hoffmann D. *The Herbal Handbook: A User's Guide to Medical Herbalism*. Rochester, VT: Healing Arts Press; 1998.

Hoffmann D, ed. *The Information Sourcebook of Herbal Medicine*. Freedom, CA: Crossing Press; 1994.

Kerr RW. *Herbalism through the Ages*. 7th ed. San Jose, CA: Supreme Grand Lodge of AMORC; 1980.

Kingsbury JM. *Deadly Harvest: A Guide to Common Poisonous Plants*. New York: Holt, Rinehart and Winston; 1965.

Kingsbury JM. *Poisonous Plants of the United States and Canada*. Englewood Cliffs, NJ: Prentice-Hall; 1964.

Krogsgaard-Larsen P, Christensen SB, Kofod, H, eds. *Natural Products and Drug Development: Proceedings of the Alfred Benzon Symposium 20 Held at the Premises of the Royal Danish Academy of Sciences and Letters, Copenhagen, 7-11 August 1983*. Copenhagen: Munksgaard; 1984.

Lampe KF, McCann MA. *AMA Handbook of Poisonous and Injurious Plants*. Chicago: American Medical Association; 1985.

Leung AY. *Encyclopedia of Common Natural Ingredients Used in Food, Drugs, and Cosmetics*. 2d ed. New York: Wiley; 1996.

Lewis WH, Elvin-Lewis MPF. *Medical Botany: Plants Affecting Man's Health*. New York: Wiley; 1977.

Liener IE, ed. *Toxic Constituents of Plant Foodstuffs*. 2d ed. New York: Academic Press; 1980.

Mabberly DJ. *The Plant-book: A Portable Dictionary of the Vascular Plants Utilizing Kubitzki's....* 2d ed. Cambridge: Cambridge University Press; 1997.

Meyer JE. *The Herbalist*. Rev ed. Glenwood, IL: Meyerbooks; 1986.

Morton JF. *Atlas of Medicinal Plants of Middle America: Bahamas to Yucaton*. Springfield, IL: C.C. Thomas; 1981.

Morton JF. *Major Medicinal Plants: Botany, Culture, and Uses*. Springfield, IL: Thomas; 1977.

Ody P. *The Complete Medicinal Herbal*. New York: Dorling Kindersley; 1993.

TABLE 2: Books

Osol A, Pratt R, eds. *The United States Dispensatory*. 27th ed. Philadelphia: Lippincott; 1973.

Penso G. *Inventory of Medicinal Plants Used in the Different Countries*. Geneva: World Health Organization; 1980.

Reader's Digest Magic and Medicine of Plants. Sydney: Reader's Digest; 1994.

Robinson T. *The Organic Constituents of Higher Plants: Their Chemistry and Interrelationships*. 6th ed. North Amherst, MA: Cordus Press; 1991.

Rosengarten F. *The Book of Spices*. Wynnewood, PA: Livingston Pub. Co; 1969.

Schauenberg P. *Guide to Medicinal Plants*. New Canaan, CT: Keats; 1977.

Simon JE. *Herbs, An Indexed Bibliography, 1971-1980: The Scientific Literature on Selected Herbs, and Aromatic and Medicinal Plants of the Temperate Zone*. Hamden, CT: Shoe String Press; 1984.

Spoerke DG. *Herbal Medications*. Santa Barbara, CA: Woodbridge Press; 1990.

Steiner RP, ed. *Folk Medicine: The Art and the Science*. Washington, DC: American Chemical Society; 1986.

Swain T, ed. *Plants in the Development of Modern Medicine*. Cambridge, MA: Harvard University Press; 1972.

Sweet M. *Common Edible and Useful Plants of the East and Midwest*. Healdsburg, CA: Naturegraph Publishers; 1975.

Sweet M. *Common Edible and Useful Plants of the West*. Healdsburg, CA: Naturegraph Publishers; 1976.

Tyler VE, Brady LR, Robbers, JE. *Pharmacognosy*. 9th ed. Philadelphia: Lea and Febiger; 1988.

Youngken HW, Karas JS. *Common Poisonous Plants of New England*. U.S. Public Health Service pub. no. 1220. Washington, DC: Government Printing Office; 1964.

Zohary M. *Plants of the Bible: A Complete Handbook... with 200 Full-color Plates Taken in the Natural Habitat*. New York: Cambridge University Press; 1982.

TABLE 3: Abstracting, Indexing, and Retrieval Services

BIOSIS, the world's largest collection of abstracts and bibliographic references to worldwide biological and medical literature. Available in several formats, including *Biological Abstracts* in print and CD-ROM. BIOSIS, 2100 Arch Street, Philadelphia, PA 19103-1399, 1-800-523-4806, http://www.biosis.org/home.html

Chemical Abstracts Service, producer of the world's largest and most comprehensive databases of chemical information. CAS, 2540 Olentangy River Road, Columbus, OH 43202, 1-800-753-4227, http://www.cas.org/

Current Contents and *Science Citation Index*, published by the Institute for Scientific Information (ISI), producer of databases of scholarly research information. ISI, 3501 Market Street, Philadelphia, PA 19104, 1-800-336-4474, http://www.isinet-.com/

Excerpta Botanica. Sectio A, Taxonomica et Chorologica, an annotated bibliography of periodical literature. International Association for Plant Taxonomy. G. Fischer Verlag, Stuttgart, New York.

GlobalHerb Software, Natural Medicine Computer Software, http://www.chiron-h.com/globalherb/

The Herb Research Foundation, a nonprofit research and educational organization focusing on herbs and medicinal plants. Library includes 150,000 scientific articles, up-to-date information on thousands of herbs, thorough files on traditional use of herbs and historical information. Herb Research Foundation, 1007 Pearl St., Suite 200, Boulder, CO 80302, 1-800-748-2617, http://www.herbs.org/

MEDLINE, MEDLARS, National Library of Medicine, index system of medical bibliographies. For access and information about these and other NLM databases, visit http://www.nlm.nih.gov/

IPA (International Pharmaceutical Abstracts), the American Society of Health-System Pharmacists, 7272 Wisconsin Ave., Bethesda, MD 20814, 301-657-3000, http://info.cas.org/ONLINE/DBSS/ip-ass.html. Database contains international coverage of pharmacy and health-related literature.

TABLE 3: Abstracting, Indexing, and Retrieval Services

Herbal newsgroup: http://metalab.unc.edu/herbmed/

NAPRALERT (Natural PRoducts ALERT) file contains bibliographic and factual data on natural products from 1650 to the present. Updated monthly. Scientific and Technical Information Network (STN), c/o Chemical Abstracts Service, P.O. Box 3012, Columbus, OH 43210, 614-447-3600, http://stneasy.cas.org.

NAPRONET, an electronic scientific forum to discuss the chemistry and biology of natural products. For more information: http://chemistry.gsu.edu/post_docs/koenwnaprone.html

Lynn Index, a bibliography of phytochemistry, Massachusetts College of Pharmacy.

Medicinal and Aromatic Plants Abstracts, Publications and Information Directorate, Council of Scientific and Industrial Research (CSIR), New Delhi, India.

Poisindex System, identifies ingredients for hundreds of thousands of commercial, pharmaceutical, and biological substances. For information, MICROINDEX, 800-525-9038, info@mdx.com or http://www.microdex.com/po-pdx.htm.

Toxicology Information Response Center (TIRC), an information center offering direct access to virtually all of the world's scientific and technical databases. Toxicology and Risk Assessment (TARA) section of the Life Sciences Division (LSD) of the Oak Ridge National Laboratory (ORNL), 1060 Commerce Park, MS 6480, Oak Ridge, TN 37830, 423-576-1746, http://www.ornl.gov/TechResources/tirc/hmepg.html.

TOXLINE, the National Library of Medicine's extensive collection of online bibliographic information covering the biochemical, pharmacological, physiological, and toxicological effects of drugs and other chemicals. Available free of charge at: http://igm.nlm.nih.gov.

Therapeutic Index

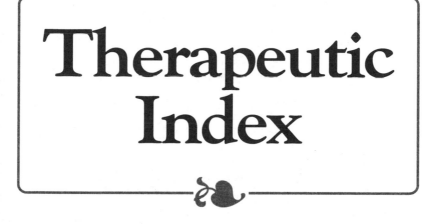

The Therapeutic Uses Index cross references the multiple applications noted within *Guide to Popular Natural Products* monographs, which are presented alphabetically. The information contained in this index is intended to be a starting point when seeking information about natural products. It is imperative to read the entire monograph before advising patients on taking any phytomedicinal or herb. Urge patients to consult a qualified medical professional for serious or long-term problems.

The Therapeutic Uses Index entries are presented alphabetically. Boldface entries refer to the condition, followed by the monograph name in which the condition is discussed. The distinction between current and folkloric uses is designated by the following key:

  C – Clinical (Physiologic effects in humans and animals. Includes data from clinical studies. Information will be found within the pharmacology section of each monograph.)

  V – In vivo/In vitro (Preliminary studies show in vivo or in vitro action. Information will be found within the pharmacology section of each monograph.)

  H – Historic/Folkloric (Reviews the historical and folk uses of the topic. Information will be found within the history section of each monograph.)

  M – Multiple (Application of topic noted in more than one category within the monograph. Example: In the Echinacea monograph, the immunostimulant properties of echinacea are cited as a folkloric application, a clinical use and in studies in vivo/in vitro.)

Please remember the uses cited in this index are not FDA approved uses. In addition, listing of potential uses are not endorsements or recommendations of Facts and Comparisons®. As a healthcare professional, use your own judgment when dispensing advice.

A fterbirth, expelling, see
  Chaste Tree, H
Aging, see Ginseng
  Melatonin, C
  Morinda, H
  Nettles, H
AIDS/HIV, see
  Bitter Melon, M
  Burdock, V
  Cat's Claw, C
  Lemon Balm, C
  Nettles, V
  St. John's Wort, C
Alcoholism, see
  Evening Primrose Oil, C
  Goldenseal, C
  Kudzu, H
Allergies, see
  Devil's Claw, H
  Dong Quai, H
  Eyebright, H
  Milk Thistle, C
  Nettles, C
  Uva Ursi, C
AMP, intracellular concen-
    trations, see
  Hawthorn, C

Anal fissures, see
  Plantain, C
Analgesic, see
  Arnica, H
  Clove, H
  Dong Quai, C
  Ginseng, C
  Lemongrass, H
  Poppy, C
  Quinine, C
  Rosemary, V
  Turmeric, H
Anemia, see
  Anise, C
  Bee Pollen, C
  Dong Quai, H
  Fo-Ti, C
  Parsley, H
  Pau d'arco, H
Anesthetic, see
  Barberry, C
  Cat's Claw, C
  Kava-Kava, C
  Propolis, H
Angina, see
  Hawthorn, H
  Yohimbe, H
Anthelmintic, see
  Cat's Claw, H

Anthelmintic (cont.), see
  Chamomile, H
  Clove, C
  Horehound, H
  Morinda, V
Antiandrogenic, see
  Saw Palmetto, C
Antiarrhythmic, see
  Betony, H
  Hawthorn, H
  Licorice, C
  Quinine, C
Antibacterial, see
  Aloe, C
  Barberry, C
  Clove, C
  Coltsfoot, V
  Cranberry, C
  Feverfew, V
  Garlic, M
  Lemon Verbena, C
  Parsley, V
  Passion Flower, V
  Peppermint, V
  Propolis, M
  Quinine, V
  Schisandra, C
  Scullcap, V
  Shark Derivatives, C

Antibacterial (cont.), see
St. John's Wort, V
Tea Tree Oil, C
Turmeric, C
Antibiotic, see
Goldenseal, C
Lemon Verbena, V
Propolis, V
Yarrow, C
Antidepressant, see
Milk Thistle, H
St. John's Wort, M
Antidermatophytic, see
Clove, C
Antidote, poison, see
Grapefruit, H
**Antidote, poisonous herbs,
mushrooms, snake-
bites,** see Fennel, H
Antiemetic, see
Clove, H
Gentian, H
Ginger, H
Lemongrass, H
Antifungal, see
Clove, C
Garlic, V
Parsley, V
Propolis, M
Sassafras, V
Scullcap, V
Shark Derivatives, C
Antigonadotropic, see
Comfrey, C
Antihepatotoxic, see
Elderberry, C
Turmeric, C
Antihistamine, see
Clove, C
Eleutherococcus, C
Antihypertensive, see
Cat's Claw, C
Gotu Kola, C
Lemongrass, H
Anti-infective, see
Echinacea, M
Anti-inflammatory, see
Aloe, C
Angelica, C
Cat's Claw, H
Comfrey, C
Devil's Claw, C
Evening Primrose Oil, C
Eyebright, H
Guggul, V
Horse Chestnut, C
Juniper, C
Milk Thistle, C
Passion Flower, H

Anti-inflammatory (cont.),
see
Plantain, H
Propolis, M
Pycnogenol, M
Saw Palmetto, C
Scullcap, C
St. John's Wort, M
Withania, H
Antimicrobial, see
Aloe, C
Anise, C
Bitter Melon, M
Black Cohosh, V
Blue Cohosh, C
Burdock, C
Hops, C
Lentinan, C
Myrrh, V
Parsley, H
Passion Flower, V
Pau d'arco, H
Propolis, C
Sage, C
Sassafras, V
Tea Tree Oil, C
Uva Ursi, M
Antineoplastic, see
Boneset, C
Chaparral, H
Ginger, H
Goldenseal, C
Mistletoe, V
Sassafras, C
Yarrow, C
Yellow Dock, C
Antioxidant, see
Bilberry Fruit, C
Chaparral, C
Garlic, C
Jojoba, C
Melatonin, C
Milk Thistle, C
Propolis, M
Rosemary, C
Sage, C
Turmeric, C
Antiprotozoal, see
Pau d'arco, H
Shark Derivatives, C
Antipsychotic, see Ginseng,
C
Antisecretory, see
Sage, C
Antiseptic, see
Clove, H
Garlic, C
Goldenseal, C
Lemongrass, H

Antiseptic (cont.), see
Myrrh, H
Peppermint, H
Sage, H
Tea Tree Oil, M
Antispasmodic, see
Anise, C
Blue Cohosh, H
Chamomile, M
Clove, C
Dong Quai, M
Goldenseal, H
Hawthorn, H
Hops, C
Lavender, H
Lemon Balm, M
Lemon Verbena, H
Lemongrass, H
Myrrh, H
Nettles, H
Peppermint, H
Quinine, C
Rosemary, H
Sage, M
Valerian, C
Antithrombotic, see
Chondroitin, C
Clove, C
Danshen, C
Garlic, C
Leeches, V
Antitrypanosome, see
Pau d'arco, H
Shark Derivatives, C
Antitumor, see
Burdock, C
Echinacea, C
Lentinan, M
Propolis, C
Anti-ulcer, see
Bilberry Fruit, C
Licorice, C
Pau d'arco, H
Propolis, H
Antiviral, see
Cat's Claw, V
Cranberry, V
Lemon Balm, C
Lentinan, C
Propolis, M
St. John's Wort, C
Anxiety, see
Betony, H
Ginseng, C
Kava-Kava, C
Schisandra, C
St. John's Wort, H
Aphrodisiac, see
Avocado, H

Aphrodisiac (cont.), see
Burdock, H
Gotu Kola, H
Guarana, H
Kava-Kava, H
Nutmeg, H
Parsley, H
Tonka Bean, H
Yohimbe, H
Appetite stimulant, see
Capsicum Peppers, H
Dandelion, H
Gentian, M
Goldenseal, H
Lemon Verbena, H
Appetite suppressant, see
Fennel, H
Guarana, C
Aromatherapy, see
Bayberry, M
Lavender, M
Peppermint, H
Rosemary, M
Tea Tree Oil, C
Arrhythmias, see
Betony, H
Hawthorn, H
Licorice, C
Quinine, C
Arthritis, see
Alfalfa, H
Angelica, H
Cat's Claw, H
Chondroitin, C
Devil's Claw, H
Ephedras, H
Feverfew, H
Glucosamine, C
Guggul, H
Horse Chestnut, H
Juniper, H
Morinda, M
Parsley, H
Pokeweed, H
Tea Tree Oil, H
Uva Ursi, C
Asthma, see
Alfalfa, H
Anise, C
Apricot, H
Bitter Melon, H
Coltsfoot, H
Ephedras, H
Feverfew, H
Ginkgo, H
Kava-Kava, H
Nettles, H
Oleander, H
Passion Flower, H

Asthma (cont.), see
Sage, H
Astringent, see
Apricot, H
Barberry, H
Bayberry, H
Betony, H
Cat's Claw, H
Elderberry, H
Goldenseal, C
Myrrh, M
Rosemary, M
Sage, H
St. John's Wort, C
Uva Ursi, C
Witch Hazel, M
Yarrow, H
Atherosclerosis, see
Eleutherococcus, H
Flax, C
Fo-Ti, C
Garlic, C
Ginseng, H
Grapefruit, C
Hawthorn, H
Athlete's foot, see
Tea Tree Oil, C
Attention disorders, see
Evening Primrose Oil, C
Passion Flower, H

Bacterial flora,
replenishment of
normal, see
Acidophilus, C
Bad breath,
Grapefruit, H
Balance of life forces, restore,
see Withania, H
Baldness, see
Aloe, H
Avocado, H
Evening Primrose Oil, C
Jojoba, C
Nettles, H
Parsley, H
Quinine, H
Rosemary, H
Bed-wetting, see
Uva Ursi, C
Bile, see
Alfalfa, V
Dandelion, H
Nettles, C
Uva Ursi, C
Bladder disorders, see
Acidophilus, C

Bladder disorders (cont.), see
Alfalfa, H
Gotu Kola, C
Hops, H
Nettles, C
Tea Tree Oil, C
Uva Ursi, H
Bleeding, see
Ginseng, H
Blood disorders, see
Alfalfa, M
Ginseng, H
Blood flow, postoperative, see Leeches, C
Blood purifier, see
Dong Quai, H
Echinacea, H
Eleutherococcus, C
Fo-Ti, C
Grapefruit, C
Milk Thistle, M
Blood vessels, dilate see
Cat's Claw, C
Hawthorn, C
Blood volume determination,
see Chromium, C
Boils, see
Fenugreek, H
Pau d'arco, H
Slippery Elm, H
Tea Tree Oil, H
Bone formation,
see Propolis, V
Bone pain, see
Cat's Claw, H
Ephedras, H
Bradykininase activity, see
Aloe, V
Brain cancer, see
Maitake, C
Breast cancer, see
Bloodroot, H
Maitake, C
Melatonin, M
Soy, C
Breast pain, see
Evening Primrose Oil, C
Breast size, increase, see
Saw Palmetto, H
Bronchial conditions, see
Comfrey, H
Ephedras, H
Eyebright, H
Ginkgo, C
Passion Flower, H
Bronchitis, see
Anise, C

Bronchitis (cont.), see
  Borage, H
  Chaparral, H
  Coltsfoot, H
  Juniper, H
  Milk Thistle, H
Bronchodilator, see
  Ephedras, C
Bruises, see
  Arnica, H
  Comfrey, H
  Danshen, C
  Parsley, H
  Slippery Elm, H
  Witch Hazel, C
Burns, see
  Aloe, C
  Chaparral, H
  Comfrey, H
  Passion Flower, H
  Tea Tree Oil, M
  Witch Hazel, H

Calcium channel
  blocker, see
  Coltsfoot, C
Cancer, see
  Apricot, H
  Barberry, H
  Bloodroot, C
  Burdock, H
  Cat's Claw, C
  Chaparral, M
  Clove, C
  Cranberry, H
  Danshen, C
  Echinacea, C
  Elderberry, H
  Eleutherococcus, C
  Evening Primrose Oil, V
  Eyebright, H
  Fo-Ti, C
  Ginseng, H
  Gotu Kola, C
  Grapefruit, C
  Green Tea, M
  Hops, H
  Lentinan, C
  Maitake, C
  Melatonin, M
  Mistletoe, H
  Morinda, C
  Myrrh, H
  Nettles, H
  Oleander, H
  Parsley, H
  Pau d'arco, H
  Peppermint, H
  Quinine, H

Cancer (cont.), see
  Rosemary, C
  Scullcap, C
  Shark Derivatives, H
  Soy, C
  St. John's Wort, H
  Turmeric, M
  Witch Hazel, H
Candida albicans, see
  Acidophilus, H
  Pau d'arco, H
Canker sores, see Mace, H
  Nutmeg, C
Carbohydrate utilization,
  see Chromium, C
Cardiac depressant, see
  Quinine, C
Cardiac disorders, see
  Evening Primrose Oil, C
  Oleander, H
Cardiac stimulant, see
  Ginger, C
Cardioprotective, see
  Eleutherococcus, C
  Guggul, V
  Hawthorn, C
  Melatonin, C
  Soy, M
Carminative, see
  Anise, H
  Capsicum Peppers, H
  Fennel, H
  Garlic, H
  Ginger, H
  Juniper, H
  Lavender, H
  Lemon Balm, H
  Lemon Verbena, H
  Licorice, H
  Parsley, H
  Rosemary, H
  Sage, C
Causalgia, see
  Capsicum Peppers, C
Cellulitis, see
  Fenugreek, H
  see Ginkgo, C
Cerebral hemorrhage, see
  Bee Pollen, C
Cervicitis, trichomonal see
  Tea Tree Oil, C
Chemoprotective agent,
  see
  Clove, C
  Green Tea, V
  Propolis, M
Chickenpox, see
  Chaparral, H
Chilblains, see Ginkgo, H

Childbirth, see
  Barberry, C
  Blue Cohosh, H
  Dong Quai, C
  Ephedras, C
  Fennel, H
  Lavender, C
  Parsley, H
  Schisandra, H
Chills, see Ephedras, H
Cholera, see
  Barberry, H
Choleretic, see
  Bayberry, C
  Turmeric, C
Cholesterol levels, de-
  crease, see
  Acidophilus, M
  Cat's Claw, C
  Evening Primrose Oil, C
  Flax, C
  Fo-Ti, C
  Garlic, C
  Glucomannan, C
  Grapefruit, C
  Green Tea, V
  Guggul, M
  Lentinan, C
  Maitake, C
  Milk Thistle, C
  Plantain, C
Cholesterol levels, in-
  crease, see
  Alfalfa, M
Chronobiotic, see
  Melatonin, C
Circulation, see
  Arnica, H
  Danshen, M
  Pycnogenol, H
Cirrhosis, see
  Milk Thistle, C
Climacteric complaints,
  see Fennel, H
  Passion Flower, H
CNS depressant, see
  Ginseng, C
  Lavendar, C
  Nettles, C
CNS stimulant, see
  Dong Quai, C
  Ephedras, C
  Ginseng, C
  Schisandra, C
  Yohimbe, C
Coagulant, see
  Boneset, C
Colds, see
  Anise, C

Colds (cont.), see
Betony, H
Borage, M
Burdock, H
Chaparral, H
Ephedras, H
Eyebright, H
Flax, H
Horehound, M
Kava-Kava, H
Lavender, H
Peppermint, M
Witch Hazel, H
Colic, see
Melatonin, C
Parsley, H
Colitis, see
Bee Pollen, C
Cat's Claw, H
Dandelion, C
Ginseng, H
Witch Hazel, C
Collagen degradation, see
Pycnogenol, M
**Colon, adenomatous
polyps** see Green Tea,
V
Colorectal cancer, see
Echinacea, C
**Congenital defects, pre-
vent,**
see Eleutherococcus, C
Congestion, see
Betony, C
Ephedras, M
Horse Chestnut, H
Conjunctivitis, see
Apricot, H
Eyebright, H
Peppermint, H
Sassafras, C
Witch Hazel, H
Constipation, see
Aloe, M
Apricot, M
Bee Pollen, C
Betony, C
Boneset, C
Burdock, H
Cascara, M
Dandelion, H
Dong Quai, H
Elderberry, H
Fenugreek, C
Flax, H
Fo-Ti, C
Glucomannan, C
Parsley, H
Plantain, M

Constipation (cont.), see
Pokeweed, H
Rose Hips, M
Senna, M
Uva Ursi, H
Yellow Dock, H
Contraceptive, see
Bitter Melon, M
Cat's Claw, M
Gotu Kola, V
Melatonin, M
Convulsions, see
Barberry, C
Betony, H
Ginseng, C
Valerian, C
Corns, see
Oleander, H
Tea Tree Oil, C
Cough, see
Apricot, H
Anise, C
Barberry, H
Betel Nut, C
Bloodroot, H
Coltsfoot, H
Ephedras, H
Eyebright, H
Flax, H
Horehound, M
Lemon Verbena, H
Lemongrass, H
Peppermint, C
Poppy, V
Schisandra, M
Tea Tree Oil, C
Counterirritant, topical,
see
Arnica, M
Betel Nut, C
Clove, H
Cramps, see
Blue Cohosh, H
Peppermint, H
Tonka Bean, H
Crohn's disease, see
Evening Primrose Oil, C
Cystitis, see
Acidophilus, C
Hops, H
Tea Tree Oil, C
Uva Ursi, H
Cytomegalovirus inhibitor,
see
Nettles, V

Dandruff, see
Burdock, C
Deafness, see Garlic, H

Dementia, see
Ginseng, H
Demulcent, see
Flax, H
Slippery Elm, C
Dengue fever, see
Boneset, H
Dental analgesic, see
Bloodroot, M
Dental caries prevention,
see
Grape Seed, C
Green Tea, V
Dental disorders, see
Anise, H
Betony, H
Clove, C
Peppermint, H
Propolis, C
Yarrow, H
Dentifrice, see
Tea Tree Oil, H
Yellow Dock, H
Depression, see
Borage, H
Juniper, C
Melatonin, C
Milk Thistle, H
Schisandra, H
St. John's Wort, M
Dermatitis, see
Aloe, C
Evening Primrose Oil, C
Feverfew, H
Uva Ursi, C
Dermatitis, atopic see
Evening Primrose Oil, C
Dermatologic disorders,
see
Aloe, C
Angelica, H
Bloodroot, H
Cat's Claw, H
Dandelion, H
Evening Primrose Oil, C
Eyebright, H
Feverfew, H
Gotu Kola, M
Pokeweed, H
Sassafras, C
Tea Tree Oil, M
Uva Ursi, C
Witch Hazel, M
Yellow Dock, H
Diabetes, see
Alfalfa, H
Bitter Melon, M
Dandelion, H
Eleutherococcus, H

Diabetes (cont.), see
Evening Primrose Oil, C
Fenugreek, H
Ginseng, H
Lavender, H
Maitake, C
Milk Thistle, C
Morinda, H
Nettles, H
Pau d'arco, H
Uva Ursi, C
Diabetic retinopathy, see
Bilberry Fruit, H
Diaphoretic, see
Angelica, H
Burdock, M
Ephedras, H
Horehound, H
Lemon Balm, H
Rosemary, H
Diarrhea, see
Acidophilus, M
Avocado, H
Barberry, C
Bayberry, H
Betony, M
Bilberry Fruit, M
Cat's Claw, H
Fenugreek, C
Goldenseal, C
Nutmeg, C
Poppy, C
Sage, H
Schisandra, H
Witch Hazel, C
Dietary supplement, see
Alfalfa, C
Evening Primrose Oil, C
Grape Seed, C
Lentinan, H
Melatonin, C
Rose Hips, M
Spirulina, H
Digestive aid, see
Betel Nut, C
Betony, C
Capsicum Peppers, H
Chamomile, H
Goldenseal, H
Ginkgo, H
Lemon Verbena, H
Morinda, C
Sage, H
Diuretic, see
Anise, H
Angelica, H
Boneset, C
Borage, M
Burdock, M

Diuretic (cont.), see
Cat's Claw, C
Dandelion, M
Elderberry, H
Ephedras, M
Ginger, H
Green Tea, M
Hops, H
Horehound, H
Juniper, M
Lavender, H
Licorice, H
Nettles, M
Parsley, H
Rose Hips, H
Saw Palmetto, H
St. John's Wort, H
Uva Ursi, M
Withania, H
Diverticulitis, see
Cat's Claw, H
Dizziness, see
Echinacea, H
Ginger, C
Gingko, C
Dropsy, see
Boneset, H
Drunkenness, preventative,
see Ginkgo, H
Dry socket, see
Clove, C
Dysentery, see
Avocado, H
Cat's Claw, M
Guarana, H
Parsley, H
Schisandra, H
Witch Hazel, C
Dysmenorrhea, see
Black Cohosh, H
Blue Cohosh, H
Chaste Tree, C
Dong Quai, H
Fennel, H
Feverfew, H
Goldenseal, H
Hops, H
Milk Thistle, H
Nutmeg, H
Parsley, H
Pennyroyal, H
Pokeweed, H
Rosemary, H
Sage, H
Dyspepsia, see
Alfalfa, H

Dyspepsia, (cont.), see
Black Cohosh, H

Ear disorders, see
Eyebright, H
Garlic, H
Ginkgo, C
Eczema, see
Nettles, H
Witch Hazel, C
Eczema, atopic, see
Evening Primrose Oil, C
Eczema-like lesions, see
Evening Primrose Oil, C
Edema, see
Bilberry Fruit, C
Boneset, H
Comfrey, H
Ephedras, H
Ginkgo, H
Horse Chestnut, C
Pokeweed, H
Pycnogenol, C
Sassafras, C
Withania, H
Emmenagogue, see
Alfalfa, C
Avocado, H
Blue Cohosh, H
Fennel, H
Lavender, H
Myrrh, H
Nutmeg, H
Pennyroyal, H
Rosemary, H
Emollient, see
Aloe, C
Fenugreek, C
Flax, H
Hops, H
Slippery Elm, C
Endometrial cancer, see
Soy, C
Enema, see Witch Hazel, C
Enuresis, see
Uva Ursi, C
Environmental stress, see
Eleutherococcus, H
Epilepsy, see
Blue Cohosh, H
Eyebright, H
Oleander, H
Estrogen release, dampening, see Melatonin, C
Estrogenic activity, see
Fennel, C
Hops, H
Saw Palmetto, C
Ethanolic tincture, see
Schisandra, H

Liver disorders (cont.), see
Gotu Kola, C
Milk Thistle, M
Morinda, C
Parsley, H
St. John's Wort, C
Turmeric, H
Liver obstructions, see
Milk Thistle, H
Liver stimulant, see
Betony, C
Longevity, enhance, see
Gotu Kola, H
Low blood pressure, see
Barberry, C
Cat's Claw, C
Hawthorn, M
Parsley, H
Propolis, V
Turmeric, C
Valerian, C
Yarrow, C
Lung cancer, see
Maitake, C
Lung disorders, see
Arnica, H
Schisandra, H
Lupus, see Licorice, C

Malaria, see
Guarana, H
Pau d'arco, H
Quinine, M
MAO inhibitor, see
St. John's Wort, C
Mastalgia, see
Evening Primrose Oil, C
Melanin production, inhibit,
see Uva Ursi, V
Memory loss, see
Kombucha, H
Schisandra, C
Menopause, see
Black Cohosh, C
Passion Flower, H
Soy, M
Menses stimulant, see
Alfalfa, C
Avocado, H
Blue Cohosh, H
Fennel, H
Lavender, H
Myrrh, H
Nutmeg, H
Pennyroyal, H
Rosemary, H
Menstrual disorders, see
Black Cohosh, H

Menstrual disorders
(cont.), see
Blue Cohosh, H
Chaste Tree, C
Danshen, M
Dong Quai, H
Evening Primrose Oil, C
Fennel, H
Feverfew, H
Gingko, C
Goldenseal, H
Hops, H
Kombucha, H
Milk Thistle, H
Nutmeg, H
Parsley, H
Pennyroyal, H
Peppermint, H
Pokeweed, H
Rosemary, H
Sage, H
Mental capacity, increase,
see
Ginseng, H
Kombucha, H
Schisandra, C
Mental illness, see
Evening Primrose Oil, C
Ginseng, M
Gotu Kola, H
Juniper, C
Metabolic control, see
Evening Primrose Oil, C
Migraine headaches, see
Evening Primrose Oil, C
Feverfew, M
Lavender, H
Mineralocorticoid, see
Bayberry, C
Monoamine oxidase inhibitor,
see
St. John's Wort, C
Monocyte, activation, see
Melatonin, C
Mouth disorders, see
Bilberry Fruit, M
Betony, M
Coltsfoot, H
Goldenseal, C
Nutmeg, C
Quinine, H
Witch Hazel, C
Mucous membrane irritation,
see
Betony, C
Bilberry Fruit, M
Witch Hazel, C
Multiple sclerosis, see
Bee Pollen, C

Multiple sclerosis (cont.),
see
Evening Primrose Oil, C
Mumps, see Pokeweed, H
Muscle pain, see
Arnica, H
Goldenseal, H
Tea Tree Oil, H
Muscle relaxant, see
Poppy, C
Muscle spasms, see
Blue Cohosh, H
Chamomile, M
Clove, H
Dong Quai, M
Goldenseal, H
Hawthorn, H
Hops, C
Lavender, H
Lemon Verbena, H
Lemongrass, H
Myrrh, H
Nettles, H
Peppermint, H
Quinine, C
Rosemary, H
Sage, M
Valerian, C
Mushroom poisoning, see
Fennel, H
Milk Thistle, C
Mutagenic, see
Cat's Claw, M
Turmeric, C
Myalgic encephalomyelitis,
see Evening Primrose Oil,
C

Nails, brittle, see
Evening Primrose Oil, C
Nasal polyps, see Bloodroot,
H
Nausea, see
Clove, H
Ginger, H
Lemongrass, H
Peppermint, H
Tonka Bean, H
Neoplastic diseases, see
Gotu Kola, C
Grape Seed, C
Nerve diseases, see
Schisandra, C
Nervous disorders, see
Betony, C
Ginseng, M
Gotu Kola, H
Hops, H
Juniper, C

Renal disorders (cont.), see
  Devil's Claw, H
  Evening Primrose Oil, C
  Juniper, H
  Milk Thistle, H
  Nettles, C
  Parsley, H
Respiratory disorders, see
  Angelica, H
  Coltsfoot, M
  Schisandra, C
Respiratory function, improve,
  see Ephedras, H
Restorative, see Schisandra, C
Retinitis pigmentosa, see
  Bilberry Fruit, H
Rheumatic disorders, see
  Angelica, H
  Cat's Claw, H
  Chamomile, H
  Scullcap, C
Rheumatic pain, see
  Chaparral, H
  Goldenseal, H
  Lavender, H
Rheumatism, see
  Alfalfa, H
  Black Cohosh, H
  Bloodroot, H
  Blue Cohosh, H
  Boneset, H
  Borage, H
  Burdock, H
  Cat's Claw, C
  Devil's Claw, H
  Dong Quai, H
  Gotu Kola, H
  Horse Chestnut, H
  Kava-Kava, H
  Lemongrass, H
  Nettles, H
  Nutmeg, H
  Pokeweed, H
  Sassafras, C
Rheumatoid arthritis
  Evening Primrose Oil, C
  Clove, C
  Pokeweed, H
  Turmeric, H
Rubefacient, see
  Capsicum Peppers, H
  Pennyroyal, H

Salivary gland atrophy, see
  Evening Primrose Oil, C
Scabies, see

Scabies (cont.), see
  Anise, C
  Pokeweed, H
  Turmeric, C
Scalp disorders, see
  Licorice, C
  Nettles, H
Schistosoma, see
  Tonka Bean, H
Sciatica, see
  Barberry, H
  Goldenseal, H
Scleroderma, see
  Evening Primrose Oil, C
Sclerosing agent, see
  Plantain, C
  Quinine, C
Scurvy, see
  Garlic, H
Sedative, see
  Barberry, C
  Betony, C
  Chamomile, H
  Fo-Ti, C
  Hawthorn, H
  Hops, H
  Kava-Kava, M
  Lemon Balm, M
  Lemon Verbena, H
  Morinda, C
  Passion Flower, H
  Poppy, C
  Schisandra, H
  Scullcap, H
  St. John's Wort, H
  Valerian, M
  Withania, H
Serotonin release inhibitor,
  see Feverfew, V
Sexual stimulant, see
  Saw Palmetto, H
  Schisandra, H
Sjogren's syndrome, see
  Evening Primrose Oil, C
Skin, aging, see
  Milk Thistle, C
  Pycnogenol, H
Skin cancer, see
  Bloodroot, H
  Pokeweed, H
Skin cleanser, see
  Burdock, C
  Tea Tree Oil, C
Skin disorders, see
  Aloe, C
  Angelica, H
  Bitter Melon, H
  Bloodroot, H

Skin disorders (cont.), see
  Burdock, H
  Cat's Claw, H
  Dandelion, H
  Evening Primrose Oil, C
  Eyebright, H
  Feverfew, H
  Gotu Kola, M
  Pokeweed, H
  Sassafras, C
  Tea Tree Oil, M
  Uva Ursi, C
  Witch Hazel, M
  Yellow Dock, H
Skin, dry, see
  Apricot, H
  Avocado, M
Skin eruptions, see
  Gotu Kola, H
  Sassafras, C
Skin irritation, see
  Aloe, C
  Jojoba, C
Skin parasites, see
  Clove, C
  Parsley, H
  Pokeweed, H
  Turmeric, H
Skin, promote growth, see
  Chitosan, C
Skin protectant, see
  Aloe, H
  Milk Thistle, C
Skin rash, see
  Schisandra, H
Skin ulcers, see
  Withania, H
Sleep disorders, see
  Danshen, M
  Fo-Ti, C
  Kava-Kava, C
  Lavendar, C
  Lemon Balm, M
  Melatonin, M
  Nutmeg, C
  Passion Flower, M
  Schisandra, H
  St. John's Wort, H
Snakebite antidote, see
  Black Cohosh, H
  Echinacea, H
  Fennel, H
Snakebite pain, see
  Chaparral, H
Sneezing, induce, see
  Betony, H
Sore throat, see
  Arnica, H
  Black Cohosh, H

Primary
Index

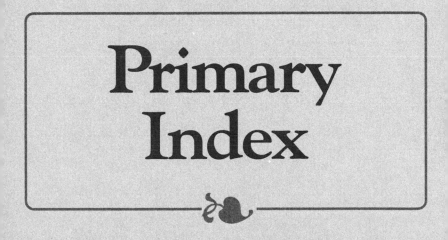

Italicized page numbers indicate botanical photographs.

Diosgenin, see Fenugreek
Dipteryx odorata, see Tonka
 Bean
Dipteryx oppositifolia, see
 Tonka Bean
Dipteryxin, see Tonka Bean
Dogfish shark, see Shark
 Derivatives
Dong Quai, 68
Dr. Caldwell's, see Senna
Dramamine, see Ginger

Echinacea, *I-5*, 69
Echinacea angustifolia, see
 Echinacea
Echinacea pallida, see
 Echinacea
Echinacea purpurea, see
 Echinacea
Efamol, see Evening
 Primrose Oil, EPO
Elderberry, *I-5*, 71
Eleuthera, see
 Eleutherococcus
Eleutherococ, see
 Eleutherococcus
Eleutherococcus, *I-5*, 72
Eleutherococcus senticosus,
 see Eleutherococcus
English chamomile, see
 Chamomile
English hawthorn, see
 Hawthorn
Ephedra altissima, see
 Ephedras
Ephedra distachya, see
 Ephedras
Ephedra helvetica, see
 Ephedras
Ephedra intermedia, see
 Ephedras
Ephedra major, see
 Ephedras
Ephedra nevadensis, see
 Ephedras
Ephedras, 74
Ephedra sinica, see
 Ephedras
Ephedra vulgaris, see
 Ephedras
Ephedrine, see Ephedras
Esculin, see Horse Chestnut
Essential fatty acids, see
 Grape Seed
Eugenia caryophyllata, see
 Clove
Eugenol, see Clove
Eupatorium, see Boneset
Eupatorium perfoliatum, see
 Boneset

Euphrasia officinale, see
 Eyebright
Euphrasia rostkoviana, see
 Eyebright
Euphrasia stricta, see
 Eyebright
European elder, see
 Elderberry
European hops, see Hops
European mistletoe, see
 Mistletoe
**Evening Primrose Oil,
 EPO, 76**
Eye balm, see Goldenseal
Eye root, see Goldenseal
Eyebright, 81

Featherfew, see Feverfew
Featherfoil, see Feverfew
Febrifuge plant, see
 Feverfew
Fennel, *I-5*, 82
Fenugreek, 84
Feuilles de tussilage, see
 Coltsfoot
Fever tree, see Quinine
Feverfew, *I-6*, 86
Feverwort, see Boneset
Finocchio, see Fennel
Flax, *I-6*, 89
Flaxseed, see Flax
Flea seed, see Plantain
Fletcher's Castoria, see
 Senna
Florence fennel, see Fennel
Flowery knotweed,
 see Fo-Ti
Foeniculum officinale, see
 Fennel
Foeniculum vulgare, see
 Fennel
Frangulin B, see Cascara
Fo-Ti, *I-6*, 91
French psyllium, see
 Plantain
Fresh water leech, see
 Leeches
"Fungus" Japonicus, see
 Kombucha

Galangin, see Propolis
Gall weed, see Gentian
Gambirine, see Cat's Claw
Garden angelica, see
 Angelica
Garden fennel, see Fennel
Garden marigold, see
 Calendula
Garden sage, see Sage

Garget, see Pokeweed
Garlic, *I-7*, 92
Gentian, *I-7*, 95
Gentiana acaulis, see
 Gentian
Gentiana lutea, see Gentian
Genuine chamomile, see
 Chamomile
German chamomile, see
 Chamomile
Gewürznelken, see Clove
Ginger, 96
Ginkgo, *I-7*, 98
Ginkgo biloba, see Ginkgo
Ginkyo, see Ginkgo
Ginseng, *I-8*, 103
Glucomannan, 105
Glucosamine, 107
Glucosamine sulfate, see
 Glucosamine
Glycine Max, see Soy
Glycoside madecassoside,
 see Gotu Kola
Glycyrrhiza palidiflora, see
 Licorice
Glycyrrhiza uralensis, see
 Licorice
Goatweed, see St. John's
 Wort
Gobo, see Burdock
Gold bloom, see Calendula
Golden bough, see Mistletoe
Goldenseal, *I-8*, 109
Gomishi, see Schisandra
Gotu Kola, *I-8*, 111
Graecunins, see Fenugreek
Granadilla, see Passion
 Flower
Grapefruit, 113
Grape Seed, *I-9*, 116
Grapple plant, see Devil's
 Claw
Greasewood, see Chaparral
Great burdock, see Burdock
Great scarlet poppy, see
 Poppy
Green arrow, see Yarrow
Green Tea, *I-9*, 117
Grifola frondosa, see
 Maitake
Ground raspberry, see
 Goldenseal
Guarana, 121
Guarana gum, see Guarana
Guarana paste, see Guarana
Guggal, see Guggul
Guggul, 122
Gum guggal, see Guggul
Gum guggulu, see Guggul